D0115141

PRAISE FOR *LEARNING TO BREATHE FIRE*

"J. C. Herz expertly debunks many long-standing fitness beliefs and shows how high-intensity exercise can yield the greatest return on your workout investment. Her *Learning to Breathe Fire* chronicles the rise of CrossFit, showing—in a way that is always interesting and insightful—how ordinary people have achieved extraordinary results following this program. **A must-read for anyone looking to maximize his or her potential."**

—Dean Karnazes, ultra-endurance star, *New York Times* bestselling author, and one of *Time* magazine's 100 Most Influential People

"Herz takes readers on a journey through CrossFit history. . . . [She] intertwines the narrative with passionate descriptions of workouts that push participants to the brink of exhaustion. . . ."

—*Booklist*

"A beautifully written mix of evocative vignettes and lucid explanations that shows us what we're capable of when we train hard and connect with our instinctive nature. This is a book about digging deep, about kindling a spirit that allows us to push past our wildest expectations. Whether your fitness habit involves going it alone or tunneling through an extreme workout as part of a group, you'll find this CrossFit journey thoroughly immersive."

—Marshall Ulrich, Badwater 146 record holder and author of *Running on Empty*

"CrossFit is a phenomenon, both as a radical way to confer fitness and as a virally successful business. **Herz tells both stories with**

exceptional insight—plus the inside lore of a dedicated CrossFitter."

—Stewart Brand, creator of the *Whole Earth Catalog*
(and CrossFitter at age seventy-five)

"The remarkable rise of the CrossFit movement is grounded and propelled by a great moral truth. Effort alone is all we may bring to life. Everything else—our genes, our talents, and our teachers—are gifts. **J. C. Herz has written a compelling book around this truth as embodied in the CrossFit culture.** As a society, we forget that we are evolved to realize our greatest strength when we are truly tested. The originators of CrossFit have rediscovered that and proved it by becoming the fittest humans on the planet. In the view of CrossFit athletes, 'the only possible sin is slacking off.' **Herz writes with sweep and depth about great characters, often racked with doubt, finding their limits and surpassing them.** This is the ultimate chronicle of how they created a training method, a championship, a corporation, and a loving community devoted to the sacred tenet of effort."

—Kenny Moore, award-winning writer for *Sports Illustrated*,
former American marathon record holder, author of *Bowerman and the
Men of Oregon*, and co-screenwriter of *Without Limits*

"I couldn't put this book down. J.C. spares no detail in helping us see into the heart and soul of a CrossFitter. Her description of what CrossFit athletes overcome is truly unbelievable. She captures the essence of the sport and what it represents, most especially the ability to push through barriers, whether physical or mental. **This is about the gut-busting journey to the last rep, but it's also about life. Whether you've tried CrossFit or just *thought* about trying it, *Learning to Breathe Fire* is a must-read."**

—Chrisanna Northrup, *New York Times* bestselling author,
CrossFit Level 1 coach, and former CrossFit Box owner

"*Learning to Breathe Fire* is a must-read for every CrossFitter and fitness enthusiast, beginner or elite."

—Dormivigilia.com

THE **RISE OF CROSSFIT** AND THE
PRIMAL FUTURE OF FITNESS

LEARNING TO BREATHE FIRE

J. C. HERZ

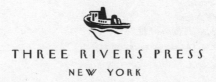

THREE RIVERS PRESS

NEW YORK

Copyright © 2014 by J. C. Herz

All rights reserved.
Published in the United States by Three Rivers Press, an imprint of the
Crown Publishing Group, a division of Penguin Random House LLC, New York.
www.crownpublishing.com

Three Rivers Press and the Tugboat design are registered trademarks of
Penguin Random House LLC.

Originally published in hardcover in the United States by Crown Archetype,
an imprint of the Crown Publishing Group, a division of Penguin Random House
LLC, New York, in 2014.

CrossFit® is a registered trademark of CrossFt, Inc., in the U.S. and/or other
countries. Images used with permission from CrossFit, Inc., are © 2008–2013
CrossFit, Inc. All rights reserved.

The views of the author are exclusively her own and do not reflect the official views of
CrossFit, Inc. Although the reader may find the practices in this book to be useful or
appealing, content is made available with the understanding that neither the author
nor the publisher is engaged in presenting specific medical, psychological, emotional,
or spiritual advice. Nothing in this book is intended to be a diagnosis, prescription,
recommendation, or cure for emotional, medical, or psychological problems. Each
person should engage in a program of treatment or prevention only in consultation
with a licensed, qualified physician, therapist, or other competent professional.

Library of Congress Cataloging-in-Publication Data is available upon request.

ISBN 978-0-385-34889-8
eBook ISBN 978-0-385-34888-1

Printed in the United States of America

Book design by Ralph Fowler
Cover design by Michael Nagin
Cover photography © MetCon Photos LLC
Lettering on front cover by Thomas Corrigan

10 9 8 7 6 5 4 3

First Paperback Edition

For Mike Hart

CONTENTS

At the peak of tremendous and victorious effort,
while the blood is pounding in your head, all suddenly becomes
quiet within you. Everything seems clearer and whiter
than ever before, as if great spotlights had been turned on. At that
moment, you have the conviction that you contain all the
power in the world, that you are capable of everything, that you
have wings. There is no more precious moment in
life than this, the white moment, and you will work
very hard for years just to taste it again.

—YURI VLASOV, RUSSIAN OLYMPIC WEIGHTLIFTER,
THE FIRST MAN TO CLEAN AND JERK 200 KG

It will feel the same. The pain is there.
Something in the head telling you you should quit.
On the other hand, something in the head tells you:
don't give up, just keep going, it's not that bad. It's the
battle in your head—to give up or just go on.

—MIKKO SALO,
2009 CROSSFIT GAMES CHAMPION

PREFACE

For the strength of the Pack is the Wolf,
And the strength of the Wolf is the Pack.

—RUDYARD KIPLING

In late winter, after an early-morning CrossFit workout, I sit quietly in my car. The next class, sprinting to warm up, races out of the gym and past my car on both sides. Each one of them is a regular person. Male and female, older and younger, larger and smaller, their gaits overlap into the unity of animals on the run. It's crisp outside, and as they gallop past I see the steam of their breath. Together, they seem less like ordinary people and more like wild creatures, a pack of beautiful animals.

I am not an elite competitive athlete—I'm one of the least strong athletes in the group: female, medium height, lean but not a great lifter or fast runner. If we were living in the Paleolithic era, I'd likely be singled out, then picked off, by a saber-toothed tiger, if no children or old people were around to pounce on. But I know what it feels like to run, jump, and move heavy weights with this pack of beautiful animals.

My aching forearm finally puts enough pressure on the ignition button to make the car start. Fortunately, I do not live in the Paleolithic era. I have all the gadgets and creature comforts of a plush, sedentary, chronically ill society. And I can't help but believe that the path out of physiological purgatory lies in the footsteps of these people who are sprinting past my car. They've found redemption in their willingness to get primal, if only for the twenty minutes it takes to blaze through pull-ups, box jumps, and kettle bell swings. Their physical power and perseverance inspire lesser athletes like me to keep going. The strength of the pack helps me dig a little deeper. There is always something left when you think there's nothing left.

UNDER THE BRIDGE

IN THE DARKNESS BENEATH PHILADELPHIA'S I-95 OVERPASS, just after dawn, a man struggles against a chain attached to a truck tire. He is in the red zone of physical effort, pulling forward as hard as he can. His comrades, straining against their chains to drag each tire forward to a predetermined line, ignore the part of their brain that tells them it's impossible to keep moving. They have learned how not to stop when the sane and obvious thing to do is to let the chain go slack. Rest is not part of the program. They do not allow it in themselves. They're CrossFitters.

Jerry Hill, the alpha wolf in this pack of hard-core fitness buffs, is always the first to appear in the shadow of the overpass. In the spring of 2006 his green Honda Civic, hunched low on its tires, crackles over shards of broken malt liquor bottles. It is the hardest-hauling compact sedan in South Philly, weighted down with truck tires, sledgehammers, kettle bells, and medicine balls that will be hurled ten feet in the air, against targets chalked onto the concrete columns of the freeway. Jerry is paid to arrive with the equipment, to sweep away the shards of broken glass, to formulate the day's ordeal, and to throw himself into it as well. It isn't the kind of fitness boot camp where the guy not exercising pretends to be a Marine drill sergeant. It's a pack of people spurring one another on, with a real Marine leading from the front.

Jerry's time in the Marines was a curious combination of training intensity and operational boredom. His training, as part of the Marine Corps 2nd Recon Battalion, was what most nine-year-old boys running around in the woods would invent as a military fantasy adventure: small teams snooping around behind enemy lines, taking notes on the terrain and counting the bad guys. Learning how to sneak onshore from a small boat moored off the coast, how to wade camouflaged through marshland, swim upriver, blow up bridges.

It was the ultimate Boy Scout adventure for a kid who'd never been able to sit down to study, or for any reason really. Growing up, Jerry lived for the moment-to-moment intensity of movement: running through the woods of his parents' ranchette in Upstate New York, jumping onto things, negotiating some kind of ridership agreement with the neighbor's pasture horse, playing basketball with himself just to burn off energy. He had wrestled for the winningest high school coach in the New York State Wrestling Hall of Fame. Coach Joe McCabe, also a Marine, had sent many restless and powerful boys into the Corps.

Being a recon Marine was a blast for guys who could take the physical beat-down of on-the-job training. A typical day might entail ten to twelve miles of running through the woods in boots and camouflage, twenty minutes to eat lunch, then an obstacle course and the run back home. Or swimming a mile in Chesapeake Bay in camouflage and fins. Or long hikes in a severe state of sleep deprivation.

On "Death Run" days, Jerry and his best friend, a skinny and wild-eyed redhead named Jason Cox (aka "Chicken Man") would tear out of their barracks on the beach in full camouflage, boots, and forty pounds of gear. A whole pack of young men kitted out in this fashion would sprint back and forth across the dunes until they collapsed. Given the code of honor and the level of testosterone, stopping short of collapse was not an option. There was no finish line. The exercise was over when only one guy was left on his feet. When they'd recovered, which at age nineteen or twenty took a negligible amount of time, Jerry and Jason would voluntarily hit the gym to powerlift. After a hard day's run, swim, or a twenty-mile patrol, a series of deadlifts, bench presses, and squats were just the thing. No one got injured. That's the glory of being twenty years old.

As if to underscore their invincibility, Jerry and Jason would vie for supremacy in feats of strength and idiocy: running at newspaper stands and tackling them to the ground. Seeing who could put the largest dent in a steel wall locker with his head. They would strategize about which head-butting technique would register the biggest impact on the lockers or on carnival boardwalk punching bags. The advantage of the carnival strongman targets was that, after five minutes, a crowd of thirty people would gather around the jarheads, cheering them on to greater heights of head-butting prowess.

But Jerry Hill didn't see any actual combat. Between 1989 and 1991, there wasn't much live fire exchanged by the few and the brave. Jerry collected weapons from Panamanian villagers, spent six months floating around the Mediterranean, and was benched for Operation Desert Storm. He loved the spirit of the Marines, the people, and the bonds between them. He hated the hierarchy. Perhaps if there'd been battles, he would have felt differently about being ordered around so much. But in the absence of any real-world need for do-or-die, the sense of being at a commanding officer's behest twenty-four hours a day, seven days a week, was stifling. He didn't want to work for anyone, ever again, if he could help it.

When he got out of the Corps, he started powerlifting competitively, to recapture the training intensity he missed from Death Run days. He could lift three times his 165-pound body weight on a bench press, deadlift, or back squat. He became a local contender, went to state competitions. Competing nationally as a member of the Pennsylvania powerlifting team, he could squat 500 pounds. But there were guys in his weight class who could squat 700 pounds. He was out of his league.

When he started running boot camps as a personal trainer, Jerry Hill's competitive powerlifting days were over, and he was doing what most aging athletes do: trying to ward off the specter of injury and decline. Just trying to maintain. He had two little girls, a baby and a toddler, to take care of at home when his wife went off to her office job. He didn't have enough money to open a gym. So he found a pack of people who were tough or crazy enough to train outdoors ten months out of the year. It was like being back in the Marines, a shot of pure testosterone before going home to change diapers.

"No machine," he'd holler in the shadow of I-95, "will ever make you this strong."[1] For a decade, he'd been railing against the idea that Cybex and Nautilus machines did anything to enhance real-world fitness. Every one of his personal training clients used barbells and did functional movements that taxed their whole bodies, not just isolated muscles. They got results. But coming up with workouts, and measuring progress, were difficult. Powerlifters were starting to buzz about CrossFit, a cult training method out of California that anyone could get for free on the Internet. At a strength training seminar, Jerry saw one of the coaches wearing an old-school CrossFit T-shirt. It was simple, declarative, truthful: "CrossFit: Mess You Up."

Jerry quizzed the guy about it and got his hair blown back by the passionate ravings of a dedicated CrossFit acolyte. He started poking around the CrossFit.com website, where CrossFit founder Greg Glassman posted daily workouts and far-flung participants posted their results in the comments field. There were detailed analyses of Olympic weightlifting technique, video demonstrations, and manifestos on the superiority of "constantly varied functional movement, executed at high intensity, across broad time and modal domains." It was all very intense—the training recipes, and the rhetoric.

Most of the movements were familiar compound functional movements. But the way they were combined was novel, and everything was timed. The clock added intensity, and the structure of the workouts, many of them named after women, provided measurable benchmarks. There was huge variation in the program—workouts were different day to day, but also week to week and month to month. The mind-numbing alternation of chest/biceps, back/triceps, common in the bodybuilding world, was nowhere to be seen.

But the obvious thing, to a trainer, was how curiously short the workouts were—five to twenty repetitions of two or three movements, for three to five rounds. It seemed almost trivial, until you tried it and discovered how diabolically intense these Workouts of the Day (WODs) could be. They weren't cardio, in the traditional sense of running or cycling or rowing, the stuff that's supposed to tax your heart and lungs. And yet the combination of weightlifting, sprints, and gymnastic movements left Jerry, who fancied himself an elite athlete, completely gassed. Here was a guy who'd been doing push-ups and pull-ups since he was thirteen, all through the Marines, and squats his whole adult life, including 500-pound back squats. And yet "Cindy"—a workout consisting of 5 pull-ups, 10 push-ups, and 15 unweighted squats, as many rounds as possible in 20 minutes—left him flattened and gasping.

A CrossFit WOD called "Fight Gone Bad" beckoned to Jerry—how could it not, with that name. The workout moves between five movement stations: (1) wall ball shots (a 20-pound medicine ball thrown to a 10-foot target); (2) sumo deadlift high pull (grabbing a 75-pound bar in the middle, with a wide stance, and pulling the bar up above the collarbone); (3) 20-inch box jumps; (4) a 75-pound push press (raising a barbell from shoulders to overhead, with momentum from the legs); and (5) calories on a rowing machine. At each station, an athlete does as many repetitions as possible in 60 seconds. One round consists of 5 minutes of work. "Fight Gone Bad" is three rounds of all five movements, with 1 minute between rounds, 18 minutes total.

At the time, Jerry had a 550-pound deadlift, so he thought a 75-pound sumo deadlift high pull would be a cakewalk. Lots of them? It was only 60 seconds. Jerry blazed through round one of "Fight Gone Bad" in his backyard and was feeling great. By round two, he was barely hanging on. Midway through the third round, he was leaning against the stucco wall of his house, watching the world spin. He didn't finish. It was terrible. It was great.

As far as he was concerned, CrossFit was obviously the way to train. The tricky part was convincing his boot camp clients that this new awful-fantastic high-intensity regime wasn't the sign of a diseased mind. But then, it's amazing what you can get people to do if you have just one other person who's willing to act as if your unconventional behavior is completely normal.

As it happened, Chicken Man lived in Philly. Whatever crazy thing Jerry had ever suggested to Jason, the answer was always, "Yeah, let's do it, Bubba." So when Jerry rolled up in his gasping green Civic to sweep away the broken glass, Jason showed up too. When Jerry had everyone throw twenty-pound balls ten feet in the air against the pillars of I-95, Jason threw wall balls as if he'd been doing it all his life.

When new people showed up wondering where the gym was, Jason would shrug. "This is it. Just do your best, and in a few weeks you'll be feeling the greatest you've ever felt. Just trust him." Some people tried it and never came back. Others stayed, abandoning the comfort and conventional wisdom of gym training for intense bursts of all-out running, jumping, lifting, and dragging heavy objects until their lungs and muscles were spent. It was terrible, in the cold and heat and darkness, to be doing this. But it was great to clock personal records doing it, to see progress, to get stronger—and to be surrounded by others who were willing to run the same gauntlet.

When it got too icy in winter, they would move into a nearby jujitsu studio whose owner was happy to sublet space in off-hours. In spring, Jerry found a more scenic waterfront location at Penn's Landing, and another prime spot by the Korean War Memorial. They lived for the moment-to-moment intensity of movement: running up and down the steps of an outdoor auditorium, jumping onto park benches, doing push-ups and squats and walking lunges that made it difficult to walk the following day. Some part of their bodies ached, all the time. But it was a good ache, the soreness of muscles rebuilding themselves. There is nothing like knowing you will be stronger tomorrow than you are today, that you will notch another gain in a month and blast past previous performance records in the space of a year. Most adults don't even remember what that's like.

After eighteen months under the bridge, in the dojo, and on the waterfront, it was time for Jerry Hill to move. His wife had found a job in Alexandria, Virginia, and the job performed indoors with air-conditioning determined the family's location. Jerry's first order of business was to find another jujitsu studio to sublet in the mornings. He hauled his kettle bells, medicine balls, and barbells into the dojo's second-floor space. Blue mats covered the floor. Pull-up bars hung by chains, like trapeze bars, from the ceiling, lending a circus atmosphere to pull-up-intensive WODs.

A few evening jujitsu students joined Jerry's morning workouts. Strangers wandered in after CrossFit.com's geographical directory identified Jerry's CrossFit Oldtown as the closest place to hit a WOD. Some of the newcomers had been lone-wolf CrossFitters following CrossFit .com WODs from their garages. Others had incurred the wrath and anxiety of health club floor managers for doing Olympic lifts in free-weight areas or handstand push-ups against the mirrored walls of local gyms. What they all had in common was this: they had abandoned the principles and conventions of mainstream fitness—what all the exercise video celebrities, magazine features, and public health authorities say is necessary to get in shape, lose fat, and build muscle. Gasping for air on the floor after eighteen minutes, sometimes after five minutes, in the best shape of their lives, they had repudiated every tenet of the modern gym and fitness industry. And none of them was looking back.

INTO THE RED ZONE
The Science Behind Maximum Effort

SO WHY DO PEOPLE FEEL SO INCREDIBLE ABOUT PULLING TIRES? Why are they so committed to this insane regime? And how do Cross-Fit's alternating combinations of strength effort and cardio stress, otherwise known as metabolic conditioning WODs, or "metcons," bring novices and elite athletes alike to their knees in less than fifteen minutes? People have been cross-training for years, switching between movements in weightlifting supersets or combining cardio with a Nautilus circuit. It doesn't leave them feeling whipped the way a CrossFit metcon of sprints and deadlifts, or pull-ups and box jumps, will leave people groaning on the ground. Beyond the punk-rock hype of an underground movement, and the competitive pressure of group workouts, on a physiological level, what the hell is going on here?

The answer boils down to two things, which combine to extract energy from the human body like nothing else. The first is intensity, and in CrossFit, *intensity* has an objective definition. CrossFit's measure of intensity is the average power output of a human body during the course of a workout,[1] and power can be expressed as a brutally simple formula:[2]

$$POWER = WEIGHT\ MOVED \times DISTANCE\ TRAVELED \div TIME\ IT\ TAKES\ TO\ MOVE$$

This objective measure of fitness—given as foot-pounds per second—informs a training regime that maximizes sheer work capacity, or how much weight a person can move by sprinting, jumping, pulling, push-ing, and lifting before he's physically spent. At weights heavy enough to completely exhaust a person (and in many workouts this is just the weight of one's own body), this doesn't take very long. Typical CrossFit workouts, named for either women or soldiers killed in action, are be-tween three and twenty-five minutes.

What they ask of the human body is essentially what you'd be asking of a truck if you hitched a moderately heavy trailer to it and told the driver to cover anywhere between twenty and two hundred miles in the minimum amount of time. The output of that engine would by far exceed the output required to haul three times the weight at maximum speed for a single mile (although the average power during that mile would be higher) or the energy required to drive ten times as far, at moderate speed, carrying only the driver. This is how CrossFit differs from quick-burst powerlifting and Olympic lifting, on the one hand, and from the aerobic universe of distance runs, cardio machines, and exercise classes on the other.

Now let's say the terrain in that twenty to two hundred miles varies dramatically. Flat stretches allow the truck to accelerate to high speed. But then comes the uphill, then the steep uphill, then downhill, then off-road, then some more asphalt with downed trees blocking the road. That requires a lot of gear switching, and if those gears are switched with too little time on the clutch, they're going to grind.

A CrossFit metcon, alternating strength efforts with cardio stress (muscle fatigue plus a jacked-up heart rate) switches the body's biochem-ical gears like nothing else, and the conscious experience of that gear shifting is a sense of agonizing fatigue.

It starts with fuel. All muscle fibers ultimately use the same fuel: ATP (adenosine triphosphate). The T stands for tri, because the molecule is a chassis for three high-energy phosphates. In a muscle cell, one of those phosphates is split off to produce energy and heat. The molecule, now with only two phosphates on it, needs to be reloaded with a third phos-phate before it can be used again as fuel.

The body has three different metabolic pathways, or fuel production systems, to reload that ATP. For intense, short-duration, high-power activities, muscle cells fire off their existing ATP, then load phosphates that are lying around (in the form of phosphocreatine) into the barrel of depleted ATP molecules to rapidly fire a big boom of effort. This is why high-power athletes take creatine supplements—they're trying to boost the amount of phosphocreatine in their cells, to maximize the high-speed boom of that fuel system.

This system of pulling phosphates off the molecular shelf is called the phosphagen system. It does not require oxygen, which is why 100% power efforts like Olympic weightlifting are called anaerobic exercise. This pathway is unparalleled for producing massive amounts of short-burst power. The downside is: the body doesn't keep a lot of spare phosphates on the shelf—it wouldn't be efficient to keep a lot of high-energy fuel lying around, given the rarity of 100% muscle effort in regular life. The phosphagen pathway depletes its fuel stocks within seconds and can take minutes to fully regenerate. Even champion sprinters cannot sustain phosphagenic effort for a full 100 meters—they reach maximum speed at about 60 meters, then slow down as the phosphagen pathway burns out.[3]

When that happens, a second fuel system takes over. With no ready phosphates on the shelf, the body breaks down blood glucose or glycogen (glucose from carbohydrates, stored in the muscle) for energy to produce ATP. This system, called the glycolytic pathway, doesn't require oxygen either. But it involves ten chemical reactions, so it isn't as fast or explosive as the phosphagen pathway. But this fuel system can sustain power output at 40% to 60% of the phosphagenic maximum for up to two minutes. A 200-meter sprint, a 400-meter run, or a 100-meter swim is a glycolytic effort.[4]

After a couple of minutes, this pathway too is depleted. Its by-products, like lactic acid, build up and begin to interfere with muscle function. At this point, the only available option is the longest-duration, lowest-power fuel system, the oxidative pathway. This system burns oxygen, which is why the activities that rely on it are called aerobic exercise. It generates a lot of energy, because it burns fat in addition to carbohydrates. But it's a long, slow, multi-stage chemical process—the energy it produces flows from a kitchen faucet, not a firehose. It produces only 10% to 20% of the power output an Olympic lift or all-out 50-meter sprint would require. But it's highly sustainable. Most marathoners only "hit the wall" of glycogen depletion at mile twenty, after hours of sustained effort. The oxidative pathway is what keeps endurance athletes going.

A CrossFit metcon, which alternates strength efforts and cardio stress, effectively drains all three tanks by forcing the oxidative pathway to function as a backup when the phosphagen and glycolytic systems recharge. Explosive high-power movements like box jumps and barbell lifts deplete the anaerobic pathways. When that energy is gone, all that's left is the oxidative generator to power through a row or a run. Then it's time for another Olympic lift. Firing from high-power pathways before they've recovered leads to lactic acid buildup and oxygen debt, so the aerobic stuff feels like it's being done on the surface of Saturn. Every gear is taxed.

These energy systems feed into different muscle types, which are similarly whipsawed by the WOD. As with the fuel systems, the body uses three types of muscle fibers for different movements. Type I slow-twitch fibers are used for low-intensity exercises like repeatedly lifting light weights or trudging on a cardio machine. These fibers aren't very powerful, but they can work for long periods of time. Type IIa quick-twitch fibers are used for activities that require more power, but less than maximum effort. They can hold out for a few minutes. Type IIb fast-twitch fibers, the third muscle type, are the most powerful of all, and the quickest to fatigue. In ten to thirty seconds, they're done, and they need at least twice that long to recover. They're also inefficient—it takes three times as much energy to do one bench press at 80% of your maximum capacity as it takes to do four bench presses at 20% of your maximum.[5]

Fibers of the same type are bundled into self-contained motor units, and each type of motor unit has a different electrical threshold for activation by the central nervous system. If an activity doesn't require much power, only Type I fibers are recruited into action. When the force required nears 20% of a person's maximum capacity, the central nervous system boosts its electrical levels enough to trigger Type IIa motor units. Only when the force requirement approaches maximum capacity—the maximum weight you can lift in a couple of seconds—does the central nervous system pump out enough charge to shock Type IIb motor units into action.

The same rotating stress that overwhelms all three fuel systems also exhausts all three mechanical systems, and the wiring system to boot. As more charge is required to fire up motor units, the neurotransmitters that perpetuate nerve signals get depleted, making it more difficult to initiate and control coordinated movements. Neurotransmitter depletion also compromises cognitive function—memory and motivation.[6] This is why CrossFitters who manipulate spreadsheets in their day jobs will use chalk or poker chips to count their rounds. They literally lack the mental capacity to do basic arithmetic in the middle of a WOD. What someone experiences subjectively as mental fog or a mustering of will is a physical process in the nervous system. But the same stress that taxes the wiring also reinforces it. The nervous system adapts to function at higher capacity. Upgraded circuits allow the body to sustain more effort, and to improve the mechanics of movement, thus increasing physical power.

To top it off, the WOD's punishing intensity has a profound hormonal effect. During high-intensity—but not low-intensity—workouts, the human body produces growth hormone,[7] which cues the body to build muscle and burn fat. Human growth hormone (HGH) has a lighter-fluid effect on physical strength and athletic performance, which is why professional athletes get kicked out of their sports for injecting themselves with it. After a CrossFit WOD, elevated growth hormone is present in the blood for a solid twenty-four hours. Other hormones and enzymes released during high-intensity exercise shift the muscles' fuel from carbohydrate to fat, and that effect persists for up to forty-eight hours after a WOD.[8] For days afterward, the body is burning additional energy and fat, just rebuilding muscle and adapting to the energetic stress of a fifteen-minute WOD.

There is a qualitative difference in the physical results of high-intensity exercise, compared with the moderate-intensity cardio sessions that are recommended by fitness gurus and public health authorities as the best way to lose fat and get healthy. This difference is partly attributable to an increase in Type II muscle fibers, which triggers a change in fat metabolism, even if a person's diet stays the same.[9] There's no Type II muscle use in anything but an all-out sprint or a maximum-effort lift. So gym members on the cardio floor, even the ones on the elliptical's "interval" or "hill-climbing" mode, aren't getting that benefit. Neither are the Nautilus folks doing sets of ten to twelve leg curls, or the guys on the bench flexing their biceps with dumbbells.

The metabolic boost of quick-twitch fibers, plus the hormonal re-programming induced by high-intensity intervals, yields some startling scientific research results. In a controlled experiment, researchers took average people and put one group in an endurance training program (45 minutes on a stationary bike at 60% to 85% of their maximum heart rate, which exceeds the typical health club cardio session), and another group in a high-intensity interval program (twenty minutes on the bike, alternating between 30-second all-out sprints and 90-second recovery periods at lower intensity). Both workouts required the same amount of energy—the calorie readouts on all the bikes displayed the same numbers. The high-intensity group, whose workouts were half as long, burned nine times as much fat as the endurance group.[10]

This finding, that short high-intensity exercise burns radically more fat than long aerobic workouts with the same calorie burn, has been replicated for men and women; overweight and obese people; young, old, and diabetic people.[11] In a study of young women, 20-minute sessions of cycle sprints (8 seconds at maximum intensity, alternating with 12 seconds at lower intensity) led to an 11.2% loss of body fat, compared with a group of women cycling for 40 minutes at 60% capacity, who lost no body fat.[12] Again, the energy required for both workouts was the same. The high-intensity group wasn't burning more calories during their workouts. But they lost a significant amount of fat in general, and abdominal fat in particular, even though they had bumped up their caloric intake by 200 calories a day toward the end of the study. They were hormonally different: their insulin resistance (an indicator of Type 2 diabetes) was lower, and their metabolism had shifted to burn more fat.

The cardio group, who lost no weight, was hormonally unchanged. They'd cut their daily caloric intake by 400 calories toward the end of the study, but had managed to gain nonsignificant amounts of belly fat. They'd improved their aerobic fitness—their heart and lung capacity— they just didn't get any leaner. The awkward consensus of well-conducted research studies is that the 150 minutes a week of moderate exercise recommended by the American Heart Association and the US Department of Health produces negligible weight loss,[13] whereas high-intensity workouts of half the duration produce dramatic fat loss.

The contrast is just as stark when researchers compare the effect of exercise on metabolic syndrome—a combination of high blood pressure, high cholesterol, high triglycerides, large waist circumference, and high blood sugar or diabetes that defines the industrialized world's health problems. On a genetic level, high-intensity exercise activates the genes that increase insulin sensitivity (thus reversing the progression to diabetes) at more than double the rate of moderate-intensity exercise for workouts with an equivalent calorie burn.[14]

A Canadian epidemiological study[15] found that among adults who met the US Department of Health guideline for moderate exercise, 30% had metabolic syndrome. Among those who did 75 minutes a week of high-intensity exercise, less than 10% had metabolic syndrome. More dramatically, people who did even 38 minutes a week of intense exercise dropped their odds of metabolic syndrome to 20%, the same as moderate-intensity exercisers who were working out 600 minutes a week. Per day, that's the same health outcome for a 6-minute sprint versus a 90-minute jog.

The evidence is clear. The only problem, researchers concede in the driest of tones, is that "some people do not like high-intensity exercise, in some cases because of low fitness."[16] People like to stay in their comfort zones. Comfort precludes intensity, unless there's something on the other side of intensity that justifies the sacrifice of comfort.

The conscious experience of a WOD is a core drill through a couple of million years of psychic sediment. In the first round of a WOD like "Kelly" (a 400-meter sprint, 30 jumps onto a 24-inch box, then 30 wall balls, five rounds), you think, "Why am I doing this? I could be watching TV on a treadmill." Your rationalizing brain still works well enough to have thoughts like this. By round four, your ability to formulate alternative scenarios is completely gone. It is a physical and psychic struggle: nerves, muscles, and will on one side and gravity on the other. You're fighting gravity, fighting all the ugly inevitabilities—decline, decrepitude, death—with all the strength you can muster. Everyone around you is in the same fight, and this makes it easier to keep going.

By round five, the depletion of every metabolic pathway, muscle fiber, and neural circuit has all internal diagnostics on the blink. There isn't even an abstract notion of heroic effort, or any abstract notion—the part of your brain that tells stories is off-line. There is only the raw impetus to finish somehow. Ninety seconds ago, it seemed impossible to keep moving. But the end is so close, and the closeness of the end unlocks a last canister of strength that your mind would not relinquish until the end. That last burst is the most terrible, and the sweetest, because its power is mined from a place that is inaccessible in the beginning. You're getting down to the good stuff, to the kindling spark of your own stronger, fiercer self.

The last wall ball reaches its zenith. It lands with a *thwump* as you take a controlled fall to the ground. In this short interval, the body produces so much heat that it radiates visibly upwards as steam, winter and summer, even in a hot room. As your lungs quench a consuming thirst for air, you can feel the kick drum of your heart, blood rushing in your ears like the ocean in a seashell. As the heat of your body rises up like an offering, every vapor droplet is shot through with light. The steam, backlit by fluorescent light fixtures, almost seems to be carrying a part of you up toward the ceiling.

We are geared for this experience, which the guidelines and caveats of modern society wall off from us. On the cardio machine dashboard at the gym, there's usually a graph divided into three shaded zones: the green not-worth-the-trouble-to-show-up zone, the yellow aerobic zone, and the dangerous-looking red "anaerobic" curve on top.

The yellow zone is where people are supposed to stay. It's the "fat-burning zone" that doesn't actually cause people to lose weight. We're implicitly instructed by this piece of equipment and the industry behind it to go faster than a walking pace, but never to really push it. To stay in the suitably safe and virtuous middle ground. People follow instructions. They stay there. And as long as they do, there is something that will always be hidden from them, which is the knowledge of what their bodies, as glorious machines, can do, and the competence and satisfaction of actually doing it.

THE MONKEY BARS

CrossFit's Genesis

Every functional exercise contains an
essential bit of human capacity.

—GREG GLASSMAN

GREG GLASSMAN, THE GUY WHO INVENTED CROSSFIT, WAS A gymnast who'd gone feral. He'd grown up in the San Fernando Valley, then a cradle of world-class gymnasts. His high school sent a sixteen-year-old, Steve Hug, to the 1968 Olympics.

What made the official programs so good—what created a deep and brilliant pool of gymnasts for coaches to draw on—was a bunch of kids teaching one another, pushing themselves, and competing against their groups. In the days before draconian consumer protection codes and liability scares, there were stainless steel high bars, parallel bars, and rings in most of the Valley's public parks. Kids would roam like packs of wild dogs from park to park to conduct informal workshops and square off against friends and rivals.

"We'd go do gymnastics in the parks, in West Valley, Lanark Park, Topanga, and Roscoe Valley, then down to Santa Monica to see the kids on Muscle Beach," Glassman recalls. "I knew when I was ten years old that I wanted to be a ring man. At twelve years old, I could do a handstand on the rings—all taught at the park. You had to earn your stripes, doing gymnastics outside."

In 1972, Glassman was in his midteens and looking to get stronger, so he could become a better gymnast. According to a story he likes to tell, perhaps the most famous of CrossFit's fireside tales, young Greg convinced his father to convert their garage into an improvised training room. As an up-and-coming gymnast in a highly competitive school program, Greg wanted to simulate the way a two-minute ring routine would leave a gymnast gasping for air. Because, he deadpans, "if you get off the apparatus and you're hunched over or you vomit or you're gape mouthed, breathing hard, wild in terror, you'll be deducted for that. So you have to get off and look as cool as a cucumber, like 'That was fun.' Or it's held against you."[1]

The problem was, none of the lateral raises and curls in the guide that came with his $19.95 Ted Williams weightlifting set from Sears would ever take him to that desperate, gasping, vomity state he needed to conquer. Standard weightlifting exercises had none of That Feeling. So, like a kid playing guitar licks in search of a song, he just started to mess around and improvise until he found it: If you bring a weighted bar to your chest, then go as low as you can into a full squat, then explode up to drive the bar all the way over your head, that's what's now called a thruster. If you do ten of those in a row, it takes you toward That Feeling.

As the story goes, Glassman did twenty-one in a row, then jumped on the pull-up bar in the doorjamb and did twenty-one pull-ups. Fifteen thrusters, fifteen pull-ups. Nine thrusters, nine pull-ups. Then he unceremoniously threw up on the floor. Victory!

As his German shepherds licked up the mess, Glassman raced across the street, vomit still on his shirt, to his friend Brian's house and banged on the door. Brian, a fellow gymnast, stared in alarm at his panting friend.

"Dude, what's all over your shorts?"

"Never mind! Come with me!"

They went to Greg's garage and repeated the workout. Brian threw up. It was awesome.

They ran across the street to get Brian's brother and bolted into his room.

"What's *on* you guys?" he asked. "You smell like vomit."

"Come on!" they yelled, the way that teenagers always do when they've discovered the be-all, end-all coolest thing ever.

"I don't think so."

Thus was born the most dreaded workout in CrossFit, later known as "Fran": 21 thrusters, followed by 21 pull-ups, then 15 of each, then 9 of each (21-15-9 in CrossFit parlance). The day "Fran" was born, Greg Glassman found his calling as a trainer. He distilled the essence of CrossFit: high-intensity full-body movements that obliterate the distinction between "strength training" and "cardio." He also encountered the binary response that people have when they see or try CrossFit. Some people get the lightning bolt: *this is what I've been searching for.* The rest think it's a sign of mental illness.

Intensity was the foundational element of CrossFit—a carryover from gymnastics. Gymnastics demands absolute physical commitment in the moment of effort. You have to stick the landing. There is no half dismount.

The flip side of CrossFit's intensity is a rabid empiricism and obsessiveness about the measurement of results. Not proxies for performance— the muscle's ability to flex or the body's ability to metabolize oxygen (VO_2 max), measured under controlled conditions—but real-world measures of athletic performance, at intensity, under fatigue, that can be clocked, counted, or put on a scale.

CrossFit's mantra of "measurable, observable, repeatable" was also rooted in Greg Glassman's adolescence. His dad was an engineer at Hughes. In the booming California aerospace industry, whose ashes gave rise to Silicon Valley, it seemed as if every dad in Greg's neighborhood worked for the defense industry. Back then, the engineering zeitgeist was all about making things fly (or blow up), and that took a lot of math and precision measurement. It was natural, then, for a somewhat hard-ass, authoritarian dad who worked for a defense contractor to instill in his son the importance of precision and measurement and the empirical derivation of mathematical formulas.

As Glassman recounts with characteristic brio,[2] his dad inculcated

this lesson by bringing home a bag of a thousand nails and a micrometer, a precision measuring tool used by engineering machinists. His dad
took the micrometer out of its wooden box and told his son to measure
all one thousand nails and record their length to the nearest thousandth
of an inch. After his father had left the room, Greg calculated that, at
the rate he'd been dutifully measuring and recording the lengths of individual nails, it'd take about eight hours to finish the project. Then he
started faking the data to speed up the process.

Eight hours later, Greg announced that he was done. His dad looked
at the data and asked his son if he had, in fact, really measured the nails.

"Yeah!" Greg replied.

"Well," said his dad, "this is bullshit." In a real bag of nails, there
are a few outliers that are significantly longer or shorter than the rest.
There are lots of nails that are a bit short or a bit long. But the bulk of
the nails' measurements cluster right around the average length. This
is the normal, bell-curved distribution that you find in most sets of
measurements—but not in data fabricated by kids. Greg had no idea
how his dad had figured out the data was fake, but he was back to measuring nails. This time, it took sixteen hours. When he was done, he and
his dad plotted the frequency of each measurement, and the resulting
graph was a perfect bell curve.

"I was taught the concept of a Gaussian distribution," Glassman says.
"That is an ineluctable essential fact of nature. Almost anything we measure in nature will show this kind of pattern. But screw the pattern—the
real lesson here was that careful observation, coupled with measurement, can reveal secrets of the universe hitherto unknown, unseen, and
undiscovered."

Which is true. The task structure of this teaching moment, however,
is apt to instill a reflexive distaste for arbitrary diktats from authority
figures, or for any form of learning or discovery that feels coercive or
by the book. If you combine a love of intensity with a passion for measurement and a psychic peanut allergy to top-down authority, you have
CrossFit's basic DNA.

Hoping to shine as a gymnast on the rings and parallel bars, Glassman enrolled at UCLA. He left, before actually taking any classes, when UCLA's program eliminated single-event gymnasts in favor of all-round competitors. He spent the next few years bouncing between a dozen California colleges. On a ring-routine dismount, he broke his leg so badly that his tibia was shoved behind his femur, an injury that left him with permanent nerve damage and a slight limp. In the summer of '78, he took a job at Hughes and hated it. He taught himself math and liked it. The problem with math, as he saw it, was that a degree in math would put him right back at Hughes, which was like the bag-of-a-thousand-nails exercise, with a pay stub.

While enrolled at Pasadena City College, he got a job coaching gymnastics at the local Y. It was the first of many facilities he'd leave, with roughly the same frequency with which he switched colleges. He worked as a trainer at Gold's Gym in Venice and left. When the Gold's Gym in Santa Cruz tried to charge him five hundred dollars a month for a 10- by 10-foot training space, he threw a temper tantrum and left. He got results out of the people he trained. That was part of the problem. Other trainers' clients would see his clients banging out sets of pull-ups and decamp to train with Glassman.

It's one thing for a trainer to make personal training clients feel subjectively better for showing up to the gym. This, plus the cheerleading and bossing around that one-on-one training typically entails, is most personal trainers' stock-in-trade. It doesn't disturb the competitive equilibrium because no one's clients get conspicuously stronger or more capable. They're not developing any skill. The minute they start developing skills and begin to display conspicuously higher levels of athletic performance in addition to their whittled waistlines, that rocks the boat.

Friendly fire from other trainers was a perennial problem. But a larger source of strife between Glassman and his health club overseers was the distribution of proceeds from personal training. When a gym member pays seventy-five dollars for a personal training session, the gym keeps half of that, and often pays the trainer as an independent contractor. In a high-tax state like California, that leaves a lot of trainers working like dogs to make a decent living while gyms mint money for providing overhead. For someone like Glassman, who considered himself a professional, the feudal business model of gym-based personal training was unjust, and this sense of injustice turned every employment situation into a ticking time bomb.

GLASSMAN'S LAST EMPLOYER WAS A HEALTH CLUB CALLED SPA Fitness in Santa Cruz. He'd moved to Santa Cruz to train officers in the Santa Cruz Police Department, and had garnered some local acclaim for whipping the Santa Cruz PD into shape. He trained civilians at Spa Fitness and married one of his clients, a strong blonde named Lauren. The two of them lived in a tiny apartment, biked everywhere because they didn't own a car, and taught spinning classes at Spa. These classes were epic interval training bouts, all-out sprints alternating with "moderate" intervals that were just as exhausting, but more sustainable.

The terrific awfulness of the workouts was catnip to a spin-class devotee named Eva Twardokens, or Eva T. as she was called by people flummoxed by the pronunciation of her Polish surname. Eva was a former Olympic skier. Her father, a Polish Olympic fencer, placed third in the 1958 World Fencing Championships in Philadelphia. At age twenty-seven, on an American exhibition tour with his Polish teammates, he slipped away from his Eastern bloc minders to seek asylum in the West. He and his wife had both been raised in the fold of Eastern bloc sports and Polish Catholicism. But in the mountains outside Reno, Nevada, the discipline of attendance at Sunday Mass was relaxed to ensure that their daughter was outdoors skiing on Sunday mornings. "Skiing is your church," Eva's mother would say. "You're outside. You're enjoying nature, and that's what God intended." Skiing was everything.

Eva was sixteen when she made the US national ski team. She made her World Cup slalom debut in 1982 at age seventeen. Three years later, she took silver at the World Cup in Switzerland and bronze at the World Championship in Italy. A six-time US champion, she blew out her knee before the '88 Olympics and missed competing in Sarajevo. But she was a top-ten finisher in the giant slalom and super G in Albertville, and in the giant slalom in Lillehammer. At age twenty-nine, she retired to become a dental hygenist and windsurf in Santa Cruz. She loved windsurfing—it gave her the flow and movement of a slalom without the joint-rattling impact.

She loved the intensity of Greg Glassman's spinning class. He was enthralled with her athletic pedigree. He offered to train her for free. And as he cobbled together the grammar and syntax of CrossFit, Eva was his high-intensity guinea pig. Her raw capacity was superhuman. But she also had vulnerabilities. She was banged up—she'd had eight knee surgeries. Their relationship was on the line if he prescribed something gratuitously extreme and stupid and busted the seam of an old injury. A lot of care went into the design of proto-CrossFit workouts to avoid hurting Eva.

Glassman shared Eva's enthusiasm for the Olympic lifts that had made her such a monster on the slopes. They were just the thing his private training clients needed to get fantastically strong. So he gathered his trainees together to watch Eva demonstrate a clean and jerk, jumping a barbell from floor to the shoulders, then propelling it all the way overhead. On the jerk, the overhead part, she missed the lift and dropped the bar, as she'd been taught. Any bar that's too heavy to lift overhead will shred shoulder muscles if an athlete tries to control it to the ground. Olympic lifters are trained to drop the bar when they miss a heavy lift. But they usually train with rubber-coated bumper plates. Eva's plates were steel, and 115 pounds of stacked steel makes a pretty explosive noise when it hits the floor.

A couple of days later, when they met for breakfast, Glassman broke the news. The clean-and-jerk incident had provided a dramatic pretext for his dismissal from Spa Fitness. And there were no more gyms in Santa Cruz to get booted out of. Every bridge had been burned.

"What am I going to do?" he asked. "I don't even know what to tell Lauren."

"It's going to be okay," Eva replied. "Start your own thing."

CLAUDIO FRANCA, A STORIED BRAZILIAN JUJITSU INSTRUCTOR and one of the first to teach Brazilian jujitsu in the United States, ran his dojo in Santa Cruz. He'd heard about Glassman's unconventional training methods. It looked like something that would be good physical conditioning for fighters. So Franca offered mat space in his dojo, if Glassman agreed to train Franca's jujitsu contenders. Glassman gratefully accepted the offer. He and Lauren ran their training business from a small patch of jujitsu mats, with high-speed sets of push-ups, squats, and other bodyweight exercises and almost no equipment. To protect the dojo's mats, athletes had to remove their shoes, which made indoor WODs with outdoor sprints a test of shoe-lacing dexterity as well as running speed.

The Glassmans had an Airdyne bike, a diabolical flywheel apparatus with pedals and arm levers, sometimes known as "the devil's tricycle." Wind resistance from the flywheel is exponential—the harder you work, the more difficult it becomes to generate additional speed. The Airdyne is Marxist in its ability to extract more energy from the strong than it does from the weak. It's kryptonite.

A sprint interval workout on the Airdyne reduced Glassman's everyday clients to quivering puddles. But the same workout would force Eva to steady herself against the wall when she tried to walk afterward. The calorie readout after Eva's Airdyne workout was higher than a non-Olympian's. But all her extra capacity had been sucked dry to achieve that marginal gain. So she was equally wrecked. Glassman loved the fact that a workout could be achievable for regular people yet also cause an Olympic athlete to nearly fall on her face.

After a year and a half, the Glassmans had enough clients to move into a dedicated space, 1,250 square feet on Research Park Drive—home base of the original CrossFit gym, or "box" in the CrossFit parlance. The Santa Cruz box was equipped with all the accoutrements a CrossFitter would recognize: Dynamax medicine balls, jumping boxes, pull-up rigs, rowing machines, dumbbells, barbells, and bumper plates. The Glassmans couldn't afford to hire a janitor, so they had to clean the bathrooms themselves. But that was okay. It was their own place.

There were a few mega-athletes in the training stable: mixed martial arts contenders paced Eva T. Garth Taylor did CrossFit for a year then went to Brazil to win the 1999 World Jiu-Jitsu Championship, justifying Claudio Franca's hunch. Professional rock climber Rob Miller trained with the Glassmans and went out to slash unassisted peak ascents from days to hours.[3] Part of the energy in that original gym came from the cross-pollination of high-end athletes—it was a place where rock climbers, surfers, cyclists, yogic contortionists, and mixed martial artists could swap techniques and learn from one another.

None of the elite athletes paid for their training. "I have always done things for athletes," Glassman says, "on the backs of software people, orthodontists, and real estate agents." But the elite athletes weren't there for marquee value. They were there to provide the outlier data in a sample that included the techies, orthodontists, and real estate agents, as well as a few grannies on the far end of the functional fitness curve. The Glassmans were determined to develop a training method that scaled from the elite athlete all the way down to seventy-somethings—this was critical to the development of CrossFit.

"The needs of the elderly and professional athletes vary by degree, not kind," he declared in an early manifesto, one of many posted to the CrossFit.com website. "Improved hip capacity will help a pro ball player's throw to first; it will also reduce the chances of grandpa falling in the tub."[4] Elite athletes need fast hips, strong torsos, and good balance to dominate their competitors, he argued. Senior citizens need those things as well, to maintain their independence. Squats were the prescription for both.

An elite athlete would be done for the day after squatting with a barbell that weighed hundreds of pounds, while a grandmother pushed the limits of her capacity squatting with a broomstick or a PVC pipe. Pushups could be done on the knees. Dumbbell shoulder presses could be substituted for handstand push-ups.

It took guts for these women to work out alongside athletes half as old and three times as strong. But there was a tremendous payoff. One frail but courageous seventy-year-old woman came to Greg Glassman in tears about her lack of functional independence—she couldn't pick her grandchildren up from the ground. After a long series of inch-by-inch improvements, she was deadlifting 100 pounds. A woman in her late fifties lost 60 pounds and could do multiple squats with a 78-pound barbell held overhead. There are a lot of twenty-something women who can't do that. Glassman had grandmothers doing pull-ups, ring dips, and shimmying up 15-foot climbing ropes. And when they slapped the ceiling, he had a roomful of elite athletes clapping and cheering for them.[5] More important, these ladies weren't helpless when they had to move a five-gallon water bottle or a bag of dog food into the house. They didn't have to ask the neighbor kid to do any of that.

There are CrossFit coaches whose main focus is building functional fitness in the elderly. "You look at what happens to people, they trip on the transition of the carpet to linoleum," says Jimmy Baker, whose clients at CrossFit Santa Cruz Central range from mid-fifties to mid-eighties. "And then, they shove their hand out there and they break something. If we just get your leg out, if we practice moving your leg out there, or back, you stand a chance at not hurting yourself."[6]

Before long, Glassman was conducting coaching seminars at the box. The curriculum for aspiring CrossFit coaches ran the gamut from nutrition and physiology to biomechanics and the principles of lifelong fitness. Glassman drew a continuum from "sickness" to "wellness" to "fitness." The idea of living a sedentary, unhealthy life until you get sick, he argued, was tragic and ludicrous. People could forestall illness and frailty simply by taking deliberate steps to move along the continuum, and it was the coach's privilege and responsibility to help that happen.

The keys to progress along the continuum from sickness to fitness were good nutrition and functional movement. The nutritional prescription was "vegetables, meat, nuts and seeds, some fruit, little starch, and no sugar." The exercise prescription was functional movement—multijointed exertion that requires the whole body to stabilize and coordinate itself. These movements—squats, jumps, lunges, pull-ups, push-ups, sprints, Olympic and power lifts, gymnastic maneuvers, and metabolically taxing movements like thrusters and burpees (dive down, do a push-up, leap up vertically with an overhead clap)—were the do-re-mi of human functionality, the kind that everyone needs to get around and make themselves useful. Lift up a five-gallon bottle of spring water (a deadlift). Put a roller bag into the overhead luggage compartment (a clean and jerk).

These movements are irreducible—they can't be trained by going from one muscle isolation machine to the next. No amount of leg extensions and ab crunches, shoulder presses and wrist flexes, adds up to snatching a barbell from ground to overhead. This isn't because the isolation-trained muscles aren't strong enough but because the nervous system of a circuit-trained gym rat isn't wired up to coordinate those nicely rounded muscles into an effective application of force. In the real world, heavy objects have to be moved and lifted without pulley cables. There are physics that come into play, in three dimensions, that require stabilization, counterbalance, and skill.

Actually lifting a heavy object overhead, as opposed to pushing up on the overhead press machine, requires a burst of explosive power—zero to 100% in a split second—that never occurs in a carefully controlled dumbbell curl. The physics also demand that you keep the load close to your body and get it directly overhead. If you don't, the cantilevered weight generates torque that shoulders can't bear, which will cause you to lose your balance and drop the weight.

Pulling the weight straight up, skimming from shins to shirt to an overhead position, means loading the large muscles of the legs and hips to generate explosive force that puts the weight in motion, upwards from the ground. As that force transfers, the weight gains momentum—it becomes easier to move up. This is when effort shifts from the large lower-body muscles to smaller upper-body muscles. Throughout, the girdling muscles of the torso provide stability. It's not a forward crunch, a side crunch, a twisty sit-up, or a back extension. It's everything, poised against everything.

This is a feat of coordination—the brain has to understand how to orchestrate all these large and small muscles into a single symphony of force. So if you've been strength-training on muscle isolation machines and you have to get something very heavy overhead, or even to your shoulders, you're out of luck, because the overhead press machine doesn't prepare anyone for that kind of real-world effort.[7] The same goes for grappling or wrestling—if you can knock someone off balance with a powerful blow (from the hips, torso, and chest), it's much easier to get them on the ground. Fighting is fighting. Leg extensions are leg extensions. They don't have much to do with each other.

As Greg Glassman formulated his über-theory of fitness in Santa Cruz, he identified ten attributes of fitness: cardiovascular/respiratory endurance (the body's ability to gather, process, and deliver oxygen); stamina (ditto, for energy); strength (the ability to apply force); power (the ability to apply maximum force); flexibility, speed, agility (the ability to minimize transition time from one movement pattern to another); coordination, accuracy, and balance.[8]

Glassman was quick to admit that there were elite athletes who could beat the best CrossFitters in any of these physiological facets. A world-class marathoner, a sub-four-minute-mile runner, or a powerlifter who could back-squat 1,000 pounds would prevail in their event. But, he argued, each of these specialists would be deficient in the other attributes of all-round fitness. The endurance runner, whose skinny frame was optimized to carry only his body weight across long distances, would lack muscular strength and power—he might not be able to do a pull-up. The powerlifter would lack speed, agility, cardiovascular capacity, and flexibility.

The closest approximation of the CrossFit ideal athlete in conventional sport is either a decathlete or a sprint triathlete. If you smooshed together a gymnast, a mid-distance sprinter, and a weightlifter, that would be an elite CrossFitter. He wouldn't take the podium in any of those sports, but he'd be physically prepared for any physical task that life might throw at him. The CrossFit rationale is that, ultimately, this is what matters in real life: the sudden dash to keep a child from running into the street, the ability to help a friend move heavy furniture into a walk-up apartment, or the lung power and stamina to enjoy a hiking vacation.

Part of what makes CrossFit distinctive as a fitness movement is this idea that life, the universe, could swerve in unexpected ways and make daunting physical demands, that your survival or success might at any moment hinge on your ability to move your body and some kind of heavy load over distance quickly. The CrossFit mantra of "constantly varied functional movement executed at high intensity" is about mental and physical preparedness to move quickly, do work, bear weight—to be a clutch player in the game of life. Every CrossFitter secretly believes that the people in their box will be the ones to survive the zombie apocalypse.

CrossFit's definition of fitness is about readiness for random physical demands. It's the triumph of the generalist. Workouts of the Day (WODs) combine all elements of fitness in an ever-changing fashion, to force physical adaptations in each of these ten dimensions, and to keep all of these elements in balance.

If you ask a CrossFitter to define CrossFit, you'll hear a recitation of Glassman's capsule description: "constantly varied functional movement, executed at high intensity, across broad time and modal domains." Which basically means, hauling yourself and heavy objects quickly, horizontally or vertically, in any one of a hundred different ways, over a period of time that ranges from seconds to half an hour. It's excruciating. But yesterday's form of torture won't be repeated for months.

If you then ask what the rote definition actually means, people will talk about being able to do things they couldn't do before. Women will talk about being able to do pull-ups for the first time. Men will talk about Olympic lifts. Anyone who's climbed a 15-foot rope will talk about that. CrossFit spurs a lot of first-time achievements and personal records. There's a thrill to doing something difficult for the first time. The more daunting a movement seems at the outset, the more satisfying it is to achieve after weeks, months, or even years. People are learning to move their bodies and objects through space in a more powerful way, and that sense of mastery keeps them motivated. It makes training seem more like play, albeit of the most exhausting sort. There are nets hanging from the ceiling. People climb. They jump up on boxes and pull-up rigs. They throw medicine balls high against the wall and drop heavy objects on the ground. The typical CrossFit box is a defoliated orangutan habitat.

The major differences between the movements in this grown-up playground and the kinds that happen at a conventional gym are the neurological elements of fitness: coordination, accuracy, agility, and balance. These capabilities require a knitting-together of nerves and muscles and adaptations in the brain. They can be acquired only through practice and are accelerated by coaching. They are entirely absent from the kinds of workouts that people do at gyms.

The modern gym has been deliberately designed to not require any coordination, accuracy, agility, or balance. The attributes of fitness that bind the body and brain together have become the exclusive province of athletes, dancers, and the few lucky children who still climb trees, pop bicycle wheelies, and hang upside down from monkey bars. The stripping-away of coordination, accuracy, agility, and balance from physical culture—from our modern notion of fitness—has made us weaker, because power, the ability to apply maximum force, requires neural circuitry that's impossible to develop on a pulley cable.

But it's worse than that. If all we lost in the transition from functional fitness to circuit-trained muscle development was power, we'd be losing something the modern world doesn't demand. Most of us can live pretty well, in a physical sense, without building huge amounts of physical power.

The problem is, the area of our brain that's responsible for full-body movement . . . that's not all it does. The brain controls movement in three areas, depending on the complexity of the movement. The primary motor cortex, the lowest-level switch box, is responsible for simple movements like tapping a finger or shifting the position of your head. Slightly in front of this area is a more sophisticated control center that's responsible for more integrated movements, like reaching for an object. In front of this is a third, even more intricate control center called the attention association area. The attention association area is the part of the brain that controls complex movements that involve the entire body. This is where coordination, accuracy, agility, and balance live. That's what it evolved to do. That's what it does in animals. When a predator leaps to latch onto a piece of prey and snap its neck, that complex coordinated pounce comes from the attention association area of the predator's brain. The neural "go signal" to pounce comes from the same place in the animal's brain that controls the physical execution of the movement.

In human beings, the attention association area, like many parts of the brain, has evolved in a way that transcends its original function. This area that controls complex movements, that generates the "go signal" to execute them, also generates goal-setting behavior and purposeful organization of thought. "To put it bluntly," writes Andrew Newberg, a neuroscience professor who researches the neural mechanisms of consciousness, "a great part of what one sees with injury to the attention association area is a loss of will and an inability to form intention. If any part of the brain can be said to be the seat of the will or of intentionality, it is certainly the attention association area."[9]

So the part of your brain that enables you to do pull-ups and squats— but isn't engaged for a bicep curl or leg extension—also gives you the discipline to study instead of watch TV, or to budget versus rack up debt on a credit card. High-intensity functional movement *requires* will power, in no small part because will power itself is what's being built in the nervous system during the workout, through the movements themselves. Every time you snatch a barbell from ground to overhead, the complexity of the movement reinforces the circuitry you need to formulate a goal.

When CrossFitters talk about how the workouts have influenced their lives by making it easier for them to get their act together, they are describing a biological process. On the flip side, the way we allow health club machines to stabilize and limit our range of movement, to literally keep us on track, leaves us less purposeful. The abandonment of complex movement and physical intensity has rendered us, in some fundamental way, less intelligent. We have been kinesthetically brainwashed by the machines that are supposed to make us fit.

RISE OF THE MACHINES
The Gym Circuit and Junk Fitness

IRONICALLY, THE PIONEER OF MACHINE-BASED MUSCLE ISOLA-
tion exercises was a guy a lot like Greg Glassman. Dudley Allen Sargent, born in 1849, was a self-taught gymnast from Belfast, Maine. He was seven years old when his father died, and as he hurtled into his early teens he became obsessed with strength training. He got hold of a popular fitness manual of the day, *The Family Gymnasium*, which recommended the use of Indian clubs—large, heavy bowling pin–shaped weights, the kettle bells of their day.

"Indian clubs became immediately necessary to my happiness," he wrote in his autobiography. Sargent convinced his uncle to convert his barn into an improvised training facility, then installed parallel and horizontal bars and began training himself and his friends to do gymnastic stunts, between bouts of Indian club swinging and weightlifting. They ganged together to start a high school gymnastics club. But the main action was in the barn, where Sargent's uncle brought friends and neighbors to see impromptu gymnastics and acrobatics performances.

After a brief stint in a traveling circus, Sargent parlayed his gymnastic prowess into a job as the physical director of Bowdoin College in Brunswick, Maine. At age twenty, in tandem with his university attendance, he ran the gym. He had to make do with a subpar space and almost no equipment. Since he hadn't been provided with funds to hire a janitor, he ended each day mopping the place up himself.

One of Sargent's job requirements was to put on an exhibition at the end of December, to show the physical progress of the students. His first presentation—a mash-up of Indian club and dumbbell drills and gymnastics routines on the trapeze, bars, and rings—was a success. His salary was doubled, and Bowdoin gave him a janitor and some money to buy additional equipment. He spent it on wooden dumbbells to augment the iron ones, and introduced "developing apparatus," pulley weight machines to build upper-body strength. The machines were simple enough to support multi-jointed exercises, and Sargent used them to simulate movements like "reaping, mowing, pitching, raking, sawing, chopping, and other kinds of labor familiar to anyone who has ever worked on a farm."[1]

Sargent's biggest problem wasn't making rugged boys into gymnasts. It was coaxing small, unathletic geeks into the gym in the first place. They were in the majority, and it was his job to get them fit.[2] He considered the machines a preparatory first step for the more delicate students, who recoiled at the prospect of strenuous exercise. The machines were his way of luring weaklings into the facility.

It worked. Gym attendance doubled, then tripled. Sargent worked with these underpowered kids to get them strong enough to pass a basic strength test: twelve chin-ups and twelve dips on the parallel bars. Once they could do twelve chin-ups and twelve dips, they were deemed "proficient" and graduated into gymnastics.

"The gratifying results seemed magical," he crowed. "The journals heaped praise on our heads for the exhibitions of our prowess which we gave in Bath and Portland later in the year. I came to regard myself as something of a magician who had drawn full-fledged athletes out of the hat with a mere twist of the hand."[3] The "developing apparatus," he came to believe, was the key to transforming reticent non-athletes into leaping specimens of athletic manhood. It seems naive, in historical hindsight. But this was an era when machines were transforming the entire economy. Relentless optimism about mechanical solutions was pervasive. It was easy for an expert trainer to undervalue quality coaching and place his faith in the limitless potential of clever devices.

After the spring term ended in 1875, Sargent went home to Belfast. While there, he flubbed a gymnastic dismount, fell to the ground, and broke his sternum—a divot in his chest marked the break for the rest of his life. He decided he'd better go to medical school, and he enrolled at Yale. With medical degree in hand, he opened a gymnasium in New York City. To promote it, he started printing up circulars—manifestos about how the medical establishment had it all wrong. Instead of waiting to get sick, he argued, people should receive expert prescriptions for health and strength at a gym! Preventative medicine was the answer to "the goblin, disease," he argued. "I wished to fortify well people rather than minister to the wrecks of humanity."[4]

The keys to warding off illness and frailty, he argued, were good nutrition and functional movement. Carbs, he argued, were the big nutritional enemy. Bread, sugar, rich puddings, pastry, and potatoes were all to be avoided, if not eliminated.[5] Sargent believed that strenuous functional movement was the ideal way of building "organic vigor," because it was how man survived in the state of nature. "All the evidence we have of the life of primitive man implies a constant struggle with natural forces, and with wild beasts and savages," he wrote. "These encounters must have severely tested his physical strength and endurance. Those that survived this trying ordeal must have been able to run, jump, and swim, to climb, push, pull, wrestle, and fight; to hurl stones, wield clubs, and to lift and carry their burdens through forest and stream, over rocks and cliffs to their mountain caves."[6]

Even in more recent times, he noted, it was necessary to clear forest, break ground, lay out roads, and build towns, all of which required full-body exertion. Division of labor represented progress in many ways but had created a class of people who worked only with their minds or their fingers. Large swathes of the population suffered health consequences as a result. The statistics, then as now, were deemed alarming. "Over fifty per cent of all the candidates who apply for admission to the Military Academy at West Point and the Naval Academy at Annapolis are rejected on account of physical inefficiency," Sargent declared. "Is this the price we are paying for our boasted civilization?"[7]

As a trainer, Sargent had nothing but ridicule for the bodybuilders of the day, who increased muscle mass with slow, grimacing resistance exercises. They might look good in a mirror, he admitted, but the ability to slowly flex single muscles in a looking glass wouldn't translate into the practical ability to control external objects. In activities that require coordination and mental alertness—tennis, boxing, fencing, and other skilled sports—the bodybuilder would embarrass himself because all he could do was pump up his physique.[8]

Instead of isolation exercises, it was imperative to engage in exercises that would tax the heart, lungs, and brain as well as the muscles: rowing, running, swimming, and riding bicycles. Sargent was a big fan of bicycles for women, particularly heavy women, who could take advantage of the leg strength they'd built just to get themselves around.

Sargent worked like a dog to keep his box running from eight in the morning until ten at night. There were adjustable-weight pulley machines in the gym, to address individual deficiencies. He did private medical consultations and one-on-one training. But the main attraction was group classes. "Class work is always better," Sargent noted. "The numbers insure cooperation and spirit."[9] Sargent's clients were the new urbanized professional class. Industrialization had made them sedentary, but had also given them spare time to exercise and money to pay for the privilege.

Even though he was working twice as hard as his medical peers for less money, Sargent believed in the results. But after running his box with a hundred members for a year in 1879, he was exhausted. He was tired of coddling "morally inert" clients who insisted on individual training, then put in half-hearted efforts and got mediocre results. As he was about to renew his lease, Harvard University recruited him to run its brand-new Hemenway Gymnasium, the largest indoor athletic facility in the country.[10] It was the same job Sargent had held at Bowdoin, with better pay, a premium facility, a fat budget for equipment, and the prestige of a quasi-professorship at the nation's most elite university. He jumped at it.

At Harvard, Sargent resumed his lifelong obsession with human measurement and the metrics of athletic performance. Over the course of his career he collected functional and biometric measurements on thousands of undergraduates. He measured everything from limb ratios and chest circumference to grip strength and the maximum number of chin-ups, dips, and push-ups an athlete could do. He multiplied the chin-up and dip counts by a tenth of the athlete's weight, "to credit each person with the number of foot pounds lifted."[11] Sargent pioneered the use of a vertical jump test, which for years was called "the Sargent test." Each set of measurements quantified an athlete's variation from the norm in a dozen different ways. Invariably, the prescription was for each person to strengthen his weakest or least developed attribute. Focusing on strengths might be more satisfying, Sargent argued. But "inharmonious development" would ultimately compromise overall fitness and health.[12]

At Harvard, Sargent conducted summer school seminars that drew physical education experts from across the country. Lectures covered everything from diet, anatomy, and the physiology of exercise to step-by-step demonstrations of specific movements. There were specialty courses on playground games for kids, and deep dives into movement and technique for specific sports. A certificate of completion for the full course required four summers' worth of seminar attendance.[13]

At the time, a "battle of the systems" was raging between physical education experts from different training factions. Sargent's seminars were a refuge from the nineteenth-century fitness wars, a place where Swedish calisthenics teachers, hard-core German gymnasts, football coaches, and Indian club specialists could cross-pollinate. More than three thousand trainers traveled from every state in the Union and fifty-three foreign countries to attend his seminars. More than a thousand schools and athletic facilities sent their staff.[14]

BACK AT THE HEMENWAY GYM, SARGENT HAD ALL THE GEAR HE could dream of. He had a soaring ceiling, a sea of mats, rings, horizontal and parallel bars, platforms, springboards, four flavors of trapeze, five climbing ropes, and extra-long ladders pitched at every angle. Many of the college's elite athletes trained with him in the winter to shape up for sports fields in the spring. They kept him busy for hours, teaching stunts or rehearsing for heavily attended end-of-term performances.

These guys were hard-core elite athletes enrolled at an elite university. "They were the most conceited, egotistical men that ever were created," Sargent wrote in frustration. "They did not tolerate or sympathize with the beginner, who had not gone through their severe initiation. They wished every one to suffer as they had suffered; they had no respect for the man whose ankles, wrists, and limbs had not been injured, and whose anatomy did not bear scars of battles won for the great cause of heavy gymnastics."[15]

"They never made good teachers, and they were the only source from which instructors could be drawn," he complained. Sargent's firebreathers were so obnoxious that lesser athletes and less intrepid beginners didn't even venture onto the gymnastics floor. They stayed on the margins of the gym, literally, and stuck to the "developing apparatus," the machines.

There were a lot of machines, because Sargent had a lot of money and very little time. Instead of 130 students at Bowdoin, he had 600 undergraduates and a mandate to whip them all into some kind of shape. He wanted to work beginners into the proficient class as quickly as he could. But they were too intimidated by the proficients' Lord of the Flies attitude. And they *liked* the machines. So Sargent bought more machines, and he designed new machines to be even easier to use. "The desire to attract as many people as possible, inexpert as well as expert," he explained, "led me to reduce my exercises to a form so simple that any child might do them."

"For a man who has previously found the feats of heavy gymnastics distasteful or discouraging," Sargent argued, the machines had advantages. "He does not have to compete with men whose superiority overawes him; he can compete with his own physical condition from week to week, and from month to month. Nor does he any longer have to worry about strain or injury. If he cannot lift his own weight, the machines can be adapted to the weight which he can lift. Moreover, they can be adjusted to develop the parts of his body that are weakest. He can work for an hour going from one piece of apparatus to another, keeping always within the limit of his strength."[16]

There were dozens of simplified "developing appliances." Foot- and wrist-flexing machines, leg extension and abdominal machines, chest developers, and such. They were a big hit. Not only did the less-proficient students flock to them, but manufacturers began to copy and sell "Sargent system" machines into gymnasiums across the country. Sargent's employment agreement precluded him from patenting anything he built at Harvard, so it was open season for commercial manufacturers to rip off his designs.

The same employment agreement that precluded patents also forbade Sargent from profiting from his inventions. So, purely in the interest of promoting the highest-quality equipment, he allied himself with the Narrangansett Machine Company, because they used the best materials and didn't cut corners. With his endorsement, Narrangansett sold beautifully crafted "Sargent system" machines into schools and gyms across the country.

Around this time, one of Sargent's former students was revamping the Young Men's Christian Association into the athletic organization we now know as the YMCA. By 1889, over 300 YMCAs were partially or entirely equipped with the "Sargent System" of developing apparatus. By 1893, the total number of Sargent-equipped gyms had jumped to 740, and 70% of newly constructed gyms were equipped with Sargent appliances. The machines were so simple to use that a facility could simply purchase the apparatus and accommodate its members without having to hire additional staff. Unlike sports teams, gymnastics, or weightlifting, the machines didn't need a coach.[17]

Once the gyms were built around machines, their physical layout was geared to move people through machine-based workouts. Gym members were conditioned to expect that exercise would be skill-free and easy. As the Sargent machines were augmented by midcentury vibrating apparatus—stand-on plates and oscillating belts that promised to minimize the hips—the idea took hold that exercise could also be passive, that you could unhook your brain and jiggle your way to fitness. Pulleys were replaced by hydraulics and later by variable-resistance cams, Nautilus's signature innovation. Rudimentary cardio machines—mechanical rowers and ski track machines—gave way to treadmills. There was a brief flicker of intensity when the Stairmaster came along—a stationary tower-climb is no joke. But Stairmaster's intensity, the fact that it made people uncomfortable, consigned it to health club Siberia when the Precor Elliptical came along.

The Precor Elliptical was a perfectly engineered instrument of junk exercise. It was built and marketed as a minimum-impact machine, just as baby boomers' knees were turning forty. Its big selling point was that it eliminated the discomfort of exercise. Whereas a treadmill runner had to propel her own body forward, and a Stairclimber user, even using the handrails, was pushing a substantial portion of her body weight up a virtual stairwell, the elliptical machine was a smooth, minimally taxing flex-and-glide movement. Unlike cross-country ski machines, each foot-push backwards on an elliptical pushes the opposite side forward. Each squirt of muscular effort is leveraged into the next movement. It has the ease and efficiency of a bicycle pedal. Except you can't go fast.

It is virtually impossible to achieve any kind of intensity on an elliptical machine. That's what makes it so popular. The pleasure principle dictates that people who don't actually want to exercise will gravitate toward the gentle zero-impact elliptical workout, which pairs so comfortably with headphones and a two-week-old copy of a tabloid magazine, or with screens that allow people to watch television while they clock their allotted thirty minutes of cardio.

One can only wonder what the world would be like if Sargent had resisted the siren song of the mechanical age—if, instead of consigning his remedial athletes to "developing apparatus," he'd made them do squats and found simple ways to lighten the load of gymnastic movements, as his functional-fitness doppelgänger did 120 years later.

"With enough rubber bands," Greg Glassman cracked, "anyone can do gymnastics." A typical CrossFit box contains a tub of gigantic rubber bands of various colors and thicknesses. They're used to provide assistance to people who can't do pull-ups. Clove-hitch a rubber band over the bar, stick your heel in the dangling end, and the tension in the rubber band absorbs some of your body weight, so you have less to lift. People who can't do pull-ups start with the thickest rubber band and switch to progressively thinner rubber bands until they can do unassisted pull-ups. With two rubber bands, one clove-hitched over the bar and another looped through the bottom end of the hanging band as a pair of shoulder supports, you can rig assistance for a handstand push-up. The idea is to get a sense of the movement, in its full range of motion, while building enough strength to wean yourself off the assistance.

Glassman's "Scaling Gymnastics" article in the *CrossFit Journal* features photos of unlikely "gymnasts" rigged up with mountain-climbing harnesses, pulleys, and large rubber bands. It was his way of proving that even gymnastic WODs could function as brilliant equalizers. He'd figured out, in a way Sargent hadn't, how to structure workouts that enabled novices and humbled elite athletes. If some alpha male got attitudinal, the CrossFit solution was easy and instant—throw a twenty-pound weight vest on the bastard and see how golden he feels on the pull-up bar. The social genius of a WOD is that it makes a world-class athlete feel a soccer mom's pain.

But Glassman had another advantage. He was living in the information age, not the industrial age. Like Sargent, he embraced the breakthrough technology of his era. But this time, it was the web. In 2001, the Glassmans launched CrossFit.com as an open-source cache of workout and exercise demos, online discussions, and the prescribed Workout of the Day posted to a blog. "Part of the motivation was to get at our clients who were traveling," Glassman told an Army audience at Fort Hood. "We had professional surfers who were all over the world. We had Silicon Valley luminaries who were all over the world, and we wanted to give them a vehicle by which they could tap into what was going on back at the gym."[18]

The only thing the Glassmans asked in return for free workout programming was for people to add their results to the comments section of each WOD post. Partly, this request was to gather data. But more fundamentally, it was to give CrossFit's online community a touchstone of shared experience—not common "likes" or links, but the sense of having survived the same trials. Every result posted to comments says, "I've been there, done that. That was frikkin' miserable. Good on ya."

In "Fran," CrossFit's evil layer cake of 21-15-9 thrusters and pull-ups, Glassman jokes, "there's that weird moment when the shuttle blasts off, where there's all this violent fucking explosion, a huge ball of fire and noise, and nothing's happened—it's just sitting there? That's how the bottom of each thruster feels like . . . *I'm going as hard as I can and not a fucking thing's happening!* And then it finally starts going . . . and then you reload and do it again, and you're like *why?* Anyone who's done that, you're part of that. That's what's in it for you: suffering and relating to the suffering, imagining yourself there. The empathy and understanding of shared experience."[19]

There's a ritual bond in the shared intensity of it. It's not just a physiological experience. Glassman recognized this. "Mind-body dualism," he says, "is a myth."

The spiritual element of virtuosity was recognized in Sargent's program as well—but not by Sargent. On the evening of March 27, 1882, noted anthropologist Frank Cushing had invited a group of Zuni Indians to one of Sargent's "meets" at the Hemenway Gymnasium. Cushing was a founding father of modern anthropology and had made his career living with the Zuni and documenting their culture as a participant observer. He thought they'd get a kick out of Sargent's gymnastic exhibitions. Arrayed in their native finery, the Zuni settled into their seats. When two students took to the double trapeze, working together to form figures and bear each other's weight, the Zuni began to shout. They were beside themselves. "They looked upon these two performers as spirit men, and treated them with a kind of religious veneration," Sargent wrote. "Spiritual was one term which I had never before heard applied to gymnasts. But spiritual the Harvard athletes were in the eyes of these Americans."[20]

THE ORIGINAL FIREBREATHER

*Firebreather—Fie-r'-brë-th-er: (n) 1. One who faces the triumphs
and tribulations of great physical opposition with an indomitable
spirit. 2. An optimistic energy associated with the heart of an athlete.[1]*

THE ORIGINAL FIREBREATHER SHOWED UP AT 6:00 A.M. WITH A
big coach-shaped hole in his life. In December 2001, Greg Amundson
was twenty-two years old, just out of the police academy and working
as a deputy in the Santa Cruz sheriff's office. He'd heard rumors of a
tiny gym on the east side of town that was churning out superhuman
athletes. If that was true, he wanted to be one of them.

Amundson was the oldest of four boys, all boisterous coils of kinetic
energy compressed by the discipline of Catholic school nuns and then
unleashed into various sports. Their dad was a chiropractor who'd seen
too many adolescent football injuries to approve of the gridiron. A former beach lifeguard and Navy diver, Raymond Amundson steered his
boys into water polo, which Greg played in high school and college.

Amundson's dad was methodical about strength training. Before his
teenage sons could touch a barbell, they had to learn the fundamentals
of gymnastics. Before they were cleared to do a shoulder press, they had
to be able to hold a handstand. Before they were allowed to bench-press,
they had to be able to do twenty consecutive dips. Bicep curls were not

on the menu. If the Amundson boys wanted to put on a gun show for the girls, they could build their biceps on the pull-up bar. As far back as Greg Amundson can remember, his dad was taking him to the YMCA to work on pull-ups.

When Raymond Amundson died of cancer, more than two thousand people showed up at his funeral.[2] Thousands of people showed up to pay their respects, because he didn't just work on their bodies. He pulled their minds and spirits into alignment. He emphasized the importance of not getting messed up in the first place. A shoulder or neck adjustment might cure symptoms. But spiritual adjustment was gently prescribed to alleviate the chronic tension that got a person out of whack in the first place. He prescribed forgiveness, a balm that alleviates pain on many levels. The ripple effect of Raymond Amundson's practice was huge, in people's lives and in their community.

And then he was gone, and there was a big coach-shaped hole in his son's life, just as Greg Amundson needed to take his physical training to a new level. As a freshly minted law enforcement officer, Amundson was convinced that physical fitness—elite fitness—was literally a matter of life or death. If he was going to face extreme circumstances out on the street, he wanted to prepare himself by training in extreme circumstances to build the mental toughness to overcome any adversary.

Adversaries in backwoods Santa Cruz could be pretty tough, because they were high on meth. In face-offs against meth addicts, cops often switch to higher-caliber guns, because meth heads are incredibly aggressive and they don't feel pain. They're relentless in a fight. They just keep coming at you. Meth makes people into superhuman zombies. So if you're going to risk altercations with them, you'd better be well armed and damned-near superhuman yourself.

For Amundson, this meant pushing his body as far as it would go, in as many ways as he could devise. He'd sprint for 1.5 miles up UC Santa Cruz's longest hill. He'd run up the hill carrying a tire or dragging his girlfriend on a bicycle. It was semi-insane. But it was purposeful. "I wasn't doing physical fitness for the sake of physical fitness," he says. "I was doing physical fitness because I knew that my body and mind were my greatest assets on the street."

What Amundson saw around him was technology displacing mental and physical toughness in the police force, weighing cops down at the same time it gave them the excuse to get mentally and physically soft. He reserved special revulsion for the taser. He hated the way a taser made it possible for the fattest slob with a badge to incapacitate someone, and how a fat cop's lack of physical authority made it almost inevitable that he'd have to use the taser. Ten years of FBI research shows that criminals attack the cops they think they can take.[3] Fat cops are their own broken windows.

When the Santa Cruz County Sheriff's Office required deputies to carry a taser, Amundson refused. "The day I need electricity to effect an arrest," he told them, "I'll turn in my badge. I'll retire."[4] He got written up a few times. When it became obvious that getting written up was not going to make Amundson carry a taser, the department stopped writing him up.

In Santa Cruz, there is a tight-knit community of high-level athletes, and elite athletes gossip like teenage girls. So it didn't take long for Amundson to hear about the crazy coach who was breeding dragons out of a stripped-down industrial space. Fringe athletes—martial artists, surfers, mountain climbers, extreme-sports types—were flocking to the guy, then decimating their peers. A friend passed CrossFit's phone number along to Amundson. He called up—years later, he still has the number memorized—and after a few rings, Greg Glassman answered the phone. In the background, Amundson could hear the sound of grunts, cheers, and heavy objects hitting the ground. It sounded like a dungeon. But more friendly.

Amundson introduced himself and asked if he could come work out.

"Sure," Glassman replied. "Come tomorrow at 6:00 a.m."

At 5:45 the next morning, Amundson pulled into a chilly six-car parking lot to see the small window in a 12-foot-high garage door already fogged with steam from the inside. Amundson knocked, then stepped inside to see Glassman striding across the room, hand outstretched. "Glad you made it!" he said. "You can call me Coach."[5]

There was only one other guy in the room—ostensibly the source of all the heat and steam clouding the window. It was Mike Weaver, one of the first Americans to win a jujitsu tournament in Brazil. Weaver was sitting on the parallel bars, and he was the fiercest-looking man Amundson had ever seen. They would be competing against each other in Glassman's Workout of the Day.

The workout started upstairs, on the mezzanine loft level of the tiny gym. The loft might have been used for storage or office space by a previous tenant. In its CrossFit incarnation, the loft was where the rowers lived. Glassman was fond of the C2 rowing ergometer as a cardiovascular ordeal that taxed the entire body. The movement echoes a squat or a deadlift, so 500 meters on the rower is a good way to bleed athletes before they move on to deadlifts or squats, so they're nice and fatigued, and also out of breath, when they start those vertical exercises. The day's workout would start with a 1,000-meter row. Then, he said, Amundson and Weaver would walk carefully down the stairs to do twenty-one kettle bell swings and twelve pull-ups. After a brief rest, they could repeat the workout if they felt up to it. Amundson wondered why he'd have to be careful walking down to the lower level. There didn't seem to be anything wrong with the stairs.

Continuing the tour, Glassman led them to the kettle bell area and explained, then demonstrated, the correct technique for swinging a bell: range of motion, correct form, do's and don'ts. The same with pull-ups. As Mike Weaver warmed up on the pull-up bar, using his hips to generate momentum—CrossFit's signature kipping pull-up—Amundson internally sneered at this more efficient version of the police department standard strict dead-hang pull-up. Using momentum to swing over the bar seemed like cheating—not a tough-guy move at all.

Amundson wasn't intimidated in the least. Pulling on a rower, then swinging a kettle bell and doing twelve pull-ups didn't seem like much work. He figured it should take him only a few minutes. At Glassman's unvarying signal to start, "Three, two, one, GO!," both men pulled as hard as they could on the rowers. Amundson's legs were jelly after a few minutes. As he leaned hard on the stair railing and wobbled down the steps, the need for careful and deliberate placement of feet and shifting of weight on the stairs became abundantly clear. Glassman cheered both men through the kettle bell swings, then watched Weaver crank through twelve kipping pull-ups. Amundson stoically completed three sets of four academy-standard strict pull-ups, then stumbled into the corner and collapsed at the foot of the stairs. He was physically devastated and psychologically blissed out. His legs were temporarily useless. But he was jumping up and down inside.

Glassman leaned over him. "Are you okay?"

"Yeah," Amundson smiled. "I love it."

"I found it," Amundson says. "It was the holy grail of what I'd been trying to create and search for myself, in my own training. And he had it."

From that day on, Amundson spent as much time as he could at CrossFit with the Glassmans. If he wasn't patrolling the city streets and back roads of Santa Cruz County, he was at the box. In those days, CrossFit workouts varied from class to class, and the classes themselves varied in character. The 6:00 a.m. class was an invitation-only, highly competitive workout for A-level athletes, "Team 6," as they called themselves. One morning, after the 21-15-9 thruster/pull-up sequence that would later be known as "Fran," the entire Team 6 cadre lay in an exhausted heap.

"It felt like I was breathing fire the entire time," Amundson groaned, struggling for enough air to speak. "It's like we're a bunch of firebreathers."

Before this, the athletes in Team 6 had referred to themselves as "gladiators," "warriors," "monsters," and "beasts."[6] But "firebreather" seemed to capture something deeper and more distinctive about what they had become and the process that had forged their physical strength, their strength of will, their rivalry, and their friendship.

They were competitors. They were teammates. They were students. And like the kids who'd taught Greg Glassman how to do gymnastics in the park, they were one another's teachers. "Coach believed that the moment you learned something, you had the responsibility to teach it," Amundson recalled in an account of CrossFit's founding days.[7] "Everyone at CrossFit Santa Cruz learned the intricacies of the foundational movements, with the expectation they would teach the skills to others. Coach had a mantra for when athletes left the gym, and it has now evolved into a piece of famous postcertification advice: 'When you get home, grab a broomstick, knock on your neighbor's door, and teach them how to deadlift.'"

At CrossFit coaching certification seminars, Glassman took a professorial tone and scrawled formulas on the whiteboard. He often used Amundson as a case in point. "When I speak of evidence," he declared, "here is what I mean: When an athlete like Greg Amundson posts a 'Fran' time of 2:48 at a body weight of 205, we can, with simple calculations, universally known and accepted by science, calculate that he has performed 54,225 foot-pounds of work in 168 seconds and that this is holding just less than 2/3 of a horsepower for almost 3 minutes."[8]

Then, to demonstrate the point, he would pit Amundson against seminar attendees in a competitive WOD. "My role," Amundson says, "was to do the workout and to win. And I had to win, because I had to prove the validity of the program. Because if a non-CrossFit athlete beat me in the workout, then CrossFit loses its merit. So there was a certain amount of self-imposed pressure. And because Coach had taken on the father figure role, I desperately wanted to win for Coach."

The two Gregs needed each other. Glassman was middle-aged with a serious leg injury. He couldn't be a living epitome of his own training principles. He needed an avatar. Greg Amundson needed someone to fill the coach-shaped hole in his life. The two men complemented each other perfectly. Glassman had (and has) a seemingly infinite capacity for conversation and discourse. He's a brilliant politician, minus the tact. Amundson is deeply observant, watchful, introspective, a doer. They amplified each other's talents and efforts. And as the seminars continued, they shared a growing sense that CrossFit was building more than physical work capacity. There was something in the movements and the intensity of effort that went deeper, that changed people.

It's not just that the workouts demanded *more* of people. The ordeal of a WOD demanded something different and gave rise to something different. Muscle-ups, for instance. To complete a muscle-up, an athlete grabs a set of rings hanging overhead and, with one powerful swing and fluid transfer of momentum, rises up to straighten his arms and push the rings down to his hips. It's a gymnastic challenge, a fusion of strength, coordination, and agility. But it's also a test of faith. Athletes have to believe, utterly, that they are going to make it all the way to the top when they grab the rings, or it won't happen.

There is nothing especially mystical about this: it's about timing. There is a difference in timing between someone who believes he is going to complete a movement and someone who doesn't. The transfer of effort from the hips and lats (the pull-up part of a muscle-up) to the triceps (the dip) has to be be swift and fluid. If the arms aren't fully primed to extend in the split-second transition between movements, the rings begin to move away from the body, and elbows drift away from the torso into a "chicken wings" position from which it's almost impossible to rise.

That moment, that split-second transition from large muscles to small muscles, also happens to be exactly when the doubting mind will interject, "Can I do this?" And in this moment of doubt, the transition falls apart. The splinter-thin time window for transition is too narrow for any hesitation. And for athletes who've never done a muscle-up before, this lack of hesitation is pure faith. They believe, in the absence of evidence, that they can do a muscle-up. Barely strong-enough athletes who can muster that faith will get a muscle-up. Much stronger athletes who lack faith in their ability to execute the movement will find themselves stuck in the chicken-wing position. When they grab the rings, they don't believe they'll make it to the top. So they fail.

There is no functional distinction between mind and body in this movement. Functional control of complex, full-body movements and the requisite strength of will and conviction come from the same part of the brain. When people get their first muscle-up, it's not just because they're stronger and quicker than they were before. There's been a mental shift as well. It can take years to get a first muscle-up. It takes a minute to get the second one. Onlookers cheer and clang the ship's bell that CrossFit boxes hang on the wall to ring in personal records. People who can do muscle-ups have a different kind of status in the box.

It makes perfect sense that at the top of a muscle-up, the pinnacle of faith and conviction, Greg Amundson looked down, noticed a particular girl for the first time, decided she was the most beautiful creature in the universe, and made up his mind to marry her. At the time, he was engaged to a different woman. He broke up with her and ardently pursued the girl he'd seen from the top of the rings. He swept her off her feet and married her. That sort of thing doesn't happen on the elliptical machine.

As Glassman and Amundson watched athletes compete at seminars, the psychological element of performance in CrossFit workouts became glaringly apparent. When two nearly identical athletes were paired off to compete at a seminar in Seattle, one of them walked up to the muscle-up rings and said, "I've never done a muscle-up before. Today I'm going to get my first one." The other admitted that he'd never done a muscle-up before either. "There's no way I can finish this workout," he said.

The first guy got his first muscle-up, then nine more. As he finished the workout, his friends came over to congratulate him. "Aw, thanks guys," he replied. "I knew I could do it." His opponent didn't even come close to doing a muscle-up and gave up. When his friends came over to commiserate, he replied, "No worries, guys. I knew I couldn't do it."[9]

Watching this scene unfold, Glassman pulled Amundson aside. "You know what, kid?" he said. "The greatest adaptation to CrossFit is between the ears." The statement seemed to hang in the air between them. It lodged in Amundson's mind. It changed the way he trained. He stopped working from the outside in—building physical strength in order to become more confident. He started working from the inside out: building courage, forbearance, serenity to boost his physical performance. He had his fiancée clock the amount of time he could submerge himself in the Pacific Ocean. He went through a phase (he's still teased about this) where he'd turn the gym shower on to cold, full blast, and test how many times he could step into it without flinching.

Every time he made improvements in these trials of will, his athletic performance spiked. He made objective gains. Faster times. Heavier lifts. More repetitions per minute. "It was more the intangible than the tangible qualities that made me faster in the workout," he says. "Let's say you do a workout like 'Fran' on week one. You do it on week two, and you're twenty or thirty seconds faster, between those two weeks? I don't think it's because you're more physically fit. I don't think that you just increased muscle mass or the contractile potential of muscle. I think it has more to do with your courage, your confidence and your determination, and your ability to persevere. Those qualities are what we attribute to good people. Good people are accountable. They have perseverance. They're determined. What you're doing in these workouts is, you're becoming a different person. Every time you're going faster, you're becoming a different person."

Amundson came to realize what every CrossFit firebreather eventually discovers: the chief competitive advantage in this sport is the ability to endure discomfort. The willingness to sacrifice comfort is what makes all the other gains possible. Anyone who's ever done "Karen" comes to terms with this. The benchmark WOD is 150 repetitions of a single movement: wall balls. The movement is not technically difficult—all you have to do is throw a 20-pound medicine ball (14 pounds for women) up to a target 10 feet in the air and catch it on the way down to a full squat. Explode out of the squat to launch the ball again. A hundred and forty-eight reps later, you're done.

With every rep, the ball shoves you down, and you have to push back, only to get shoved down again. The essence of a shove, what makes it so demoralizing, is that you have to absorb force from something that's not working very hard to generate that force. That's why bullies shove. And while you're being repeatedly shoved by a twenty-pound ball falling from ten feet in the air, your heart rate is maxing out. Your body wants a lot more oxygen than it's getting.

The shortage of oxygen, plus the experience of being shoved, produces a groaning sense of awfulness. Not pain, in the sharp sense that pain is acute and local. It's a global awfulness, a misery, like flu. The mind responds to this awfulness with a loud, dissonant drone of "just make it stop." The only way to finish "Karen" in a reasonable amount of time is to mentally compartmentalize the horrifying totality of the task, ignore the mental imperative to stop, and just concentrate on the next few reps. When you can do that, you've learned how to keep moving past the siren song of comfort and relief to the finish. The benchmark time for "Karen" is a pretty good proxy for a person's general ability to suck it up.

But this was exactly why Greg Amundson loved "Karen." "On a spiritual level, I would actually look forward to that discomfort," he says. "I would beckon it. I would seek it out. I knew it was the best thing for me. It's like a hot bath that you have to melt into, one foot at a time. If you were just to jump into that temperature of water you would probably injure yourself. But if you melt into it one limb at a time, ease into it, all of a sudden you're up to your neck in that water and it feels great. That's what I would do with the workout."

"It sounds crazy," he says, "but I felt like when I really pushed it, I was getting closer to God, that I was getting closer to spirit. The harder I went, the faster I got, the stronger I became, I just felt like every time, it was closer and closer to a place of stillness and truth and spirit. . . . If you read about Roger Bannister when he was running his four-minute mile, it's beautiful. He's writing about it like poetry. He was spending more time in the air than on the ground, like he was flying. There were some workouts that were like that."

For Amundson, these transcendent moments of intense discomfort and cosmic calm always involved squats, weighted or unweighted. But then, most of CrossFit involves squats—with a barbell, with a medicine ball, with dumbbells, or with body weight. Amundson would be moving his weight from very near the ground to full vertical extension, over and over, revving into oxygen debt, and suddenly become aware of how his thoughts were affecting the functional capacity of his body. He wondered if it was possible to reprogram his mind, to silence the thoughts that were interfering with his performance.

And as he wondered this, a Bible verse unspooled from his Catholic school childhood. It was from the Gospel according to Mark, when Jesus teaches people how to pray. He says that if someone tells a mountain to throw itself into the sea with absolute faith, the mountain will be cast into the sea. The visual image is so arresting that it's easy to skip over the very odd thing He says next. He says that people should pray as if their prayers have already been granted. What a person wants should be so solidly conceived and constructed in his mind that it seems to have already happened in the past. This twist in tense, changing a wish into a memory, He says, is the way to get things done, prayer-wise. It's a very strange idea.

But to Amundson, it made a sudden kind of practical sense. "Don't talk how big the mountain is. Just cast the mountain into the sea," he says. "Rather than entertaining the self-talk about the pain, the discomfort, how much more I had to do, I started praying and thinking the solution. And so my mantra became: one more rep, stronger as I go. Healthier, stronger, every round. I would pray the solution, and my mantra became the solution, rather than the workout or the problem."

Amundson was just as attentive as the other athletes to technique and mechanics. He didn't discount the importance of physics when it came to hauling ass or moving a barbell. But he spent more time on the metaphysics of hauling ass and the metaphysics of moving a barbell—how the reality of foot-pounds per second is constructed in the mind, before it occurs in time and space. He was intensely deliberate about his mental and physical preparations for the WOD. He had an unvarying warm-up routine: foot shuffles, overhead squats, and giant upside-down arcs on the GHD sit-up rig. The GHD (glute-ham developer) is a padded metal frame that transforms ordinary sit-ups into a movement most commonly seen on the flying trapeze: you hook your feet into the foot anchors, lean back onto a bench that supports the hips, and hang your torso, upside down, over the edge. Then, with one strong flex of the quads, you whip your entire torso from the upside-down hanging position, up and over, to touch your toes. Large leg muscles generate most of the physical momentum, but the movement also engages the lower abdominals. A few dozen of these, for a beginner, can transform the entire area between hips and sternum into one big ache.

Once Amundson had dialed into his preparatory ritual, his body was warm. His mind was focused. He was ready to win, and he was almost impossible for the other firebreathers to beat. After losing to Amundson over and over, one of the fiercest athletes in Team 6, Dave Leys, asked him what he was *doing* to keep getting faster.

Amundson searched for words to explain how he'd crossed over, how the physical intensity of the WOD was a chassis for spiritual and psychological conditioning, in a way that wouldn't seem crazy. "Dave," he said, "I just pray harder."

Amundson was the first firebreather to realize what the WOD really was, because of the way he'd grown up. You can't listen to nuns lead daily prayers from kindergarten to sixth grade and not recognize ritual for what it is. Rituals, across time and cultures, have some very distinctive qualities. They have the quality of invariance: a specified choreography and rhythm, a deliberate and disciplined set of actions.[10] It's this deliberateness that distinguishes ritual from habit. Habit is absentminded—it's something you do repeatedly without thinking. Bring full presence and attention to that same behavior, and it becomes ritual. Physical intensity enforces full presence and attention. The alternative is having a twenty-pound ball fall, ten feet down, onto your face.

Ritual has a structure and a language that sets the activity apart. CrossFit WODs have a codified vocabulary that's used only within the context of a WOD. Numerical progressions, rhymes and verses in the rep schemes, give WODs a formal beauty, a poetic or musical structure, even if performing the compositions is hellacious. AMRAPs (As Many Rounds as Possible within a fixed amount of time), Rounds for Time WODs (a fixed number of repetitions in an open-ended amount of time, i.e., a WOD "for time"), and chippers (a litany of different movements, each completed before moving on to the next type), are the product of aesthetic conventions and constraints, like haiku and sonnets.

WODs have names. Initially, this was for the sake of convenience. Instead of having to explain what a thruster was, and that a workout started with twenty-one of them, then twenty-one pull-ups, fifteen thrusters, fifteen pull-ups, nine thrusters, and nine pull-ups, it was easier for Greg Glassman to explain the workout once and give it a name, "Fran." He borrowed the female naming convention from the National

Weather Service's system of designating tropical storms (although he also joked that "anything that left you flat on your back, looking up at the sky, asking 'What the fuck happened to me' deserved a female's name.")[11] The *CrossFit Journal* published the first six benchmark "Girls" in September 2003:

"Angie" (100 pull-ups, 100 push-ups, 100 sit-ups, 100 squats, for time)

"Barbara" (20 pull-ups, 30 push-ups, 40 sit-ups, 50 squats, five rounds for time, with 3 minutes between rounds)

"Chelsea" (5 pull-ups, 10 push-ups, 15 squats, each minute for 30 minutes)

"Diane" (225-lb deadlifts and handstand push-ups, 21-15-9)

"Elizabeth" (135-lb barbell cleans and ring dips, 21-15-9)

And last but not least, "Fran."

"The crushing charm of these ladies lies in their magnificent capacity to root out weaknesses and humiliate you with them," Glassman noted.[12] The Girls, like all rituals, take you back to the last time and the first time. Every birthday cake, Christmas morning, and midnight kiss on New Year's Eve connects to the ones that came before. Every benchmark WOD takes you back to previous encounters with the same beautiful bitch who knocked you on your ass the first time. It never gets easier. Your times just get faster.

In the ritual of a WOD, opposites clash and fuse: "Measurable, Observable, Repeatable" binds to "the Unknown and Unknowable." The experience beckons to people who love structure and rules. It sings to people who thrive in chaos and live to see how far they can push it, whatever "it" is. On the whiteboard, the WOD is all about clarity, measurements, statistics, calculation, and analysis. At "Three, two, one, GO!," all hell breaks loose. People who love order can fight to restore it, and put their shoulder to the wheel. People who feed on chaos can set themselves loose and ride that chaos all the way down to the Dark Place. The ritual genius of a CrossFit WOD gives both kinds of people exactly what they want, swirled into its opposite. The hero is also the dragon.

When each 6:00 a.m. WOD was done, Amundson would shower, put on his uniform, his badge, his sunglasses, and drive away. He did the same thing on patrol as he did in the box: put himself in an uncomfortable situation, then master the situation by controlling his own thoughts and emotions.

Amundson would drive up to the remotest part of Santa Cruz County and look for the most intimidating person he could find walking on the street. He would look for a car that screamed "Stop me" and pull it over. "It was like stepping in front of the cold water," he says, "or that moment in a wall ball workout where you make a choice to either step forward and continue or step back and stop. I would have repetition of contacting just the gnarliest, biggest, baddest people I could find."

"There was never a struggle. They would always just succumb. And a lot of the other deputies were like, *Greg, these people are what we would call Three Deputy Calls. These are the type of people that require three deputies to apprehend.* They thought I was some ninja, and I'm like, I'm not even putting my hands on these people. They're putting themselves into handcuffs. There is just something very powerful about commitment that I think, in people's deep psyche, in the deep primal mind, people can sense when someone is fully committed, and it's the most powerful thing in the world. When you commit to a workout, it's the most powerful thing in the world. There is no stopping that person that's willing to commit and willing to pay the price. When I committed to making those contacts, I was willing to pay the price. I was willing to die."

It wasn't just attitude. Amundson was physically imposing: 200 pounds of muscle, shaved head, sharp jaw. You would have to be high on meth to dream of taking the guy down. Rational troublemakers, the ones who weren't high on meth, instinctively sized him up and responded to his air of absolute assurance. His former partner, John Shepard, remembers, "It was kind of a martial arts thing, this command presence.

If you have the command presence, because you have that inner mental confidence that you are physically capable of handling whatever's thrown at you, your demeanor changes. You're calmer. If you don't have that, you overreact."[13]

Amundson and Shepard would joke that if they had their way, they'd patrol the West like Wyatt Earp, with a gun on their belts and nothing else. They wanted their guns, if it came to that. But they knew that the assurance of hard training would reduce the chance of having to fire a shot. They trained in martial arts, drilled defensive tactics, leveled up, joined the SWAT team. Amundson pulled Shepard into CrossFit. He pulled a lot of cops into CrossFit by virtue of his own impressive physical performance. In 2004, he and a female Santa Cruz police officer from the gym, Naomi Silva, went to the Police and Fire Olympics and crushed the competition. They both won the Toughest Cop Alive event, an eight-part gauntlet of a 5K run, shot put, 100-meter dash, 100-meter swim, 20-foot rope climb, bench press, pull-ups, and an obstacle course. Amundson set a world record in the event. He'd never run a triathlon, but he took third in that event with a knobby-tired mountain bike. He finished second in the open-water swim. He hadn't been training for that either. It was a dramatic proof of CrossFit's claim to put athletes in a ready state for any physical challenge.

Cops took notice. They wanted to get some of that mojo. Amundson started teaching a law-enforcement-only class at Glassman's gym. He gave seminars to police departments across the country. In many police departments, there's no real physical fitness requirement for cops after they graduate from the academy. Obesity rates are higher among cops than in the general public.[14] It takes a lot to convince a room full of overweight cops to take their fitness seriously.

But Amundson gave cops a different way of thinking about themselves. "You, my friends," he would say to a roomful of deputies, "are professional athletes."[15] Football players and mixed martial arts (MMA) fighters train hard because *it's their job*. But MMA fighters have an advantage over cops, he argued. MMA fighters know when, where, and whom they're going to fight. A cop on the beat doesn't even know how many opponents he may have to fight, and whether they'll be carrying weapons, much less when and where that fight's going to happen. Cops have to be ready for the fight of their life at any moment, Amundson would say. So they should think of themselves as professional athletes, and train for the sport of "protect and serve" as hard as they can. Cross-Fit's inroads to the law enforcement community can be attributed, in no small part, to the way Greg Amundson's seminars put cops in the same category as their sports heroes.

But the sermon he preaches to civilians is largely the same. "That workout gives people a chance to get primal, to access that inner warrior that's there, in everybody," he says. "We're so sheltered and protected that it doesn't live very well in people. But it's there, and we need to access it and become comfortable with it." Every time people show up to do a WOD, they have a serious fight on their hands. It's not literally a fight for their lives. But it can feel that way, if you do it right. "Every time I worked out," Amundson says of his early CrossFit years, "I questioned if I was going to live."[16]

A decade after he showed up at Greg Glassman's gym to crumble at the foot of the steps, Amundson distilled what he'd learned, to help people bring themselves into alignment, physically, spiritually, and socially:

> Pursue virtuosity in functional movement.
>
> Believe unconditionally in yourself and the ability of others.
>
> Learn new skills—Teach them to a friend.
>
> Forge an indomitable body and spirit.
>
> Apply character traits learned in the gym to life:
> Perseverance—Honesty—Integrity—Resilience—Courage—
> Loyalty—Respect and Service
>
> Be humble.
>
> Encourage others.

This fifty-word summation, half chivalric code and half Bushido, has come to be known as "The CrossFit Way." Most CrossFitters have seen it online or on a T-shirt or on the wall of their box. Not everyone who hits a WOD fashions their life after these principles. But there is undeniably a feeling in the average CrossFit box that the ritual of a WOD is about more than working up a sweat. The willingness to struggle through it is tacitly understood as a test of character and a shared ordeal.

This is why CrossFitters tend to trust one another, even if they've never met, more readily than they trust strangers on the street. At a CrossFit box, people buy T-shirts on the honor system—take a shirt and write your name and shirt size down. The front desk often becomes a drop-off and pick-up space for labeled items and envelopes. At a regular health club, if someone you knew only from spin class asked for help getting his car started, you'd probably feel reluctant, even suspicious. At a CrossFit box, people who barely know someone will help jump-start his car if he's stuck with a dead car battery. These are small gestures of trust from people who consciously train themselves to be useful, if not heroic.

It's difficult to disentangle the physical aspects of CrossFit training from its moral undertones. There's an earnestness to it. Some people love this. Others find it distasteful or ridiculous, depending on how much of themselves they're willing to invest in a workout. A group of CrossFitters finishing a WOD has not, after all, ascended to the base camp of Everest or survived a firefight. They just feel that way, and it magnifies their sense of purpose, and their loyalty to fellow members of their expedition.

NASTY GIRLS

THERE WAS GLEE IN GREG GLASSMAN'S HEART EVERY TIME A female CrossFitter walloped some unwitting male in an athletic competition. It was such dramatic proof that his training methods were superior. Even before he had his own gym in Santa Cruz, when he was still a personal trainer and spinning class instructor at Spa Fitness, he'd invite clients to ride bikes with his wife, Lauren, and Eva T. As a trainer in the gym, his focus was on other people's performance. But outdoors on a bike, he was competitive. "You haven't had the bike-riding experience," he'd quip, "until you're riding with a handful of people who would die today to get their wheel in front of yours. *That's* bike riding."[1]

"Hey, we're going on a bike ride up Main Street," Glassman would say to a few personal training clients. "You guys want to join? We'll have breakfast after—come on by!" It sounded so friendly and casual. The sun was out. The girls were fresh faced and leggy. Everyone would meet at the bottom of a climb and take off. At that point, it became apparent that the pretty girls were viciously strong riders. He'd sprint forward to spur them on, then drop back to watch them compete with one another and smoke the guys. It was his favorite hustle.

At CrossFit coaching seminars, aspiring trainers could always look at Amundson and say, "That dude is just stronger and tougher—he'd be a beast regardless of how he trained." But to see a petite blonde or Asian girl, maybe 110 pounds, beat a firefighter, a cop, or a Navy SEAL at some bodyweight workout with sprints and pull-ups, that got people's attention.

This was especially true on military bases. At a seminar for the 1st Special Forces Group at Fort Lewis, Washington, Glassman pitted his best men and three of his best women against a pack of Army Rangers. He was warned by the captain, going in, that "this isn't exactly a lady-friendly environment."[2] The workout was "Fat Helen," upping the standard three rounds to five rounds of a 400-meter run, 21 kettle bell swings, and 12 pull-ups, for time. "The CrossFit men wore body armor. The women wore no body armor. We beat everybody," Glassman recounts. "We got down in the dirt and kicked their asses with girls. The Rangers were unable to hide their tears in the rain after being publicly beaten by women."

The athletic dominance of these tiny women completely sold the idea that CrossFit had some kind of special sauce, because there was no way that these pint-size females started out stronger and faster than the macho men they beat 98% of the time. "You've got something to learn," Glassman would tease a Special Forces operator or SWAT team officer. "You just got beat by a pottery teacher from the hippie high school."

Nicole Carroll was the pottery teacher from the hippie high school. She looked the part: a whisper over five feet tall, huge hazel eyes, and a big blonde mane of pre-Raphaelite curls. She had a degree in cultural anthropology and taught yoga at a meditation retreat in the redwood mountains above Santa Cruz. Before diving into CrossFit, she'd been on her way to graduate school in ceramics. She was the last person you'd expect to see in the midst of CrossFit's Fight Club brotherhood, much less winning an athletic throw-down.

And yet, joining Glassman's traveling troupe of lifter-gymnast-sprinters was a kind of homecoming for Nicole. Her father was an old-school bodybuilder, of the Arnold generation. Free weights. Barbells. No machines. Tagging along with him to a series of Long Island strongman gyms, her whole childhood rang with the clank of steel plates, dumbbells, and bars, the sound and scent of guys pumping iron. She was comfortable with it. She was game for it. "Hey," her father would yell to his buddies, "check out my twelve-year-old daughter's back squat!" It was fun to impress her father's muscle-bound friends. But she'd seen the female bodybuilders at those gyms. She didn't want to look like them. If upper-body strength meant looking like a Ms. Olympia contestant, she wasn't interested.

So when she'd walked through the doors of Glassman's gym in Santa Cruz, after scaling down CrossFit's website WODs on her own for six months, she was shocked to see so many women doing pull-ups. In bodybuilding gyms, as a kid, she'd seen women doing strict pull-ups. But those women were extreme specimens of musculature. She'd always assumed that in order to do pull-ups, you'd have to be on steroids. But these women doing pull-ups in Santa Cruz didn't look like professional athletes. They were just regular professional women, doing tons of pull-ups.

Seeing normal-looking women spring up and over the pull-up bars, she felt shock, and then a kind of competitive outrage. It was as if she'd been denied some kind of basic literacy, and it pissed her off. The fact that she couldn't do a single pull-up became unacceptable. "I want to be able to do it, and I should be able to do it," she thought. "There's no reason I can't do that."

She fell in with the 7:00 a.m. crew. After the SWAT team and MMA badasses were done with their throw-down, there were more women in the box. Eva T. was the strongest female in the original gang. She'd been training with Glassman since CrossFit was in its infancy. Even the toughest firebreathers were in awe of her unrelenting strength and pale-eyed Slavic beauty. She was an Olympian, the daughter of an Olympian. She had nothing to prove, and a lot to invest in the female athletes who gravitated toward her and emulated her. Her mere presence in a WOD made female athletes feel like members of an elite women's team.

One of the women Eva brought into the gym was a surfer chick named Annie Sakamoto. Unlike most of the people showing up to Glassman's classes, Annie hadn't been much of an athlete in school. She'd tried water polo, basketball, swimming, soccer, track. She stayed on the junior varsity team as a mediocre eleventh-grader, after all but a handful of her classmates were playing varsity. She liked playing sports and being on a team. She just wasn't focused enough to excel. After one year of college, she dropped out of school to surf in Costa Rica, then Kauai. Surfing wasn't sports, the way moving a ball around a field was sports. It was just pure movement, body awareness, and fluidity—the fluidity of motion and the fluidity of water, and how a body in motion can ride on top of the water. She was in her element on the waves. She was dialed in.

Eva knew Annie from the surf scene, and from a hip-hop dance class they took together. She'd seen how well Annie could move, the animal grace that took her smoothly through the water and across a dance floor. This girl belongs with us, Eva decided. Annie Sakamoto could be amazing. She just had to be roped in. So Eva kept plying her to try CrossFit when they saw each other. She wouldn't let up.

IT WASN'T AN EASY SELL. ANNIE WAS A SPARKLING FREE SPIRIT, happily employed at a seafood restaurant on the beach. She wasn't a hard-core type A personality, and she didn't want to get overworked or hurt. "I've heard people puke," she told Eva. "I don't want to puke." Eva gave assurances that no puking would result from an introductory workout. They did a light-lifting and gymnastics WOD, three rounds of ten sixty-pound deadlifts, ten pass-throughs on the pommel horse, and a 400-meter run. It was fun. There was no puking. *That wasn't so bad*, Annie thought.

Her next CrossFit WOD was a 7:00 a.m. workout with Greg Glassman, and it was a wild ride: three rounds of a 500-meter row, thirty kettlebell swings, a bunch of air squats, three climbs up a cargo net up to the ceiling, and twenty-five GHD sit-ups. GHD (glute-ham developer) sit-ups are about ten times as forceful as regular sit-ups. But there's a curiously long lag time between exertion and the ache of recovery that follows. Athletes can do seventy-five GHD sit-ups and walk away feeling fine. The next day, they're a little sore around their lower abs. The second day after the workout is when the mule really kicks.

"I couldn't sit down, stand up, walk, laugh, fart, or anything," says Annie. "I thought I had a hernia. As soon as I recovered, I was hooked.

With the cargo net and everything, it really challenged me in a way I'd never been challenged before, physically and mentally as well." GHD trunk pain notwithstanding, Annie excelled, because she could move so well. Anything the Glassmans demonstrated, she could pick up. She could see complex technical movements and just flow into them, the way a surfboard cuts into a wave. "Greg was completely enamored of her," Eva remembers, "because she could do everything well."

For Nicole and the other women, working out with Eva felt like track practice or volleyball practice, where everyone was moving together, each testing her own limits of agility and speed. On a high school track or field, there is a galloping moment when a pack of ponytails, flying with breathless energy, flashes across the line. The girls have not yet reached the crest of their physical strength. They are still growing, and the extravagance of youthful energy comes from a physical sense of getting stronger every day, and testing that strength against the other girls. The physical process of growth bathes young bodies in the elixir of quick recovery: the more you burn now, the more you will be able to burn tomorrow. That is what the prime of life feels like, in the rhythm of girls' feet tearing together down a track, and the arcs and leaps of movement, in training and competition.

The women doing pull-ups in Santa Cruz felt, in those morning WODs, the way they did when they were teenagers burning energy to get stronger, racing against one another. And in the physiology of that effort, the cells of their bodies were reprising the biochemistry of those golden sweaty afternoons. At 90% to 95% effort, cells shift their chemistry to produce HGH: human growth hormone. It doesn't happen at moderate intensity, only at a gallop. HGH signals the body to burn fat and build muscle. It gets the body closer to the biochemistry of a body that's still growing. It changes the way a person feels, as well as the way she looks.

When women are pulling themselves up on bars and throwing down some serious weight, there's an energy in the room. It spurs the men—it leaves them without excuses—but in some deep way it juices the whole group.

It is difficult to describe the ambience to someone who's only seen women doing choreographed cardio classes or jogging together. In moderate exercise, there's a decorum of always holding something back, being poised, conversational, looking good. There's an element of display, of women gazing at themselves in a mirror, or at one another, that is comfortably and conventionally feminine. It's easy, in an aerobics class, to evaluate and compare body parts. Health club voyeurism is accentuated by the gender segregation of health club activities. In the free-weight area, men do bicep curls and stare down their reflections. In mirrored studios next door, women do the latest-fad workout class and survey the girth and consistency of their hips, butts, and thighs. Women rarely venture to the bench press. Men rarely join the harem in Zumba, yoga, or step class. In addition to the ogling that goes on, as members of the opposite sex walk past each other's workout areas, there's a lot of same-sex compare/contrast going on, in the mirrors.

CrossFit is coed, and there are no mirrors. When women first show up, they look at trainers like Eva and Annie, the cuts in their shoulders and the V's of their backs, and say, "I don't want to bulk up." But then two months go by, and these women decide they want to climb a rope or deadlift their bodyweight. They start to diet for performance, because if they drop five pounds, the pull-ups will be that much easier. They start to eat more protein, less starch, less sugar. Food becomes fuel and stops being a pacifier. The women's legs get stronger. Their waists shrink. Their backs broaden. They get faster. They lift themselves up. Their bodies become a by-product of what they're able to do. In a conventional fitness club, women are trying to turn back the clock on their physical appearance, to tone their arms and flatten their tummies with small repetitive movements. In a CrossFit box, women are honing athletic performance and functional movement. Form follows.

Six months go by, and these women are pulling weight over their heads with a fierceness of effort some of them have never known. Sometimes, at the launch point of force, toward the end of a WOD, when the women are dredging the dregs of their strength, from one corner of the room or another there's a wild kind of yell, a Maria Sharapova tennis scream, the unintentional sound of sudden compression blasting air out of a woman's rib cage. It isn't casual or conversational. It isn't feminine. It is deeply female. The women absorb the crackling undercurrent of their own battle energy when this happens. The men do too.

And though they are together, and men's shirts are off and standard female attire is knee socks, tank tops, and booty shorts, it's not a sexually charged environment. Partly, it's because these people are not strangers—CrossFitters see each other sweaty and stinky with no makeup and messed-up hair, almost every day. They're familial. But beyond that, the effort they plow into a WOD is so total and so earnest that it's a little bit sacred. There is a real vulnerability to people when they are not sure they're going to lock out a big lift or get through the next set of box jumps. The intensity of the effort humanizes them.

The differences between men's and women's bodies are eclipsed by the fact that they are all engaged in the same intense effort—the body parts they have in common are aching the exact same way. So when they see each other, they see the whole person moving: some bit of virtuosity that leaves them in awe, or a glitch or miss that makes them flinch or remember their own early struggle for mastery. They see their own aspirations and weaknesses. After the WOD, out for beers, there may be flirting and shenanigans. But in the box, as the clock ticks and the weights drop, everyone is a brother or sister.

GIRLS ON FILM

In December 2005, on the day CrossFit's fabled "Nasty Girls" video is shot, Eva T., Annie Sakamoto, and Nicole Carroll are competitors. They don't just want to sweat. They want to win, and in the box they can unequivocally own the desire to come out on top. Not "win-win" or playing a supporting role to help everybody win, but faster-than-the-others, leave-them-in-the-dust, highest-score victory. A CrossFit box is one of the few social settings where it's admirable, sexy even, for a woman to unequivocally and aggressively compete for score, for time, physically, against other women or against men. On benchmark WODs named after women, female pacesetters regularly out-compete men. Local boxes pride themselves on the strength of their elite females.[3]

It takes Lauren Glassman two weeks to perfect the composition of the "Nasty Girls" workout, to balance its demands against the relative strengths and weaknesses of Eva, Annie, and Nicole. Greg and few of the elite male athletes have given her grief about the difficulty of the WOD. "Bullshit," she tells them. "My girls can do it. This is it."

Videos of elite athletes facing off in brutal WODs is chum in the water for CrossFit's online community. It gets people excited to do the workouts, to try to best the firebreathers at CrossFit HQ. Greg and Lauren's production method is to call a couple of firebreathers a day in advance, or the morning of a workout, and say, "Hey, we're going to shoot a video—just be ready." Most of the time, the athletes have no idea what they'll be asked to do. It's part of the mystique, the Unknown and Unknowable: Here's the mission, "3-2-1-GO!," camera's rolling. Athletes show up mentally and physically ready for anything, to compete. The challenge might play to their strengths or reveal the chink in their armor. No one ever questions the tasks.

Lauren loads up three 95-pound barbells as she describes the workout: three rounds of 50 squats, 7 muscle-ups, and 10 hang power cleans (jumping a loaded bar up from hip height to rest on the shoulders). On paper, the WOD doesn't seem that bad. Squats certainly aren't bad, even though there are a lot of them. It's just a question of pace. Three sets of 10 power cleans seems like a reasonable number. Eva isn't crazy about the muscle-ups, especially up against Annie and Nicole, whom she affectionately calls "the midgets" when pitted against them in gymnastic workouts. Eva is five feet five, around 140 pounds of slalom-pounding muscle and sinew. The midgets are five inches shorter and 20 to 30 pounds lighter. Competing against them in bodyweight workouts is like chasing squirrels. At least there's a bar that weighs almost as much as they do, to slow them down.

Where Lauren has set up the rings, the ceiling isn't tall enough for gymnastic rings to hang at the standard height of eight feet. So for muscle-ups, instead of being able to catapult up with a strong swing of the hips, the women have to start from a dead hang with their knees bent, power themselves over the rings without the benefit of momentum, quickly transition into a dip, then straighten their arms and push the rings down to their hips. It's make-do, less elegant than a full range muscle-up. But that's part of the challenge.

Nicole has never done muscle-ups in a workout before. She's tried one or two in practice, just to establish it's possible. But never in a WOD, much less in competition. She has no idea how to string them together, and three sets of seven is completely uncharted territory. She is nervous as hell.

Annie Sakamoto, as always, is good to go. She's never done a 95-pound hang power clean before. But there's nothing about the movement her body doesn't understand. She flows through the first set of squats and muscle-ups like it's nothing, and she's the first to pick up a bar. She deadlifts it to her hips and jumps it up. "Oh my God," she thinks. "*Wow*, that's heavy." She turns to Lauren. "What the hell is this?"

"Just keep going," Lauren says, from behind a video camera. "You'll be fine." Annie knows the power cleans are going to be tough. Eva is on her heels, jumping up the bar with mechanical efficiency. The deep dorsal and ventral ridges of Eva's exposed midriff ripple and flex to stabilize her body under the load. "What did I sign up for here?" she wonders. But the camera's rolling. Lauren is taping this face-off, and whatever happens will be posted on the CrossFit home page. Bite the bullet, get it done.

Nicole, last back to the bar, shakes out her hands. Holy crap, that was hard. The power cleans are no picnic, but they're a respite from the rings. It is not clear how the second set of muscle-ups is going to happen. By the time Nicole chalks up her hands, she knows the second set will gut her.

The second of three sets in a CrossFit WOD is the Valley of the Shadow of Death. The first set is all fresh energy and exuberant charge. The third set is the leap to freedom, the last few heroic reps with the clock ticking down. It has the propulsion of pushing through to the finale. But in the middle set, there's no light at the end of the tunnel. It's just tunnel. All you can do is gird yourself to the task. This moment at the beginning of the second set is the most predictably miserable part of a three-round WOD. But in a strange way, the repetition of this experience makes it a familiar marker, even a necessary component of the ritual: this is the second set—this is where I get through the suck even though the end is not in sight. Bear down—get it done.

By the time Nicole gets back to the rings for her third round, Annie and Eva are halfway through their last set of muscle-ups. As Nicole struggles up her fourth rep, the other two are off to the barbells, racing to move steel from hip to shoulder through the finish. Annie pulls herself under the barbell for the last time in just under ten minutes, and Eva chucks down her last power clean twenty seconds later.

Nicole is still on the rings, failing. This is the special reckoning of gymnastics workouts: when shoulder muscles run out of juice, there's nothing to do but wait for them to recharge. It creates a frustrating and powerless sense of urgency, when nothing can be done but wait to try again. And in this trough of waiting, there is a punishing psychological and kinesthetic calculus. You need to wait long enough for the muscle to recover, or else a premature attempt will result in failure and drain the shoulder again, leaving you in the same place, only more fatigued. But you don't want to wait too long and burn time on the clock. There is no indicator light on your shoulders to tell you exactly when they have enough charge to get over the next hurdle. So you have to reach into a physical sense of your body, to gauge its readiness. It is an animal sense that barely exists in us. Our nerves tell us where our limbs are, and if part of us is in pain. But gauging whether we have enough power to spring from one place to another, under fatigue, is like shining a flashlight into the fog. We can only grope for a sense of blood flow, watch the second hand on the clock, and guess.

Nicole guesses wrong and fails, expensively. Hands on the rings, with one muscle-up left, she leans back and hangs her head. Tears pool in her eyes, because she's always been able to muscle through anything via sheer will. But mental toughness is not going to spark her shoulders into action before the meat in them is ready to bear up her weight. There is no way to push through. It is crushing her to realize this, and the pain is salted by Annie and Eva's having left her behind. She's always been close at their heels in any workout. Now she is losing by a mortifying three-minute margin, on camera, and the thought of this gashes her emotionally.

Gripping the rings, Nicole lowers herself to a hang and looks up as if she's begging the ceiling to intercede on her behalf. Leaving one foot on the floor, she wrenches herself up, crosses her ankles and compresses her entire body. Her face tilts back in a grimace that any midwife would recognize. Struggling to extend her arms above the rings, she can't straighten them completely. If this were a competition with judges calling no-reps, this agonizing last push wouldn't be counted. But as imperfect as it is, this is the real last limit of her strength.

She releases herself from the rings, takes seven steps to the bar, and deadlifts it to her hips. Relying on the rested strength of her legs, she does five cleans unbroken. She puts down the bar, shakes out her hands, and resets her feet. Breathing hard, she picks the bar up and jumps up another two cleans in quick succession. She launches the bar up again, but this time the weight of it lands heavy on her shoulders and her knees give way. She folds down into a squat before powering 95 pounds up to a stand. She lowers the bar and holds it for a moment against her legs, leaning over. It seems like a waste to let the bar drop all the way to the ground, when she'll only have to deadlift it up again for two more reps. She grits her teeth and squinches up her eyes as she jumps the bar, but she can't launch it high enough to get under, and finds herself in a full squat with the bar below the shelf of her shoulders. It tilts, tumbles down, and bounces off the ground. She picks up the bar and muscles up the second-to-last rep. Almost collapsing under the final power clean, with one knee an inch off the ground, she keeps her balance and her footing to stand up with the bar. Finally done, just shy of thirteen minutes, she chucks the bar to the floor and walks into the parking lot.

Nicole is crying even harder now, with embarrassment. Coming in last, by a long shot, stings. But having melted down so badly, and knowing that meltdown was recorded on video and will be posted to the CrossFit main page is almost too wretched to contemplate. This isn't just friends and people who feel like family, although that would be bad enough. It's her career. CrossFit's online community is all of her professional peers. These are the people who show up to training seminars where she's supposed to be an expert. How is she going to convey any kind of authority when everyone has seen her reduced to tears, failing and staggering to finish a WOD that Annie and Eva tore through like wildcats. She's let herself down, badly. She feels that she's let down Greg and Lauren. The shame of it leaves her sobbing in a friend's arms.

She is, to say the least, not interested in viewing the video online. Posted as a benchmark WOD with 135 pounds as the prescribed weight for men, "Nasty Girls" (set to Nitty's hip-hop tune by the same title) goes viral in the CrossFit community. As far as Nicole is concerned, its runaway popularity only compounds the humiliation. Greg Glassman nudges her online to check out the comments. They go on for pages, from guys who have to substitute pull-ups and dips for muscle-ups and take double the girls' time to finish the workout.[4]

In the online comments where the CrossFit diaspora post their workout results, Jerry Hill posts the third-fastest time on the board, nine minutes and seven seconds, bending over backwards not to sound like he's bragging. "Wish I had an answer to this performance, plays into my strengths—reps were short enough for me to be able to take advantage of my speed." Only a handful of athletes manage to finish the WOD in less than twelve minutes, as prescribed. The vast majority are simply in awe of what they've seen, and verbally bow in homage to Nicole:

"Wow, if anyone wants to know the secret of [CrossFit]," one says, "it's right there in that video. Nobody in my gym, nobody, pushes themselves that hard. Inspiring."

"Those girls humbled me," says another. "25:00 using 115 lbs for cleans and subbing 3 dips/3 pull-ups for muscle-ups."

"If I trained with half the intensity of those three women, I'd be twice the athlete I am today."

"I was cheering out loud for Nicole at the end! (anyone else do that?)"

"Way to gut it out Nicole. You've got some Heart."

Even Greg Glassman is surprised by the unanimity of response from the die-hard brethren online. "Who'd have thought," he asks Nicole, "that last place would become the hero of the whole thing?"

CHRISTMAS IN IRAQ

CHRISTMAS ABBOTT WAS NODDING OFF IN HER MOTHER'S trailer when she heard her first incoming mortar. She'd been told it was an occupational hazard in Baghdad's International Zone. By 2004, the fortified administrative district, once home to Saddam Hussein's ministries and palaces, had become a nexus of command, control, and creature comforts for the Coalition Provisional Authority and the US military's host of private-sector and non-governmental remoras. Steel-reinforced concrete walls, barbed wire, and armed checkpoints girded the perimeter.

For this reason, the I.Z. was called the Green Zone, or even "the bubble." But it was more of a doughnut. Mortars and rockets regularly flew over the blast walls. A muffled *thmmpp* was the first sound. Then a whistle, as the munition traced an arc through the air. The loudness of the whistle, like the lag between lightning and thunder, told you how close the boom was going to be. Then, if the rocket or mortar wasn't a dud, came the explosion.

Christmas, twenty-two years old, was no stranger to trailers. She'd grown up in a trailer in rural Virginia. Her parents had slept in one room of their wood stove–heated home. Her brother slept in the hallway, and Christmas shared a bed with her older sister, Kole, in the other room. The two girls went to Young Life once a week and church once a week. At night, they'd sit up in bed and read Scripture to each other and try to understand it, until their mother shushed them to sleep. They were close, the way little girls can be when their nights end with whispers and giggles in the dark.

One night in November, when Kole was sixteen, the girls were in a car accident that rolled their car seven times. The concussive jolt of impact, torn metal, and shattered glass left Christmas physically unscathed. But Kole was knocked into a coma. Two of her lumbar vertebrae were broken. She would die within days, they said at the hospital. Then they said she wouldn't wake up. Then they said that, even though she'd woken up, she'd never walk again. Kole's body did heal, perhaps out of sheer stubbornness, for which the women in her family were well known. She became the exception in her physical recovery. But something inside of her would not heal.

"Her spirit had been damaged a little bit," Christmas says in a voice that gets tighter and tighter as she recalls Kole rendered immobile.[1] Once fiercely independent, athletic, and a straight-A student, Kole hated her own helplessness. It made her angry. Christmas, at age thirteen, could not understand why her sister's love seemed to have burned away. Christmas's parents couldn't fix it. God wouldn't solve it. The pillars of her life were incapable of protecting her from destruction and pain. So, why bother. With anything.

Her grades dived. She started smoking, which wasn't easy for her parents to thwart since they both smoked. She started drinking and consorting with people who condone fourteen-, fifteen-, and sixteen-year-old girls smoking and drinking and all that entails. She did go to work, when she was old enough, as a project manager's assistant at a construction company. She squeaked through high school, left home, and ran wild. She moved to Richmond and took a few college classes. Working three jobs to pay for them didn't seem to interfere with hard living. When you're twenty-one and working as a cocktail waitress at an all-night bar, drinking makes it easier to smile, and smiling does wonders for tips. "It was pretty incredible money to make," she says. "I was still paying for school out of pocket, up front. I didn't want to go into debt. Debt scares the crap out of me."

At the time, her mom was working in Iraq, doing the same kind of purchasing work she'd been doing as a local school administrator. But without electricity, in a war zone, for Kellogg, Brown and Root (KBR), a global engineering and construction company that does a lot of business in dusty places. On television, people saw night vision footage and embedded journalists in flak jackets. What they didn't see was the vanguard of procurement managers air-dropped in to ensure that all those tip-of-the-spear types and State Department nation builders were hewing to Defense Federal Acquisition Regulations—hundreds of pages of procurement policy specifying everything from accounting systems to the contracting clauses for laundry and dry cleaning services.[2] For this, war zone bean-counters were paid handsomely, compared with what they'd be making in places like Lynchburg, Virginia.

For Christmas's mom, the KBR gig was a chance to get out of debt in a single year of work and see some sites from the Old Testament. Babylon lies in ruins in Iraq. Abraham was buried there. Nineveh, just off the road east of Mosul, is where an Assyrian king is said to have heard Jonah preach and then covered himself in sackcloth and ashes to forestall the divine destruction of his city. The rolling destruction of Iraq, often ascribed to God, has been executed for thousands of years by the best-trained and best-armed empires of the day: Persians, Arabs, Mongols, Ottoman Turks, the British, the Americans.

Christmas worried about her mom working in a place where bombs were going off on the road. At the same time, it was damn impressive. "My mom works in a war zone" can put a bit of swagger in your step. On phone calls, her mom kept trying to convince her daughter to come over. "I think you would just love this," she'd say. Twelve-hour days, seven days a week, for four months, then two weeks off. Money to pay for school. An adventure that could set them both up for a different kind of life.

When an innate streak of backwoods stubbornness takes hold of a woman like Christmas, or her mother or sister, whatever's in the crosshairs may as well lie down and die. Every week, when KBR posted its new job openings, it received a relentless return blitz of Christmas Abbott's résumé, submitted in response to any job that vaguely corresponded to her skill set. This went on for six months.

On December 22, 2003, two days after her birthday, three days before the holiday she was named after, Christmas got a morning phone call from her dad. Her parents were getting a divorce. They'd been married twenty-six years, so they were supposed to be safe in happily-ever-after. The news left Christmas feeling gutted, the same way she felt after Kole's accident. She called in sick and went over to her best friend's house to watch movies and fall apart. That afternoon, her phone rang.

"May we please speak to Christmas Abbott?" asked a business-like voice on the other end.

"Yeah," Christmas snapped in rare moment of audible pique. "Who's *this*?"

It was KBR recruiting. Without waiting for her to respond, a quota-chasing human resources drone laid out a pay package and requested that she leave for Houston the following week.

"I'm sorry," she said. "Back up for a moment. What's the position? Where am I going? What's happening?" She'd responded to so many postings, she had no idea what job she was about to take, even though she knew she was going to take it.

What came out of the cosmic hopper was laundry. She had just agreed to become a laundry attendant in the mother of all war-zone wash-and-dry facilities. The I.Z. laundry complex, run strictly according to Defense Federal Acquisition Regulations on the contracting of laundry and dry cleaning services, was a 10,000-square-foot facility. Christmas's job was to sit at the counter. When people brought in their laundry, she would count out the laundry items and give them a ticket. When they came back with their ticket, she'd find their laundry. That was it: taking in and issuing laundry, twelve hours a day, seven days a week, in the desert.

She fell in love with the job. In a desert war zone, soldiers and Marines get filthy, and so do their clothes. When they get inside the wire and bring in their laundry, they are exhausted, and everything they own is covered in dust. When they come back showered and see their clothes clean, folded, and smelling of fabric softener, it visibly lifts their spirits. When a unit came in, matted in mud after a month in the field, she'd grab their bags. "I will see you boys first thing in the morning. We will get this down to you right away," she said. "I special-treated the guys who were out in the field—it's so much more rewarding to put on clean clothes when you're always dirty."

STILL, THE FIRST MONTH AWAY FROM HER FAMILY AND FRIENDS she cried. Her mother had relocated to Basra, so Christmas got to sleep in her mother's trailer instead of a dorm room with ten other girls. She went to sleep with her pay stub on the night stand, to remind herself that things were going to get better.

And then, a few weeks in, came the *thmmpp*, and the whistle, and the boom—a rattle and crash, like the sound of two cars slamming into each other. Christmas jumped clear across the room, as if that would be somehow safer. She had no idea what to do. All she knew was that she was suddenly very, very awake and alert and aware of her own pounding heart and panting lungs, which were singed with cigarettes and the mystery smoke from the I.Z.'s burn pits. It dawned on her how absurd and idiotic it was to smoke in this environment. She quit cold turkey.

A couple of weeks later, she tried to run a mile. She'd never run a mile in her life, and halfway through, she felt like she was going to die. Her inability to move much faster than walking pace for such a piddling distance was a grim reminder that if something catastrophic were to happen, she'd be helpless. She'd be one of those victim-y little girls that has to get rescued by some big brave strong person. She'd be a burden. That thought, in itself, was repugnant.

Bouncing between Kirkuk and Mosul, working her way up the hierarchy from laundry attendant to regional assistant manager of laundry facilities in northern Iraq, she found out where the gyms were. Her workouts were cobbled together, the usual fitness-club movements, hard work but nothing unconventional. In Al Asad, a Marine came up to her in the gym, a friend of a friend. He'd brought his laptop.

"Hey, Christmas," he said, "I think you would dig this." The video had taken him half an hour to download over a dial-up connection. It was Annie Sakamoto, Nicole Carroll, and Eva T. doing muscle-ups and squats and power cleans—the "Nasty Girls" video.

Christmas could barely wrap her mind around it. "Those girls were *so amazing to watch*," she marvels, even today. "They were doing something I had no idea could be done. And then to see their struggle with it. I could relate to it, instead of it looking like it's totally easy the entire time. And in the end, Nicole's fight to complete it was mesmerizing. She didn't cry because it hurt. She cried because it was such an overwhelming experience, and *that's* what spoke to me. This girl could have stopped. But she didn't. She kept going. It didn't matter. The other two girls were done, and they were cheering her on. She had a couple of failed attempts that didn't count, and she got the work done finally. When you push your body to that limit, that your only choice is to cry— that was so amazing, and I had never seen anything like that before. I hadn't been part of anything like that. It mesmerized me. It still does. It's my favorite video ever."

When she could pick up her jaw and speak, she asked the Marine what those girls were doing. He said it was CrossFit. She didn't know what that meant. "Well, whatever it is," she declared, "I want to do it. I want to work out so hard, and it's so intense, that it makes me cry." She had no access to the Internet. But she started improvising ways to achieve red-zone intensity, to follow Nicole into that place. When she watched the video, she couldn't see the rage and frustration in Nicole's tears. She could only see release.

At the end of her first year overseas, Christmas was in much better shape. She had also reached the upper echelons of laundry management in Iraq, and there wasn't much climb left in that trajectory. So she applied for a job as the assistant to a camp operations manager in the I.Z., making sure food trucks came in, making sure contractors were getting their vacation time coordinated and had all their travel documents, purchasing supplies, and generally helping to make sure the camp had everything it needed to sustain life.

But this wasn't a regular camp filled with active-duty military or war zone bureaucrats. It was a sector run by and for private security contractors, and specifically, Blackwater's private security contractors. Six hundred alpha males earning multiple times what they'd been paid as Special Forces operators, Green Berets, Army Rangers, or in the elite units of foreign militaries. All living literally on top of each other in stackable modified shipping containers, for three to six months at a time, with only a couple of dozen female contractors in camp.

Every day, as she traversed "the boulevard" that connected the chow hall, camp offices, and the camp's largest building—the gym—Christmas was a walking lamb chop within sniff distance of highly competitive wolves. She had tactics for successful navigation of this environment. The first was a Blackwater boyfriend, a Marine Force Recon vet, that nobody much wanted to mess with, even though he was deployed to a different part of Iraq. The second was the same confidence and incandescent friendliness she'd projected from behind the laundry counter. She never looked at the ground. When some ultimate warrior said hi, she smiled and said hello, as if it were some white-picket-fence fantasy of small-town Main Street America. Lastly, she did Cross-Fit with brutal intensity at the gym. She fought ferociously with every WOD, which made her seem less of a tender morsel than she might have first appeared.

There were two other guys in camp who did CrossFit, Chazz Rudolph and Ray Bily, both former Marine infantry. Chazz was twenty-five. Ray was just into his thirties and had been a cop after he left the Corps. They were both on the American ambassador's protection detail.

In the Marine Corps, Chazz's favorite book had been *Gates of Fire*, about the Battle of Thermopylae, and when the film *300* came out, the studio released workout videos of the actors doing CrossFit. Wanting to look like a Spartan, Chazz went from Gold's Gym in Plano, Texas, where he was in the top 1% according to the trainers' assessments, to a CrossFit box. His first WOD was five rope climbs, thirty wall balls, and thirty box jumps, five rounds. He had never done a wall ball or a box jump, and his only rope-climbing experience was on the Marine Corps obstacle course. He got to the second round of the workout and imploded. Like Amundson at the foot of the steps in Santa Cruz, Chazz was wrecked, and completely smitten. After three months at the box, he deployed to Iraq and became the crazy weirdo doing kipping pull-ups and kettle bell swings alone in the Blackwater gym and raving about CrossFit to anyone who would listen.

The only person who would tolerate his ravings was Ray. But barely.[3]

"Dude," Chazz said, "you've gotta do this." Chazz demonstrated some kipping pull-ups.

"That's gay," Ray said. "Get away from me."

"I know you!" Chazz picked up, a week later. "This is totally your personality."

"Get away from me!" Ray repeated. "I'm not doing that."

This went on for a couple of months.

"All right," Ray said finally. "I will give you two weeks of my unbridled discipline—let's do this. But then, if I don't do it, you have to leave me alone."

"Okay, deal." They shook on it.

Two weeks went by, and Ray got what Chazz had been saying, about the physical gains. But there was something else that twenty-five-year-old semi-invincible Chazz may not have realized, that Ray could sense in his bones.

"It just woke something back up inside of me," he says." You know how sometimes, something will grow stagnant inside of you? And you just go on with life? And as life progresses, you remember how things used to be, and the things you used to be able to do? When I was first in the Marine Corps, I could run 3 miles in under eighteen minutes, no problem. As time had gone by, I was thinking, I used to be able to do this. I used to be able to do that. The high-intensity stuff you used to beat your chest about, especially in an alpha male community such as Marine Corps infantry, you remember those things.

"I was like, oh my gosh, I'm really doing work here. Then you see guys sitting there yelling at other dudes doing one curl, or watch guys who could bench-press 480 pounds and could barely run from here to there. I started looking at things, thinking, I'm doing something that's above and beyond what other people are doing. I saw myself being able to increase strength and endurance at the same time. All of a sudden, doing a two- to three-mile run in body armor was nothing."

Ray's mental focus began to sharpen up, toward the end of a WOD when he was pushing through oxygen debt and muscular fatigue. He knew that if his mind fogged, if he stopped paying attention to the details of form or technique, with the loads he was moving, he'd injure himself. And if that happened, in this environment, he'd turn from an badass into a liability, and leave an elite team short one man. He couldn't afford to throw out his back or blow out a tendon, a ligament, or a rotator cuff. So his mind was tuned in to the nerves that ran along his lower spine and through his limbs, signaling the slight misalignment of an ankle or elbow, or a dangerous rounding of the lower back.

Outside the wire, heightened attention to detail was an absolute requirement of his job. His unit didn't have the luxury of the president's Secret Service detail, to rope off a whole neighborhood and post security on every rooftop. Their job was to move a high-value individual from point A to point B through Baghdad while monitoring every threatening detail in the environment: the hands of every merchant and pedestrian they passed, a soda can on the road, suspicious potholes, shoes in trees, anything out of the ordinary that might allow someone on a rooftop to push a button and know where the bomb would go off. The ability to suss out anomalous details is a war zone bodyguard's stock-in-trade. Out the window of an armored vehicle or on the fifth round of a heavy metcon, it was a feat of mental discipline to dial in to the details, to finish the work without injury. To Ray, it all felt like the same thing.

And now, this little girl wanted to join Chazz and Ray's secret society. They'd been eyeing her kettle bell swings and well-executed deadlifts at the gym—she was obviously watching the same YouTube videos that they were. She'd seen Chazz hitting a few WODs and mustered the gumption to walk up to him at the chow hall. "I know you're doing that crazy CrossFit stuff," she said. "I'm doing it too. It'd be nice to have a workout buddy."

"Holy shit," Ray exclaimed when Chazz told him. "That girl wants to do *this* stuff?" It was like Eliza Doolittle suggesting to Henry Higgins and Colonel Pickering that she could learn to speak like a lady. Ray had to give it some thought. He did not think highly of what most women in camp did by way of a workout. "Those girls always smelled like they'd just walked out of the friggin' perfume department at Macy's. They'd go in their little spandex and run on the treadmill for a while or maybe lift some light weights. They were very feminine and dainty about it," he says dismissively. "Christmas wasn't dainty, dabbing the sweat of her freshly made-up brow. She was doing straight work."

"Okay," he decided. "Let's see how far we can push her. Let's see if we can make her cry. Let's do it. Why not." Thus was Christmas Abbott adopted by two trained killers as their fitness guinea pig and personal project in the summer of 2007.

Christmas had said she wanted to cry. She was about to get her wish.

"They just thrashed me left and right whenever they could," she recalls with great nostalgia. "They took no mercy on me."

The first time she broke down in tears was on a workout called "Chelsea": 5 pull-ups, 10 push-ups, and 15 squats every minute, on the minute, for 30 minutes. But it wasn't a helpless cry—it was the sound of pain being driven out of her body. "When I've pushed my body so physically far that my body has no choice other than to release it emotionally," she says, "it's pretty incredible." Every time she cried, she'd think of the moment when she saw the "Nasty Girls" video for the first time. It was helping her, on some primal level. It left her with a sense of pride.

In any case, Ray and Chazz weren't going to scale the workouts for her, other than for Olympic lifts. They used the 20-pound medicine ball, so that's what she was going to use—there were no 14-pound women's medicine balls. They used a 24-inch box for jumps, so that's what she was going to use.

The only problem was that, even though her legs were strong enough to manage the jump, the prospect of launching vertically onto a 24-inch box scared the bejesus out of her. It took fifteen minutes of intensive coaching to get Christmas over the mental barrier. But after her heels landed on the box, she wouldn't stop. Ten minutes later, Chazz declared, "You're doing 'Kelly' now." Christmas had gotten a 24-inch box jump.

That meant the three of them were now ready to do 150 of them, 30 at a time, between 400-meter sprints in the blazing Baghdad sun and 30 wall ball shots to a 10-foot target with a 20-pound ball. It took her 45 minutes. "I finished it, and they were right beside me, cheering me on," she says. "They allowed me to get into that mindset of there's nothing you can't do."

Ray had a habit of not letting a WOD lay him out on the ground—it was part of his discipline, not giving into the tunnel vision of exhaustion. Christmas began to mimic him, refusing to collapse. To this day, she says, "Every time I work out, I literally walk around the gym and have my lioness chest out. I put my foot on top of the ball, my foot on top of the bar, because I own it. In the wild, you fall out on your back, that's surrendering—that's an animal surrendering. I'm not going to surrender to the workout. It's mine. If I'm on my back or my knees, I've surrendered. I'm not going to surrender. I will not fall down. I will crawl to stand back up. It builds mental fortitude."

Pretty soon, Ray and Chazz's little experiment began to match and even outpace them on bodyweight workouts. The dynamics of their triumvirate shifted into an escalating spiral of bravado: Christmas was determined to hold her own against the men. Ray and Chazz's innate high-octane male competitiveness was amplified by the drive to impress an attractive female, or rather, to not lose to the other guy in front of her. The fact that Christmas was off-limits or that Ray was married only intensified the athletic competition that left all three of them feeling like they were about to die on a daily basis. There were no more Stop signs. It was a three-way game of chicken.

All three of them ached constantly and knew exactly where the others were physically hurting. "Your lats would be completely trashed, or your quads would be trashed," Ray remembers. "We were always squeezing somebody's traps or something, and be like, 'Oh my God, you son of a bitch, what is the *matter* with you?' You'd grab somebody's leg in chow and watch the person completely buckle. It was almost a sibling rivalry, poking fun, best friends."

Workout design was a game of liar's poker crossed with Russian roulette, with a bullet in every chamber. CrossFit.com's prescribed WOD was simply a point of departure for the day's keelhauling. The challenge was how to take the regular ordeal and bend and twist it into some un-dreamt-of torture, something with flair and originality. The only question was who would play the final trump.

"Okay, this is what we're supposed to do," Chazz would say. "But, oh man, wouldn't it be *evil* if we did *this*?"

"We *could* do it that way," Christmas would reply. "But then we could do it *this* way, and it'd be *horrible*."

"Oh God!" Ray exclaimed. "You're *horrible*! Let's go do it!"

In practical terms, this meant insanity like "Fran," but with pull-ups on gymnastic rings instead of bar, with as many unbroken pull-ups as possible on the rings. Or the "Painstorm" workouts first devised as a monthly competitive face-off between CrossFit London and Cross-Fit Central Scotland, with some displaced US Marines thrown into the mix. Seven hundred years of Anglo-Scottish enmity were clearly evident in the design of these WODs, many of which lasted an hour.[4] Chazz was incredibly excited to find them online and excitedly ushered Ray and Christmas into a WOD called "Fight Gone Crazy."

The CrossFit benchmark, "Fight Gone Bad" is 5 movements, as many repetitions as possible in 1 minute for each movement, moving station to station. Rest a minute, and do the whole series again. Repeat. Fifteen minutes of work, 18 minutes total. It guts people. "Fight Gone Crazy" is 20 movements, some bodyweight, some involving a 95-pound barbell or a 35-pound kettle bell, as many repetitions as possible in 1 minute for each movement, with 1 minute of rest between every 5 stations. Twice in a row. Forty minutes of unmitigated sprint, broken up by seven 60-second rest periods to reflect on the insanity of the exercise.

"I was twenty-five. I can no longer do that," says Chazz. "I would never do that workout again."

"He would never do it now, on his *own*," says Ray, now pushing forty. "But I promise you, if I walked into his gym and said we're doing 'Fight Gone Crazy,' he'd go, 'You're an asshole.' But he'd do it. That's just how it is."

Life in the I.Z., as in all war zones, fused intensity and boredom in a way that blurred the lines between exquisite adaptation and idiocy. Ray, Chazz, and Christmas were more physically powerful than they'd ever been, faster than they'd ever been, sharper, and hungry to test themselves. They would go for incredible runs with no body armor or helmets, take a long swim in the pool, and then back to camp. A *thmmpp* would signal incoming mortar or rocket fire. Still running, they'd mentally gauge the distance from the *shoooo* sound that followed, and ditch into a bunker as the boom went off. Then they'd dust themselves off and keep running and think it was funny.

They could play, immersed in their own skein of rituals and lingo. It was, as Chazz puts it, "like starting a little family of CrossFitters." Chazz had been awarded some kind of protection-detail employee-of-the-month stipend of fifteen hundred dollars. Instead of taking the cash, he asked his manager to buy a C2 rower and some bumper plates for the gym. Some of the more open-minded Blackwater guys saw what Ray and Chazz (and, most stupendously, Christmas) were able to do in the gym and asked to join their group. Within a few months, Ray, Chazz, and Christmas were coaching two classes a day for a group of fifteen people who also donated or chipped in for equipment: slam balls, kettle bells, rings, everything a small group of people needed to run their own box.

"Back in those days, Chazz, Christmas, and I, we were a community. We were a family," Ray reflects. "Like-minded individuals came together at the right space and time. It was magic."

As the roasting summer cooled into balmy winter, the bomb-spiked idyll came to an end. Christmas's contract was up. She moved back to the States to get her CrossFit coaching certification and open a box in Idaho with her Marine Force Recon boyfriend. As a permanent and visible testament to the distance she had traveled, Christmas had her entire right arm tattooed with the image of a barefoot goddess surrounded by fairy-tale woodland animals and flowers. One of the goddess's hands is delicately raised in greeting, and the other carries a sword.

"Come ready, be nice, but always be prepared to protect yourself," Christmas says. "She's walking on the red brick—her path—and it is what she wants it to be."

FALLUJAH, FOR TIME

Sprinting Wars and the Next Generation of Combat Training

BY THIS TIME, CROSSFIT WAS PROLIFERATING ACROSS TWO WAR zones and infiltrating military bases around the world. It was cheap, improvised, and time efficient. It didn't break in heat or dust. And it made soldiers physically more powerful than they'd ever been, in a new era of military conflict that demanded heavy loads be hauled as quickly as possible from point to point. Counterinsurgency in Iraq and Afghanistan was not a game of long marches and precise campaigns. In a landscape of steep hillsides, hot stairwells, and dangerous corners, hazard boiled up in sudden twenty-minute bursts of load-bearing cardiovascular suck. It was CrossFit as a live fire exercise, and any soldier with half a brain knows to train as you fight.

On the CrossFit main site, favorable reports from Navy SEALs resounded with a strong message: give us more—this shit works. One SEAL's perspective on functional fitness, published in the *CrossFit Journal*, listed a dozen ways that CrossFit training mapped to the rigors of special operations in Iraq: lifting heavy objects and people off the ground (deadlift, cleans); pressing heavy objects over a wall (clean and jerk, push press); standing up while bearing weight (squat); pulling oneself up over a railing or wall or into a window (kipping pull-ups, muscle-ups); stepping up with weight (box jumps). Digging and carrying awkward-shaped objects for unknown time and distance; sprinting in forty to sixty pounds of gear; wrestling and subduing enemy combatants on stairs, on a hillside, or in enclosed spaces. All these activities required the explosive power that special operators cultivated in their daily CrossFit WODs.[1]

In response, CrossFit HQ published a series of how-to guides, developed by special operators and regular grunts, for adapting CrossFit training to austere environments. The Canadian Infantry formalized a nine-week series of programmed WODs designed to enhance combat fitness "anytime, anywhere," using large rocks, light armored-vehicle tires, and ammo cans and soccer balls filled with sand in place of the Olympic weights, kettle bells, medicine balls, and other trappings of a conventional CrossFit box.[2] Most of CrossFit's "Girl" WODs could be adapted this way.

Jim Decker, an Army Special Forces soldier stationed in Japan, published his recipe for a go-anywhere CrossFit workout kit: a set of gymnastic rings, a small pair of parallettes, a fifty-five-pound dumbbell, and a stopwatch, along with a notebook containing a few months' worth of WODs from the CrossFit.com archives.[3] About half the "Girls," he observed, were body weight only. "All you really need is something to pull up on, and an observant CrossFitter can find that practically anywhere." Observant, in the sense of being aware of your surroundings—and also, perhaps, in the sense of keeping kosher fitness-wise, hewing to ritual and custom, even in foreign places.

The magic of these nomadic fitness survival guides was how they cast each athlete as a hunter-gatherer explorer, a childhood fort-builder, alive to the environment and its wealth of ready materials. Once you were determined to hit the intensity of a daily WOD, all it took was imagination. "Take a walk around," Decker advised. "Root through scrap piles, barns, and tool sheds, and start collecting apparatus for your primitive gym." Any tree was a potential pull-up bar or handstand push-up support station. Rocks and ammo cans were fodder for heavy lifts and carries, power cleans, and kettle bell swings. Buckets could be weighted and used as dumbbells for thrusters, weighted box steps, and Turkish get-ups (rising from a prone to a standing position with one arm raised above your head). Even a stick could be used to refine Olympic lifting technique and speed under the bar. Dross was treasure. Industrial wreckage was a gold mine. Just think, Decker mused, of an abandoned auto and the trove of exercises you can concoct with the equipment lying there: axle thrusters, leaf-spring Olympic lifts, bumper dips, tire flips and carries. The possibilities were endless.

For a special operator or a grunt on the ground, post-9/11 conflicts epitomized the Unknown and Unknowable. Any convoy could be flipped by a roadside bomb, creating casualties to haul to safety. Afghan soldiers could turn around and strafe their American trainers. Urban landscapes and mountain patrols were primed for treachery and ambush. Worst of all, the kind of physical training that had been standard drill for decades was woefully inadequate for the physical demands of combat in the urban heat of Iraq and the mountains of Afghanistan. The Army's test of physical fitness consists of 2 minutes of push-ups, 2 minutes of sit-ups, and an unencumbered 2-mile run. The Marine Physical Fitness Test (PFT) is a little more strenuous, with a perfect score consisting of 20 consecutive pull-ups, 100 crunches in 2 minutes, and 3 miles in under 18 minutes, blissfully free of kit and gear.

The problem is, no enemy in a modern war zone is ever going to challenge a soldier to go jogging. The long runs favored by drill sergeants aren't weighted with the kinds of loads a typical soldier is humping around on patrol. And running with heavy loads—or sprinting with heavy loads, when you're being shot at—isn't like running in shorts and sneakers, but for longer. It's a different metabolic ball game.

Captain Brian Chontosh, a decorated Marine who led troops into the second assault of Fallujah in 2004, was one of the loudest spear rattlers for CrossFit in the trenches and one of the more savage disparagers of the light-load aerobic regime blessed by the military's training czars. "I've got guys that max out at PFT, 300 points," he fumed before the American Society of Exercise Physiologists at their annual conference.[4] "They're crazy fast, they're doing it all. They're running sixteen-and-a-half-minute three miles. They knock out their twenty pull-ups, and they knock out their hundred sit-ups in about a minute forty-five. They're crazy fit. They'd be successful in combat, correct? Their performance failure in a combat scenario has cost lives. I've seen people fail physically in combat that were perfect 300 PFTers, because they couldn't handle load for duration while being stressed by physiological, psychological, mental, environmental, and operational stressors."

As technology advances, he explained, "I'm required to carry more gear. I become heavily encumbered. I've got weapons that are bigger and badder. I've got optics. I've got communications equipment. I need to be able to shoot, move, and communicate. I've got protective armor. The average soldier ready to close with the enemy is already about seventy-five pounds heavier than his average weight, and he's carrying this on an encumbered body. It takes eleven days to clear the city of Fallujah, and you've got Marines carrying a hundred to a hundred fifty pounds because we're going to add explosives, breeching equipment, grenades, the first aid kits, and all the medical supplies. So why not put loads onto our body that are typical in this situation and train to them?

"This is what combat boils down to: A guy gets shot, I need to go over there, pick him up, move him about a hundred meters, two hundred meters to safety. I need to negotiate obstacles along the way, avoid getting shot. He weighs approximately three hundred pounds with all his kit and gear. I might have a couple of minutes to take off his helmet and his body armor, if I need to. But maybe I don't want to, because as I'm transporting him, he could get shot again. So I keep his body armor on. So, jack up a dude that's three hundred pounds, get him on my shoulder, move him a distance to safety so I can save him before his life blood seeps out. He's got thirty minutes to live. Where do you find that muscle pattern anywhere, in anything that we've done or experienced in any type of workout regime? I find it in CrossFit. It's called deadlift, clean, snatch, clean, run, sprint, negotiate obstacles, and we're doing it. For me, it's a no-brainer. It's done. I'm sold. That's what we do on the battlefield."

WHAT CHONTOSH FOUND IN CROSSFIT WAS MORE THAN AN AC-
celerated physical adaptation to the reality of urban warfare. It was
a psychic adaptation as well: the stress of high-intensity sprints under
heavy loads could be harnessed to steel a soldier's mind to endure other
stressors—heat, cold, elevation, hunger, darkness, sparse and irregular sleep, and the hormonal spike and crash of adrenaline, all of which
shove human consciousness closer to the yawning chasm of I-just-can't-
anymore. Exercise physiologists, lab-based academics, don't account for
these factors in a sanitized training environment. "But I'm telling you,"
he said, "I can start doing it. I can start simulating some of these effects.
Environmental stressors, psychological stressors. I can fight these things
off. I can fight off injury. I can fight off how the mind drifts and closes.
I can maintain mental agility, so they can focus and concentrate and
perform, and again in combat."

Chontosh's method for doing this was to engage his men in the middle
of a high-intensity couplet or triplet, to see if they had the mental clarity
to count their own reps and control their breathing. Between rounds, in
the fog of exertion, they might be given a leadership scenario, and at the
end of the WOD they'd have five minutes to articulate a response about
the decision they'd make. There was no separation between physical
and mental training. It was all under fatigue, learning to breathe and
think in the heat, under loads, under duress. Learning how to exert the
hauling force of draft horses while gaming out the next tactical move.

Forged into CrossFit firebreathers in the 120-degree deserts of Jordan
and Kuwait, these men suffered no heat casualties and no injuries on
four-hour training exercises in full kit and gear. In their assault on Fallujah in November 2004, in the nastiest shooting gallery of a hot urban
war, only 3 of Chontosh's 158 Marines were killed in action.

In the unremitting pressure cooker of Fallujah, Marines would literally step into the night to hit a CrossFit WOD during lulls in the action.
A typical Fallujah workout might start with weightlifting exercises in a
makeshift tent, then move on to Tabata-style drills. Tabata workouts,
named after a Japanese exercise physiologist, consist of twenty seconds
of all-out effort alternating with ten seconds of rest, for a total of four

minutes. In his research, Tabata found that athletes who trained at high intensity for short periods of time increased their aerobic capacity as well as their anaerobic strength, whereas athletes training at moderate intensity for longer periods of time built only aerobic capacity, with no anaerobic gains. His namesake interval scheme looks easy on paper. In practice, it wrecks you.

After weightlifting and Tabata drills, it might be time for sprints in body armor. "Incoming fire usually deterred running," one Marine conceded in a post to CrossFit's online journal. "Aside from the obvious environmental factors—heat, dust, danger—the experience was memorable because it was so varied and random. I adapted rather quickly to the unpredictability. I expected it, knowing CrossFit's theory."[5]

Unsurprisingly, these Marines crushed the PFT upon their return, despite not having done any crunches or run 3 miles in months. They were all, in a sense, extreme athletes, under the command of a captain who viewed combat as the ultimate test of functional fitness. "CrossFit is combat," Chontosh declared, quietly devastating his audience, who considered CrossFit edgy before being told it was the physiological distillation of human warfare. "Combat is CrossFit."

The Marines, the service that always does more with less, nurtured a special affinity for CrossFit in these years, and not just because it made them tougher. There was something about CrossFit that was so harmonic with the ethos of Semper Fi. CrossFit demands courage and an appetite for discomfort. It presses the whole person, mind, body, and spirit, against the whetstone of strain and fatigue, and people must choose to stay there until they are sharp. It changes people. It alters their identities, and binds them. The Marines are hierarchical, where Cross-Fit is decentralized and tribal. There are plenty of tattooed and pierced CrossFitters who'd bristle at military command and control, and lots of moms and white-collar professionals who couldn't handle a rifle. But in the way CrossFitters train, and the way Marines are forged, there is a resonance that was instantly recognized and embraced by CrossFitters and Marines alike.

In January of 2008, Greg Glassman ran a CrossFit certification course at Camp Pendleton, West Coast home of the Marines' School of Infantry. Civilians paid the regular fee, but there were twenty free slots for Marines to learn how to train the fundamental movements of Cross-Fit. At the customary social evening between two days of high-intensity coaching, exposition, and competitive WODs, Glassman sought out Dan Wilson, the officer who'd been CrossFit's chief proponent at the Infantry School.

"Dan," he said, "I'm getting rid of the original CrossFit gym in Santa Cruz and all that equipment. If you guys come and get it, we'll give you all that equipment."

Glassman, a raging libertarian, was growing weary of California. His father lived in Arizona, where he and Lauren could afford to buy a house. More important, CrossFit had outgrown its original incarnation as the Glassmans' mad science laboratory of high-intensity fitness. They had proven out their methods in the clubhouse. Now it was time to scale, and that required a single-minded dedication to expanding the cadre of CrossFit trainers.

At a thousand dollars per person for a one-weekend CrossFit Level 1 seminar, the trainer certification business was more profitable than running a gym. More important, it was a force multiplier: every new Cross-Fit trainer, armed with all the videos and articles on the main website, was either going to start a CrossFit affiliate or improve the training level at an existing CrossFit box. Low cost of entry and the decentralized affiliate model meant that new boxes could pop up anywhere a certified CrossFit trainer wanted to hang out a shingle, with no central coordination or top-down management.

What held it together was the culture: the methodology, the website's daily WODs, videos, articles, and manifestos, and the Level 1 seminars, where the knowledge but also the spirit of virtuosity was enacted and transferred to newly minted coaches. Every coach autonomously set the tone for an entire tribe of CrossFit athletes. So it was critical to evolve the Level 1 seminar—the entry-level accreditation of CrossFit coaches—from a traveling throw-down into a repeatable ritual that encapsulated the core of CrossFit coaching: attention to technique, the combination and interplay of movements and metabolic pathways, nutritional philosophy, and scaling techniques that make each WOD equally grueling to athletes of wildly different abilities. But also the social conventions and cues: cheering on the last athlete, celebrating any personal record, not just the top scores on the leaderboard. Going out for beers instead of everyone heading their own separate sweat-soaked way. If the goal was to spur a movement, Glassman's place was on the road. So the Santa Cruz lease was up.

But here, at Pendleton, were a bunch of Marines with an empty warehouse. Who better to inherit the original Santa Cruz pull-up bars, rowers, and bumper plates? The gear was guaranteed to give dozens and hundreds of jarheads a beat-down, and vice versa. They were worthy of each other.

On March 19, 2009, Wilson pulled onto Research Drive with a tractor-trailer and nine Marines. They did the gym's last WOD ("Fran," of course) and loaded every last bar, plate, rack, rower, rope, kettle bell, plyo box, and dumbbell into the truck.[6]

Inside CrossFit's nursery, now almost vacant, Glassman addressed the inheritors of the first firebreathers' teething toys. Reflecting on his legacy, he sounded a lot like Knute Rockne in a halftime locker room, or Mel Gibson before the climactic battle scene in *Braveheart*. "We changed the world from in here," he said. "I'd always thought that taking this apart would be a sad day for me. It's not. I don't feel a thing other than the fiery optimism of knowing that this thing's going to resurrect down the road four hundred miles and continue to live on forever. God bless you boys and everything you do. It's an absolute honor, from CrossFit Santa Cruz to CrossFit Camp Pendleton."

As a token of appreciation, the Pendleton Marines presented Glassman with a bottle of sand from Iwo Jima, where, said the sergeant major, "much blood was spilled to overpower the Japanese defenders. The flag raising during the battle of Iwo Jima represents the fighting spirit and tenacity of Marines. You also have made an important and historic contribution to the Marine Corps. Your donation will be instrumental in preparing warriors, both physically and mentally, for the rigors of combat. We thank you, Coach, from the bottom of our hearts."

The truck doors were closed and bolted. "Done," said Wilson. "Tomorrow morning, we'll meet you at CrossFit Camp Pendleton." The next day, Wilson's Marines packed out the gear into the Warehouse, as they called it, and with its inaugural WOD, "Fat Helen" (three rounds for time: 400-meter run, 21 kettle bell swings, 12 pull-ups), CrossFit Camp Pendleton was born. And there the equipment remains to this day.

Wilson caught some flak for the whole affair. The overseers on some corner of the base, perhaps the ones running Pendleton's treadmill center, were incensed enough to trigger an investigation into whether accepting a gym full of beat-up CrossFit gear was illegal according to military rules about accepting gifts on behalf of the Corps, or whether it had been insubordinate to take the truck or the nine Marines to Santa Cruz. But Wilson had been granted permission for all of it. To the degree that rules had been unknowingly bent, it was all to improve the fighting fitness of Marines, and no one up the Corps chain of command will punish a lieutenant colonel for that, even if he's stepped on some toes along the way.

As he transferred out of Pendleton, en route to his next post at the National War College, Wilson motorcycled to Greg Glassman's house in Arizona and spent a couple of days there. They reminisced, and talked about what was next. "If you're going to Alexandria," said Glassman, "you need to CrossFit with Jerry Hill." He picked up the phone and called the former Marine, whose rented jujitsu studio was an echo of his own first training space.

"Jerry," said Glassman. "I've got Dan Wilson coming down. I want him to CrossFit with you."

THE BLUE ROOM

Martial Arts Sublets and the Forbidden Pleasure of Dropping Barbells

WITH A FEW BARBELLS, MEDICINE BALLS, PULL-UP BARS, BOXES, and kettle bells, and a nominal fee to CrossFit HQ, any certified Cross-Fit coach could become the proprietor of a CrossFit affiliate. In the economic hangover from the dot-com crash, this meant guys like Jerry Hill could sublet space, often from martial arts dojos, before they had enough athletes to afford a dedicated space. From Glassman's early years in Santa Cruz to today, there's been a symbiosis between CrossFit and martial arts, especially jujitsu, mixed martial arts, and Krav Maga.

Part of this compatability is cultural, and part of it is architectural. The cultural part is a fundamental embrace of functional fitness. In martial arts, it doesn't matter how beautifully curved your biceps are, or if you have six-pack abs. If you can't hit hard, or if you're easily winded, someone's going to mess you up. Any kind of conditioning that makes you hit harder or breathe better in the middle of a round makes it less likely you'll get messed up. So people who do hard-core-combat martial arts (as opposed to the beauty-of-grace-and-form varieties) are serious about high-intensity training.

The time domain of a martial arts match, a single-digit number of minutes of all-out effort, is on the same order as a WOD. The type of effort required—violent bursts of explosive effort under fatigue and time pressure—is exactly what CrossFit cultivates. It's competitive, high discipline, heavily male (along with a certain type of seriously kick-ass female). It demands the ability to suffer, and develops an athlete's capacity to suffer and keep going—the quality of relentlessness.

CrossFit, in its early days, attracted MMA fighters with a geek streak. Guys like Josh Newman, who went to Yale, built and sold tech companies, and spent time getting his teeth knocked loose in Connecticut MMA arenas, invariably stumbled onto the CrossFit website and caught the bug. After winning the state MMA championship in his weight class two years in a row, Newman was looking for an edge. As he says, "There's nothing like getting the crap beat out of you to keep you honest at the gym."[1]

When he checked out the CrossFit.com site, Josh thought the Workout of the Day was a joke: 400 meters of walking lunges. Then he tried it and, about 100 meters in, realized, "Oh yeah—I'm fucked." The next day, he missed his stop on the subway because he literally could not stand up. He had to wait until the next stop, when a lady near the pole got off, so he could slide across the subway bench, grab the pole, pull himself to a standing position, and hobble onto the platform. If something so simple and time efficient could incapacitate him, he thought, this was clearly the way to go.

Before long, he'd roped in a buddy who did Brazilian jujitsu (and later founded CrossFit Virtuosity in Brooklyn) to work out in Central Park. They showed up with medicine balls and kettle bells and did pull-ups on the playgrounds. People joined, and pretty soon ten of them were getting in trouble with the park police for doing box jumps on benches or stringing gymnastics rings up on the trees. This went on for six months, until it got cold. Then they moved into, and got kicked out of, six gyms in the space of two years. Because they did things like rig treadmills to see how fast they could run without shooting off the back. Or bang out so many pull-ups in a personal training gym that clients would simply abandon the hardbody trainers who'd brought them there to Feel the Burn and maybe move the peg down one notch on the machine. At a Chinatown kickboxing gym, the manager saw Josh and his pals doing high-volume barbell WODs, marched over, and barked, "What you guys are doing looks really dangerous." Ten feet away guys were punching each other in the face, which was, apparently, not really dangerous.

The absurdity, and the hassle of it all, was just too much. So in 2007, Newman rented a 1,000-square-foot place in the Garment District, "The Black Box," which refers to CrossFit's empirical discipline of measuring inputs (the workouts) and outputs (athletic performance) from the training method. In a lovely stroke of irony, the term is also drama-world jargon for a small, bare-bones experimental theater.

Newman needed thirty members to cover the rent, and he had twenty people. "There are not thirty people in New York City who are going to do this CrossFit thing," he thought. "This is just going to be an expensive gym membership for me." That year, the Black Box grew from thirty members to over a hundred. Newman got kicked out of his first Garment District space when, during a WOD, a barbell someone dropped from overhead crashed straight through the floor into the space below. It was after hours, but the landlord wasn't so thrilled. When the Black Box decamped to a larger space, also in the Garment District, Newman and his people pulled up the mats to move. They had broken literally every tile.

The tiles were broken because CrossFitters, left to their own devices, regularly dump heavily loaded barbells from overhead onto the ground. There is a legitimate reason for this: safety. If an athlete is going for maximum effort with a load he's not sure he can propel all the way up to his shoulders, or all the way overhead, it's essential that he be able to fail safely. And failing safely on a one-rep-max Olympic lift or overhead squat means dropping the bar.

Also, it's fun to drop barbells. The ability to instantly jettison a serious amount of weight gives strength workouts the quality of play, no matter how strenuous the effort. If you can't do the lift, you can eject. And if you do manage to launch a heavily loaded barbell over your head, and your heart is pounding with the hot-damn-I-did-it victory beat of a personal record, it is sublime to simply release your fingers from the bar and have all those bumper plates suddenly not compress your body. The spine springs back to its full length. Muscles no longer brace. *There, I did it—I'm free.* That sense of victory and freedom, the sudden lightness of releasing a heavy burden, is like getting a cast taken off. It's like getting a cast taken off your soul.

When it's synchronized, the ritual of dropping barbells is even more intense and satisfying. So for instance, in an every-minute-on-the-minute set of heavy snatches, every sixty seconds a clock ticks down, and your coach bellows, "Three, two, one, GO!" The lightning of electrical impulse courses through each athlete's nerves and muscles at the same moment. Every barbell flies toward the ceiling. There's a slight variation in speed, depending on each athlete's height and strength. Then, within a few seconds, all the barbells come crashing down, and the boom of dozens of twenty-five- and forty-five-pound rubber bumper plates hitting the ground is like war drums. Thunder. It's beautiful. This is why every tile in the Black Box was broken. It's also why CrossFit boxes outside industrial areas tend to have unhappy neighbors and grouchy landlords.

So Josh Newman was sent packing by his first Garment District landlord. He was also nearly arrested in Times Square for sprinting up 41st Street wearing a weight vest—the kind of vest that's black nylon, with rows and rows of tiny pockets to hold one-pound lozenge-shaped weights, and looks exactly like a suicide bomber vest. Seconds into his full-speed dash into Times Square, Newman was being shouted down by ten police officers, two of them with guns drawn. "But then," he recalls, "they realized I was too small and Jewy looking to be a threat. They just said, 'I don't know what you're doing, but *never do it here again.'"

Around the same time, a police car on Eisenhower Avenue in Alexandria, Virginia, slowed to a stop, its red-and-blue lights flashing in the pre-dawn darkness. Jerry Hill lowered his wheelbarrow and raised his hands. The wheelbarrow was loaded with two hundred-pound dumbbells and an engine block, and he'd been sprinting with it, to build grip strength, on his way to the jujitsu studio where he trained athletes. Grip strength is essential when you're moving a lot of weight with a barbell, or stringing together dozens of pull-ups, and the best way to build grip strength for these activities is by holding on to something heavy for as long as possible, preferably while you're also winded. Hence the wheelbarrow, the dumbbells, and the engine block.

"I'm a strength coach," Jerry projected his voice to the police car. "These are weights. It's strength. And conditioning." The lights kept flashing. The cop got out of his car.

"I'm a strength coach," Jerry repeated with conviction. "These are weights. It's strength. And. Conditioning." The cop scrutinized him, calculating the odds that this wiry little white guy was telling the truth versus running down Eisenhower Avenue with a stolen engine block in a wheelbarrow.

"You look suspicious," the cop growled, got back in his car, and drove away.

Jerry and his wheelbarrow trundled off to the dojo. Same as in Philly, here was a jujitsu gym whose owner was happy to earn some extra cash by time-sharing a facility with CrossFitters. Aside from the cultural kinship between CrossFit and martial arts, they have similar real estate requirements. Both disciplines tend to occupy marginal space, often industrial space: warehouses, converted light-manufacturing buildings, former auto body workshops. Space needs to be cheap, open to accommodate sparring, and easy to equip with basic training apparatus: mats, weights, punching bags, maybe a drinking fountain. Adding some kettle bells and medicine balls doesn't screw up this kind of floor plan.

More important, the diurnal rhythms of martial arts and CrossFit were, at least initially, a perfect counterpoint. Martial arts athletes tend to work out in the evening. CrossFit's early adherents were morning people, rising before dawn to hit an o'dark thirty WOD. Jerry's classes started at 5:15 a.m. and ran every forty-five minutes through 8:15 a.m. Then it would be time for him to go home and be Mr. Mom. But for three hours in the morning, he was king of the Blue Room, so named for the color of the jujitsu mats. "It was on the second floor," he remembers. "Everyone was asleep. It was like a speakeasy."[2]

It wasn't ideal. Because the jujitsu studio was, in turn, subletting space from a conventional gym downstairs, there were constraints on how Jerry's gang could use the equipment. There weren't fixed pull-up bars, only bars hung on chains from the ceiling. So people learned how to time the kipping motion of their hips, generating momentum in tandem with the pendulum swing of the bar, to get up and over. There was a knack to it, as with any acrobatic trick.

There weren't boxes to jump on, so they stacked mats to 24 or 30 inches, to jump on. Shoes weren't allowed on the mats, so when it was time to run outside, people had to quickly lace up their shoes, run downstairs, do their sprints, then run upstairs and kick off their shoes for the next WOD.

Worst of all, they couldn't drop weights on the floor, which meant that heavy Olympic lifting WODs were out. For a powerlifter like Jerry, this made every barbell WOD into an unconsummated love affair. Bars would be loaded with less weight than he knew his athletes could handle with their mightiest one-time efforts. They'd string together barbell movements from the floor to hips, from hips to shoulders to overhead, and then, in a controlled sequence, back down to the ground. They never got to throw their whole selves into one skilled and mighty pull from the ground.

But there are different ways to build strength, and the early core of Hill's CrossFit Oldtown gang built their strength with pull-ups, push-ups, and tons and tons of air squats. They did muscle-ups on gymnastic rings. Dan Wilson had trained with Greg Glassman in Santa Cruz and with the Marines in Pendleton, but he got his first muscle-up in the Blue Room. "Get up there and fight it, Dan," Jerry hollered as Wilson swung from a pull-up to the transition. "You're there, brother!!!" From the top of the rings, Wilson, graying, buzz-cut, whooped for joy. "Was that good?" he asked.

"Yeah," Jerry laughed, "that was awesome." They got it on video. It's one of the best middle-aged "still got it, baby" moments ever recorded.[3]

The Blue Room gang did a lot of air-sucking metabolic conditioning, or metcons, alternating strength efforts with the cardio stress of box jumps, wall balls, or sprints in the stifling humidity of northern Virginia. Before long, men's shirts were off, and the habit of ripping shirts off during a WOD was well ingrained.

A statistician named Harold Doran was the chief instigator of the shirt-taker-offers. Perhaps it was the heat and sweat, or the high intensity, or a touch of OCD, but when Jerry yelled "Three, two, one, GO!" to kick off a heavy metcon, Harold's shirt had only moments to serve its intended purpose before it was jettisoned to the floor. It became an inside joke that leavened the heaving intensity of summer WODs. Harold had a way of making deadpan remarks about his shirt removal that made it okay for everyone else to laugh—he deftly controlled the joke. He began to spin a thread of self-deprecating humor that pervades CrossFit Oldtown to this day—a mixture of absolute seriousness about physical effort and mock seriousness about yourself. It's the sensibility of absolute commitment to a fast 800-meter sprint or a set of unbroken pull-ups, then making yourself ridiculous with a put-on remark. *Yeah, I'm a serious athlete, check out these abs.*

After his morning stint as class clown, Harold would hit the showers, change into a suit, and drive north over the bridge into Georgetown as an absolutely different, stone-faced, stressful grown-up. He's a psychometrician, which means he analyzes student test data: all the standardized tests that Congress mandated in No Child Left Behind, that teachers complain about, that teachers' unions scream should never be used in teacher evaluations. State commissioners of education pay guys like Harold to churn those data into statistical results that show embarrassing long-term differences between great teachers and the ones who stunt students' learning for years. These statistics invariably trigger political attacks, from local school boards all the way up to Capitol Hill. Managing these projects and their blowback is all serious, all the time.

"When I go into the office," Harold says, "I'm swamped. Swamped. There are real grown-up issues. They're complicated. They're stressful. They're hard, and they're taxing. But guess what? CrossFit is everything that my real world is not. I get to walk into the gym, and I get to be silly and crack jokes and be friendly and not be stressed out. I don't think about work when I'm in the middle of 'Fran.' I don't think about a client deliverable when I'm in the middle of a back squat. It is pure complete absolute absence of all that other stuff in my life. It's so amazingly therapeutic, because all of that stuff is set aside. CrossFit people don't know anything about my real world, about my work world. They know my family. They know my back squat, and they know my deadlift. But they don't know my nine to five, and I love that."[4]

In the Blue Room, the proverbial "What do you do?" was displaced by "What can you do?" It was a question everyone asked themselves as they walked through the door to discover what crazy challenge Jerry was going to throw at them on any given day. No one knew in advance. If they had, they might have stayed home. It was always a surprise and a test of mettle and aplomb to discover that today's WOD was something you were particularly bad at, or hated.

It was competitive—you can't put a bunch of type A personalities, athletes, in a room with a physical challenge, a whiteboard, and a stopwatch and not get competition. By definition, every movement in a CrossFit workout is measurable, repeatable, observable, and timed. The results are all benchmarked. There are thresholds for intermediate and elite performance, or "Pro" and "Pack," as Jerry differentiated scale levels for a WOD. For anyone hitting a WOD after the dawn brigade, there was the implicit gauntlet of whiteboard results, scrawled in dry-erase marker, to be scrutinized by near-peers. *That's my time to beat.*

Competition was fierce but ephemeral, the way it is in rugby. Mike Hart, a Catholic high school wrestler, had majored in philosophy at Wheeling Jesuit University and minored in rugby. Or maybe it was the other way around. But he understood this: when the clock is ticking, your whole purpose in life is to crush your opponents, and the minute the game is over, you go drinking together. In his college days, Mike played a rugby tournament in Ohio, called Sevens in the Snow because the fields were so blanketed with snow that it was hard to know where the bounds were or if you were over the line to score. Hurtling through the snow with the ball, he got hit by an opposing player and kept going. He got hit by a second guy and kept running. A third player slammed into him, and he pushed the whole straining pack of three guys five yards to touch the ball down. The drama of knowing it was all up to him, outnumbered in a last-ditch effort that required all-in berzerker commitment, left him completely unaware that he was only midfield.

Mike was to CrossFit Oldtown's competitive spirit what Harold was to its sense of humor. It was all fight and scrum and claw in the brief interval of a WOD, then kudos and respect. It was rugby.

In a gym, there are members and instructors. In fitness boot camps, there are clients and trainers. People sweat, disassemble, and go home strangers. The Blue Room gang was something else. There was an Us: a team and a coach. It wasn't just a team because people were sacrificing all the energy they had. It was a team because that outlay had a purpose: progress. Measurable progress, real achievement, more power, more speed, more skill. For everyone. Beating a PR, a personal record, wasn't just a source of personal satisfaction. It made the group better. It made the pack stronger.

Every time someone beat their record, or got their first muscle-up, or pull-up, or joined the "20 pull-up club" or the "30 pull-up club," there was an attaboy on Jerry's Blue Room blog, with pictures of people on the bars, or laid out on the floor, or grinning with ripped calluses held up like badges of honor. There were videos of regular people with the kind of voice-over expert performance analysis most people hear only when they see Olympic diving events broadcast on TV. Every day, there was a picture of the whiteboard results with postgame commentary. "I'd always rather watch a Winner than hear one talk," Jerry would write above a set of posted results. "Saw 16 of them in action today."[5]

On a day where athletes chose one of six WODs listed under the rubric "Epic Pain," Jerry noted that a newcomer had "left one of the biggest pools of sweat I've ever seen. I think *we'll keep* Aaron around! Welcome to the Team, brother."[6]

On a day when nobody in the Blue Room could do the "Nasty Girls" workout as prescribed, Jerry pointed out that many had tackled heavier power cleans than they'd ever attempted before. How many, he wondered, would be doing the WOD as prescribed in three months, six months, or a year? Two years? "Yes, you will stumble; yes, you will occasionally fall short of personal expectations you placed on yourself.

Strive on. Pick yourself up. It's failing that leads to success. CrossFit Oldtown is a tough lot, a rare breed.

"Now, who's ready for 'Murph'?"[7]

"Murph" may be the hardest workout in CrossFit's cornucopia of ordeals. It's a Hero WOD, named after Michael Murphy, a twenty-nine-year-old Navy SEAL who died in Afghanistan. As recounted in Marcus Luttrell's *Lone Survivor* and elsewhere, Murph's four-man reconnaissance team helicoptered into the mountains to capture or kill a Taliban leader. Once there, they were discovered by a group of local goat herders and had to decide whether to kill them. Murphy had been nicknamed "The Protector" as a teenager for defending a homeless man who'd been attacked while collecting cans, and for defending a special-needs kid who'd been shoved into school lockers. Murph looked at the goat herders and determined that there was nothing especially hostile about them, so he left them alive. Before long, the SEAL team was surrounded by armed Taliban, possibly alerted by the goat herders they'd let pass. The Chinook helicopter Murphy called in for reinforcements was shot down with a shoulder-fired missile, killing all sixteen people aboard. With no radio reception to send another distress call, Murphy left his protected position to relay his team's location back to base, scrambled back to cover, and kept fighting until he died from his wounds.

He had a favorite CrossFit workout: a 1-mile run, then 100 pull-ups, 200 push-ups, and 300 squats, then another 1-mile run, all in a ballistic vest. He called it "Body Armor." That's "Murph," with a 20-pound weight vest substituting for combat Kevlar. A month after he died, CrossFit.com posted the workout on the main page as a Hero WOD.

Hero WODs are ten times harder than regular CrossFit workouts. They're fallen soldiers' favorite workouts, a sacrifice of human energy to the glorious fallen dead. What some battle-trained soldier did, to get tougher, to test himself, is re-enacted push-up by push-up, power clean by power clean, sprint by sprint. What a fallen warrior did, at the peak of his physical powers, regular people do, or struggle to do, in his memory. Hero WODs are meant to take an athlete outside himself. They're supposed to put you in the Hurt Locker. They put you on the ground.

You feel like you're about to die. Then you get up, and remember some incredibly strong, brave young guy who didn't.

The first Hero WODs were posted as a gesture of respect to armed forces doing CrossFit in the field. But they were less of an invention than a haphazard archaeological discovery, as if some fitness freaks in Santa Cruz had gone out to drill a well and cracked into some long-forgotten temple. This kind of ritual barely exists in modern society, aside from prayer and Civil War re-enactment. Hero WODs are physical action as a form of remembrance. They commemorate special days: the anniversary of a fallen soldier's birthday, or an athlete's own birthday. September 11. "Murph" has become a Memorial Day fund-raiser for military charities. Jerry put it on the whiteboard the week after Michael Murphy was posthumously awarded the Medal of Honor. Josh Newman was doing "Murph" when he was forced to a halt by New York's finest with guns drawn.

Two of the Blue Room boys finished "Murph" in under an hour, an impressive accomplishment considering that a minute was lost every time they had to lace up their shoes and run downstairs, or run back upstairs to do pull-ups, push-ups, and squats. Chriss Smith, an actual Navy SEAL working out at the Blue Room, did not break an hour and finished only four minutes ahead of a petite woman named Andrea, who roasted beans at a local coffeehouse and later became his wife.

After three hundred crushing WODs, Monday through Saturday, Jerry posted a chokey reflection on the Blue Room's first year, his pride in the the pack, and hopes for the future. "I'm sorry," he wrote, "but I gotta share a story about my 5 year old Anna. Several months ago I bought a climbing rope and hung it in our basement (right next to the rings). Now Anna is pretty talented. She excels at a lot of things and has done so since an early age. . . . She is also pretty tough on herself, tougher than I'll ever be on her. With her tough self-expectations I've also seen a tendency for her to shy away from things she can't initially do, to get frustrated. I want her to experience the unknown, not to fear the possibility of defeat and then be paralyzed by it—to persevere through adverse situations, to feel the victory of picking herself up off the mat after a fall and have at it one more time. So what's a dad to do?"[8]

In Jerry's case, it was hang a rope next to his desk, and never suggest that his daughter climb it, or ask her to climb it. There were a few rules: no swinging on the rope—it was there to climb. No jumping from stacked-up boxes so she could get near the ceiling rafters and quickly reach the top (the first thing she'd figured out). While he was doing grown-up "computer work," she took a few attempts, got frustrated, and wanted nothing to do with the rope for a month. That was okay, he reassured her. It was good to have a challenge. Then something changed. She stopped saying "I can't" and "I'll never be able to do this." She started having fun tackling a lofty but do-able challenge, trying different things, keeping at it, until she climbed the rope.

"What a look of pure joy on her face. It's all a Dad or a Coach can ever hope for."

And this was the difference between the Blue Room and "fitness boot camp": there was a Marine in charge, for sure. But no one was getting yelled at, or bossed through one more set or three more reps. That sort of drill sergeant behavior is considered unseemly in CrossFit. It implies that the person doing the work is too weak-spirited and lazy to push themselves, that they are so resigned to their own lack of drive that they pay someone to intimidate or herd them through their discomfort. Most CrossFit athletes would be insulted if a coach implied they needed to be bossed through a WOD. Most of them, like Anna, push themselves harder than their coach ever would. It's part of the ethos. The challenge is there—everyone has to seize it for themselves.

It would have been understood without Jerry telling stories like this on the blog. But by telling these stories, by always commenting on team performance, not just individual milestones, by articulating his philosophy, he gave the pack an identity and a leader. The blog defined a set of shared values about what to strive for. It also defined the pack as a pocket of resistance against a big, dominant, malign Enemy: the fitness industry itself.

Today's culture, Jerry argued in the wake of major league baseball's steroid scandal, encourages us to pursue fantasy ideals. "We can ask each other if the bar is set too high for our professional athletes, but a better question might be if the fitness image set for you and me is even more unrealistic. A main villain in perpetuating these much sought after images is the health and fitness industry. Everyone is led to believe there is an easy way to get fit. . . . So, is it news that baseball players are looking for the ultimate quick fix, or is it more shocking that we are?"

For all this passion, Jerry was still struggling to build a following large enough to leave the jujitsu studio and move into a space of his own. CrossFit Old Town was a precarious small business with only a couple of dozen paying members. So when one of his athletes stopped showing up regularly, Jerry started to worry. Trying to sound more concerned than nervous, Jerry called the guy up. "I've noticed you haven't been showing up lately. Is something wrong?" he asked.

"Actually," replied the truant athlete, "I'm the chief of the fire department here in Alexandria. I've been scouting your program. I want us to start doing this."

THE FIREFIGHTER CHALLENGE
Five-Alarm Fitness

ADAM THIEL HAD TAKEN THE ROAD OF THOUSANDS OF FIRE-fighters before him, from winning plays on a high school football field to hauling unconscious people out of burning buildings. In high school he was a middle linebacker, which meant being powerful enough to take a hit from a lineman and fast enough to chase down a receiver. Football conditioning required a lot of conventional weightlifting. Thiel could squat five hundred pounds and bench three hundred.

In the spring, he joined the track team even though he hated running, which meant throwing discus and shot put by default. In the raw cold and dark of what passes for spring in Chicago, Thiel's track coach had the team jumping on boxes and swinging a set of salty old Russian kettle bells. The coach, "Crazy Joe O.," was generally considered to be out of his mind. "We thought it was crazy and ridiculous. But it really did work, with vertical leap, lateral quickness, and a lot of other things," says Thiel. "We only did it when we were forced to do it, because we thought it was a bit loony. But it definitely helped us be strong and quick in three dimensions, when you're being beat up in the middle."[1]

When Thiel got into firefighting recruit school in the '90s, he hewed to the fitness regime of the academy, lifting weights and running on alternate days. He still hated running, and the prevalence of running injuries among his fellow recruits didn't make it any more attractive.

There were always four or five people in the academy limping through runs with shin splints, hurt knees, and plantar fasciitis. As far as he knew, it was just accepted that recruit schools always had those kinds of injuries, and it was up to recruits to simply suck it up and get through the distance.

After recruit school, he realized that, as much as he loved pumping iron, aerobic capacity was a core part of his job. But an aerobic regime of running and more running seemed dismal. So he got into triathlons, which meant spending hours in the pool and on the bike. His days off were consumed by epic cycling bouts and the long, slow distance-triathlon running regimen. He whittled down his six-foot frame from the meaty composition of a middle linebacker to a wiry 162 pounds. He finished an Iron Man. The triathlon time-suck escalated as he pondered double- and triple-distance events. "I realized it was insane," he remembers thinking. But how else was a competitive guy going to notch progress?

On September 11, 2001, he showed up for his shift at the Alexandria Fire Department, and went home seventy-two hours later. Over the days and weeks that followed, he worked thirty-six-hour shifts at the Pentagon, and then went to New York City to assist with recovery efforts at the World Trade Center. A week after 9/11, letters containing anthrax spores were mailed to media outlets and congressional offices, killing five people and infecting seventeen others. So firefighters shifted their time and efforts to buildings where the anthrax scares were going down, and Thiel was plunged into liaison meetings with the FBI. It was a grinding marathon of crisis response. It incinerated the surplus time and energy Thiel had spent running, swimming, and cycling. Like everyone in the department, he was mentally and physically exhausted.

He quit the department and took an administrative job. Running firefighter training programs for the state of Virginia meant driving up to a thousand miles a week. Lack of exercise and highway fast food ballooned his weight to 235 and tanked his annual physical results. In two and a half years, Thiel went from iron man to fat man. Looking at blood work that had gone from stellar to a disaster, his doctor told him he was killing himself. So he quit being a bureaucrat to become deputy fire chief in Phoenix, Arizona.

Thiel would have gotten back into triathlon training. But now he had kids and was going for a PhD on nights and weekends. Multi-hour training sessions were not feasible. As a former triathlete, his whole idea of a good workout was calibrated to epic endurance events. "If I don't have a minimum of an hour to work out," he thought, "why even bother?" With this mental model of training, up against tight time constraints, it was impossible to translate good intentions into commitment.

Toward the end of 2006, as he was getting ready to leave Arizona to become fire chief back in Alexandria, he heard some of the Phoenix firefighters talking about CrossFit. Greg Glassman's gospel of high-intensity functional fitness had spread from California eastward and was starting to blaze up in the first-responder community. Fire departments in Orange County, Oakland, Washington State, and Colorado were already using CrossFit, officially or unofficially, as their fitness regime. Phoenix firefighters were starting to catch the fever, and urged their deputy chief to check out the CrossFit website.

Looking at the WODs and videos online, Thiel had a weird flash of recognition. "This is a lot like what crazy Joe O. had us doing back in the day with those crazy boxes and Russian kettle bells. This is some kind of retro, steam punk-ish, back-to-the-future thing." The idea of getting an elite athletic workout in ten minutes, or even twenty minutes, was loopy, he thought. "You couldn't just do *that*."

But some of the firefighting community's über-elite athletes were converts. These were the guys who not only set benchmark records in their own firehouses but competed in the Firefighter Combat Challenge, an event originally designed to predict whether recruits were physically ready to run into a burning building and carry out people trapped inside.[2] Each competitor has to carry a 42-pound hose up six flights of stairs, then hoist a 42-pound hose up from the ground, hand over hand. From there, it's a race to slam a 160-pound steel beam down a track with a 9-pound sledgehammer, to simulate the challenge of chopping through a door or wall. The next segment is a 140-foot sprint to pick up a hose that's pressurized with water and drag it 75 feet through swinging doors, then open the nozzle to blast a target with water. Finally, a 175-pound dummy must be grabbed from behind and dragged backwards for 100 feet.

When the event was set up at the Maryland Fire and Rescue Institute in the 1970s, its creator, Dr. Paul Davis, noticed two things. The first was that firefighter performance varied wildly. The second was that the fitter firefighters were intensely competitive. Almost immediately, the blackboard near the drill tower was transformed into a leaderboard listing the names and times of the competitors, who pushed themselves to their limits to improve their rankings. Ten years later, Davis was marketing the event as a national competition, and by the '90s it was televised on ESPN.

By the time Thiel's firefighters started proselytizing him, CrossFitters were dominating the Firefighter Combat Challenge and similar competitions across the country. Given CrossFit's emphasis on moving heavy loads as quickly as possible, this isn't surprising.

But there was one aspect of the CrossFitters' performance in these firefighting challenges that was very odd: they were using less oxygen than their competitors.[3] As part of their full kit and gear, competitors had to wear masks and breathing systems that measured their oxygen consumption, and the CrossFitters were pulling less out of the tank.

Lon Kilgore, a professor of exercise physiology at Midwestern State University who'd been analyzing CrossFit's methods and metabolic pathways for a few years, was struck by this weird finding. It flew in the face of accepted wisdom about aerobic performance. The conventional understanding is that high-level athletes consume more oxygen than lesser athletes—a higher VO_2 max allows them to process more oxygen to power movement. Oxygen fuels effort, so doing the same amount of work in less time should require more oxygen, or at least the same amount of oxygen, not less. So why were the CrossFit firefighters pulling *less* oxygen out of the tank? Had they somehow become better at oxygen handling? Was there some kind of elaborate respiratory adaptation that improved their aerobic capacity?

"It is really tempting to look for some elegant explanation involving gas transport kinetics, enzymatic energy of activation, and a whole bunch of other scientific jargon," Kilgore wrote in a paper posted to the *CrossFit Journal*. "It's not nearly that complex an explanation."[4] The answer wasn't chemical. It was neural.

The CrossFitters *were* doing less work than their competitors, even though they were moving heavy loads faster. They were simply wired better, in terms of how their brains controlled their bodies. This made them more efficient by eliminating a lot of extraneous work that didn't actually contribute to strength or speed.

"Think of it this way," Kilgore explained. "Remember your first ring dip? Remember how wiggly your arms were and how much anterior, posterior and medial-lateral movement there was? Now fast-forward to today and your mastery of the ring dip. How much wiggling is there now? The movement is more coordinated and each repetition takes less time than those first few brutally hard and spastic dips. Regular Cross-Fit training has eliminated the extra work you used to do when you used a bunch of extra muscles to stabilize your body on the rings. Reducing the amount of working muscle reduces metabolic cost (calories burned and oxygen consumed). This will result in either the ability to perform an activity for a longer period of time or, in this instance with firefighters, in consuming less oxygen per unit work."

Pulling a weight from the ground to overhead, or holding a weighted bar overhead while sinking into a deep squat, or carrying a forty-five-pound plate over your head for 100 meters develops more than strength. It reinforces neural pathways that make all movement smoother, more efficient, and more stable. Beneath the threshold of consciousness, the circuitry that binds the brain to abdominal and back muscles, shoulders, wrists, the soles of the feet is more integrated. There is less shifting of weight and strain to compensate for lack of balance: more signal, less noise. Whether intensely strenuous or only moderately taxing, work comes at a lower metabolic cost because the wobble is gone.

This nerve-network adaptation isn't triggered by long, straight runs on flat surfaces, or working out on machines that permit movement only in a single plane. An overhead press machine or leg extension machine puts the body on rails. There is nothing for the nerves to learn. When someone who trains on those machines suddenly has to haul ass up six flights of stairs with a weight on one shoulder, the muscle isolation rails are gone. Compensating for the lack of rails is tiring. CrossFit's demand that athletes move in multiple planes, using different metabolic pathways, in constantly varied ways, forces the development of tensile control.

When we perceive animal grace, it is because certain creatures have this kind of control, a smoothness and lack of wobble in their movement. A cat, or a gliding bird, has what CrossFit athletes unwittingly build in every WOD. Perhaps, in our evolution and history, human beings have traded body control for cerebral horsepower. As the front of our brains came to dominate our consciousness and our survival depended less on hunting than on the ability to plant and plan, and later to read, type, and make phone calls, our animal intelligence fell away. Our body control atrophied. We began to wobble and become clumsy. Perhaps this is what makes us marvel and yearn to see athletes in motion: our own lost animal grace.

There was a second factor at play in the CrossFitters' paradox of lower oxygen demand: as counterintuitive as it sounds, strength training increases running performance without increasing VO_2 max (the capacity to transport and process oxygen). Stronger muscle, Kilgore reasoned, means that fewer motor units are required to accomplish the same amount of work. Less-active muscle requires less cellular fuel, and therefore less oxygen. So more oxygen stays in the tank.

As the people trapped in burning buildings get fatter and fatter, the job of carrying them out becomes more and more taxing. It requires more oxygen and more strength. But the cruel irony of an obese society is that the firefighters faced with these escalating metabolic demands are increasingly obese themselves. While the Firefighter Combat Challenge gets airplay on television, the reality is that the obesity rate among firefighters is higher than it is in the general public. Between 73% and 88% of American firefighters are either overweight or obese,[5] and less than 40% of them meet the minimal standards of physical fitness.[6] The leading cause of on-the-job death for firefighters isn't heroic battle against a fatal blaze. It's heart attacks, which account for about half of all firefighter deaths each year, double the on-the-job heart attack rate for police (22%), other emergency medical service providers (11%), and on-the-job deaths for all occupations (15%).[7]

Why are firefighters, whom most people visualize as heroically strong male calendar models, so out of shape? For one thing, their sleep schedules are disrupted by shift work, which is correlated with obesity. More perniciously, the food culture of a typical firehouse revolves around competitively large portions of starchy foods (pasta, pizza, biscuits and gravy) that are guaranteed to send insulin levels soaring, and an abundance of sugary snacks. The starchy food is driven by preference and pocketbooks, since firefighters typically split the cost of all their meals. Anyone who wants to eat healthier food, which is more expensive, has to put pressure on everyone else, lest he alienate himself from the bonding ritual of a shared meal. The ever-present sugary snacks are often provided by well-meaning members of the community who send candy, cookies, and cakes as a gesture of civic appreciation. On top of that, there are no widely enforced standards for physical fitness in fire departments. Recruits have to pass a fitness test, but once they're part of a crew, they don't get fired or suspended for inability to meet the physical demands of the job.

In Alexandria, Virginia, a city that predates the Revolutionary War, fire department response means paramedics hauling 250-pound citizens from the top floors of Old Town row houses while doing CPR on the way down the stairwell. It's a high-intensity effort, and having first responders huff and puff around corners and up and down stairs has life-or-death consequences. A deconditioned workforce with higher health-care costs and disability retirement rates also has financial consequences for a financially strapped municipality.

This was the reality that Adam Thiel faced in his new job as Alexandria fire chief. There were a lot of overweight people in the department, including himself. There were other, uglier elements of department culture that also needed to change. Racial issues and unsubtle resentment of female firefighters in the firehouse created palpable tension in the force. Fire stations were split into factions that barely spoke to one another. "People associate fire departments with being paragons of teamwork," Thiel says. "That was not the case here."

Thiel was working 80- to 100-hour weeks, and the stress of the job demanded the mental release of physical exercise. As he hit the gym for twenty minutes on the treadmill here, thirty minutes on the bike there, he tried to figure out how to allay the department's social tensions and boost fitness in an environment that was nutritionally geared for obesity.

By happenstance, CrossFit came onto his radar screen again, via Jerry Hill's website. Hill's CrossFit blog was more of what Thiel had seen back in Arizona—the crazy stuff that his track coach made him do in high school. This is ridiculous, he thought. On the other hand, he'd done plenty of ridiculous things in his time, on a dare. He'd done the Polar Bear Plunge, and CrossFit wasn't nearly as insane as wading into Chesapeake Bay in January. Besides, he says, "When I'm skeptical about something, I have to try it."

So in the freezing cold, he drove to the Blue Room, took off his shoes in deference to the dojo's prohibition of footwear on the mats, warmed up, and hit an eleven-minute WOD. He cannot recall the exact movements—the memory is blacked out. "I remember laying on my back after eleven minutes, looking at the ceiling. Flayed. Done," he says. "And I remember feeling as bad as I did after the Iron Man, when they had to pump two thousand cc's of IV fluid into me." For a triathlete, training with a group was a foreign experience. "But," he thought, "this might be a good thing for the Alexandria Fire Department. Maybe this'll be a good part of this organizational transformation package I'm putting together."

After he 'fessed up to Jerry that he'd been scouting CrossFit for the fire department, they cooked up a plan to introduce CrossFit to fire department employees. Over the course of a week, thirty or forty people learned how to do kipping pull-ups, wall balls, kettle bell swings, and other foundational movements. The fire department fitness volunteers were ethnically diverse, male and female. Some were hook-and-ladder firefighters. Others were administrative staff. They were all over the map, in terms of their fitness levels.

The coaches running them through the gauntlet—Jerry, Chriss Smith, and Andrea Seward—were a muscular white guy, a wiry black guy, and a woman with the compact frame of a former gymnast. "It was important for them to see the different physicalities," Thiel says. "It made it accessible to people."

The fire department's battalion chief, a former Marine, was instantly hooked and started prosyletizing the rest of the department. Thiel converted half a truck storage bay into a CrossFit box. He let firefighters get their CrossFit coaching certifications at the department's expense. The firefighters who took him up on this offer were, like the Oldtown coaches, an ethnic mix of different body types: tall, short, buff, skinny, male, female. They worked out at CrossFit Oldtown and trained firefighters in the converted firehouse truck bay.

There were holdouts. Plenty of guys were happy to sit on weight benches at the YMCA instead of getting their heart rates up. The EMS guys were particularly skeptical. "What is this?" they asked. "You're going to get people hurt."

"Have you tried it?" Thiel asked. "Why don't you try it?"

SHORTLY AFTER THEY TRIED IT, THE EMS SKEPTICS BEGAN NUDG-ing and nagging the department to pay for their CrossFit coaching certifications.

By this time, a new recruit class was entering Alexandria's firefighting school, and a couple of them were already CrossFit trainers. Thiel decided to overhaul the recruits' fitness program. Instead of the conventional regime, physical training was CrossFit-centric, with running on alternate days and yoga for flexibility. Other firefighting schools had flipped to CrossFit and seen improvements in strength and endurance, reduction in body fat percentages, and a dramatic drop in lost time due to injuries.[8] The first batch of Alexandria recruits on the CrossFit PT program had no lost-time injuries at all, which was unheard-of. Injury rates in the next three recruit classes were also dramatically lower than they'd been with conventional physical training.

There were a couple of injuries. Someone's head hit a barbell that was on the ground. A recruit tried to deadlift more than she should have, strained her lower back, and had to take it easy for a few days. Lower-back strain is probably the most common CrossFit injury. It gives the program a bad rap among critics. It is true that if you pull a loaded barbell up from the floor and round your back on the way up, you might strain your lower back. It's also true that if you load more weight onto the bar than you're strong enough to lift, because you see the other guys are loading their bars heavier than yours, and you insist on hoisting the weight up with a rounded back because you're trying to keep up with them, you'll probably torque your lower back.

Doing CrossFit without injuring yourself requires three things: knowledge, skill, and judgment. You have to know how to do the movements correctly, which is why nearly all CrossFit boxes have a ramp-up course for beginners, who are explicitly shown the right way and the wrong way to perform each movement before they're allowed to join the regular classes. Injury-free CrossFit also requires skill: you have to master the movements with light weight before you increase the weight. Some of the movements, particularly Olympic weightlifting movements, are fairly technical, so this can take a while. Which means that you have to check your ego while you build muscle memory and skill. Most important, avoiding injury in a high-intensity workout requires judgment: you have to be aware of your body, and if you can't maintain good form, you need to slow down or ratchet down the weight.

If injury-free CrossFit requires knowledge, skill, and judgment, the "CrossFit causes injuries" critique relies on one condition and one big assumption. The condition of this critique is that CrossFit athletes are not given enough knowledge to avoid injuring themselves. CrossFit's certification of trainers and its cultural obsession with the subtleties of technique minimize this risk. But it's possible that somewhere, there's an affiliate whose coaches don't bother to properly instruct beginners or who spend more time coaching elite athletes than keeping a hawk-eye on newcomers. This would be unprofessional practice and a violation of trust, like a doctor not taking the time to explain treatment options and side effects to a patient. In a medical context, this failure to educate a patient means the practitioner is not meeting the standards of his profession. But it doesn't mean the practice of medicine is dangerous.

More fundamentally, the argument that CrossFit is "dangerous" hinges on the assumption that skill and judgment should not be necessary to engage in a fitness activity. After all, there is no skill or judgment required to safely train on an elliptical machine or a Nautilus circuit. There is no technique to master on a variable-resistance machine. If you can't push the weight all the way to the end of a predetermined arc, you retract your limbs, and the apparatus clangs back into place. It may not deliver the benefit of functional movement, but it also carries near-zero risk.

Therefore, the critique goes, CrossFit is dangerous, because people with no skill or judgment are more likely to hurt themselves doing it. By the same logic, bagels are dangerous, because two thousand people a year injure themselves so badly trying to slice a bagel that they end up in the emergency room.[9] But we don't characterize bagels as dangerous or malign bagel bakers because their product causes injuries. Instead, we admonish bagel consumers who slice vigorously toward their hands because of their lapse of skill and judgment.

Torquing your back on a deadlift hurts. It might even take you out of commission for a couple of days or weeks. But it does have a sterling quality that chronic sports injuries like shredded long-distance knees, plantar fasciitis, and tennis or golf elbows lack. It gives you a very strong memory that the coaches were right, and that improper barbell technique is a Bad Thing to Avoid in the Future. You learn not to do it again, and you avoid repeating the experience. It drives the acquisition of skill and judgment. It doesn't just get worse and worse and worse, little by little, over the years until you creak too much to engage in the activity. Chronic injuries don't give you that moment of "ooh, don't do that again." Because they happen over time, rather than on a single day, chronic impact injuries may not even be characterized as injuries. They're *issues*—a knee issue, or a shoulder issue. Whereas if someone strains their back on a deadlift, it's an injury.

But aside from the semantics of chronic versus sudden injuries and the politics of personal responsibility, there is a curious discontinuity in our perception of risk, depending on whether we categorize an activity as "fitness" or "sport." When we think about sports, all kinds of risks to ourselves and our children seem implicitly acceptable: basketball ankle sprains, baseball ligament tears (and ensuing surgery), soccer concussions, cracked ribs from judo, ice hockey tooth loss. In sports where feet do not directly touch the ground—skiing, skating, tobogganing, cycling, skateboarding, snowboarding—we gleefully engage despite the fact that we're one skid away from orthopedic catastrophe.

If we instead think about "fitness," it seems outrageous that someone would get hurt just trying to lose weight or "firm and tone." If someone gets injured in cardio step class, the instructor might be fired. If people hurt themselves using a piece of home exercise equipment, this can trigger a Consumer Product Safety Commission recall or even a class action lawsuit. Even the innocuous-seeming Nintendo Wii was hit with a class action lawsuit claiming Nintendo was liable for injuries because people were not warned to adequately warm up before playing Wii Fit games.[10] Fitness injuries are someone else's fault. As a society, we consider ourselves entitled to burn calories in a risk-free bubble.

Our risk tolerance for sport is higher than our risk tolerance for fitness because we perceive the benefits of sport to be more substantial: the experience of team play, the development of coordination, and the acquisition of strength and skill. In sports, we strive for progress. Sport gives us aspirations we can visualize: a fast finish, a goal scored, a perfect hit or pitch, the completion of a 10K or marathon or triathlon.

With fitness activities, we're mostly trying to forestall or reverse physical decline. The benefits, aside from reduced pant or dress size, are mostly invisible: a decrease in the likelihood of diabetes, osteoporosis, Alzheimer's,[11] depression,[12] and a host of other ailments. There are no skills to build. On an elliptical machine, there's no meaningful sense of progress, especially when people's pants aren't feeling any looser. After six months, moderate-intensity aerobic exercise doesn't lead to fat or weight loss.[13] So it's understandable that any risks associated with it would be unpalatable.

CrossFitters don't consider themselves to be engaged in "fitness," the way conventional gym members do. They don't show up out of a sense of guilt or obligation or because they don't like their thighs. They walk through the door determined to get stronger, faster, more skillful, to beat personal records and elevate the performance of a team. Anyone who's been on a sports team knows what it's like to practice and race with your group, wanting to do your best alongside friends and sometime rivals.

The fact that WODs are scaled, with stronger athletes more heavily weighted or challenged, eliminates the psychological barrier that keeps less athletic kids out of sports in the first place: there are no obvious laggards. Unless you carefully scrutinize the loads and decipher the whiteboard annotations, everyone looks to be doing pretty much the same thing in pretty much the same amount of time. It might be physically impossible for the bottom third to perform as quickly as the top third. But the top third are lifting twice the weight, or doing muscle-ups instead of dips, or chest-to-bar pull-ups instead of regular pull-ups. They're not coasting across the finish line to bask in their virtuosity while exhausted stragglers catch up. They're struggling just as much as the weakest people in the room—perhaps more, because they have a higher tolerance for discomfort. Everyone fights to finish. Everyone belongs.

CrossFit athletes assume the risk of injury in the context of sport, rather than the context of what mainstream exercisers consider to be a fitness activity. This explains why gym-oriented fitness experts and CrossFit defenders talk past each other about injury and flame each other online. One group views CrossFit through the lens of Pilates and Zumba and bicep curls, and the other views CrossFit through the lens of gymnastics and basketball and NASCAR. CrossFit calls itself "the sport of fitness." It really matters which of those words comes first.

The flash point of these conflicting perspectives is rhabdomyolysis, or rhabdo. Rhabdo isn't the garden-variety soreness or stiffness that gym rats feel the morning after a hard workout. It's an acute disintegration of muscle tissue that floods the bloodstream with muscle dust, a protein called myoglobin, that turns urine red or brown. Rhabdo isn't something that health club members (or their trainers) are generally aware of, because health club exercise isn't intense enough to give anyone rhabdo. If you can carry on a conversation in the middle of a fitness activity, you won't ever get rhabdo doing that fitness activity.

Emergency room doctors are familiar with trauma-induced rhabdo from car crash injuries. Exercise-induced rhabdo happens when an athlete executes so many strenuous and repetitive movements that muscle fibers literally break down into the blood. It's been documented in high-intensity exercise and endurance sports, from marathons and triathlons to cross-country skiing[14] and ultimate Frisbee.[15] Rowers[16] and swimmers[17] have also fallen prey. In mild cases, rhabdo causes muscle soreness, tenderness, weakness, and swelling. In rare but severe cases, rhabdo can put a person in the hospital for multiple days on an IV drip and cause kidneys to fail.

Exercising for long periods in hot weather heightens the risk of rhabdo, because elevated body temperature and dehydration both make it harder for the kidneys to clear myoglobin from the blood. This is one of the reasons why mild and moderate rhabdo is endemic in hot-weather NFL training camps,[18] and why overzealous college and high school football coaches have sent kids with rhabdo to the emergency room by the dozen.[19]

The prevalence of preseason football rhabdo reveals another reason why some athletes, including CrossFitters, get rhabdo in the first place. In most cases, the athletes have taken time off from their training. They're a little out of shape, and may have gained weight. They show up and hit a long, strenuous workout as if they're in peak condition.[20] They're strong enough to exert an impressive amount of effort. But by picking up where they left off, when their capability has actually dropped, they are grinding their muscular gears, and the ground dust of muscles in the blood is rhabdo.

Certain movements are more likely to trigger rhabdo in athletes who are at risk: pull-ups and GHD (glute-ham developer) sit-ups crank large muscles from full extension to full contraction under constant tension, and high-volume sets of these movements can seem deceptively doable. The oh-my-God-what-was-I-thinking soreness, even the garden variety, can take a full day to hit you. Weak or beginning athletes with low muscle mass can't do enough of these movements to get rhabdo. CrossFitters who've been hitting three WODs a week for months or years are protected by their level of conditioning. The athlete spoiling for rhabdo is a guy who *used* to run triathlons, and therefore considers himself a badass underneath the spare tire, who comes back from an extended break and matches the intensity of three-days-on, one-day-off CrossFit veterans.

This is exactly what happened to Adam Thiel. The day before he was scheduled to fly to Tokyo for a conference, he hit a WOD that contained a hundred pull-ups. He did half of them as prescribed, then clove-hitched an oversized rubber band around the pull-up bar to do the other half with assistance. "That's probably what did me in," he admits. "I should have stopped." By the time he got on the plane he was swollen and hurting, but figured that if he ended up needing medical attention, there were hospitals in Tokyo. He guzzled water, grimaced his way through the conference, and returned to CrossFit with a recalibrated sense of when to push through and when to ease off. He didn't get rhabdo again. In the grand scheme, he decided, a dramatically higher fitness level was worth the risk that a type A out-of-shape guy takes at the outset of his CrossFit career.

Ultimately, the (mostly online) sniping and countersniping about rhabdo boils down to a fundamental disagreement about risk in general. Is risk something to be driven out completely (assuming this is possible), or is it something to be managed? If risk is something to avoid, then it's rational to eliminate activities that might carry risk, regardless of their benefit. Risk avoidance has a comfort factor, because it walls off the prospect of bad things happening. But it takes a lot of activities off the menu.

If risk is something to manage, then the rational behavior is to weigh risks against potential benefits and take steps to minimize the impact of the things most likely to go wrong. Risk management isn't as comfortable as avoidance, because it dwells in the day-to-day assumption that bad things sometimes do happen. But because it's based on resilience, not insulation, it's more robust.

What Adam Thiel chose for himself, and for the Alexandria Fire Department, was an approach to risk that was less comfortable but more robust. All the fire stations are equipped with C2 rowing machines, wall balls, kettle bells, and pull-up bars. The newest station has space allocated for a 5,000-square-foot CrossFit box with racks and Olympic bars and plates and ropes, a significant improvement on the converted truck bay that accommodated the department's early CrossFit converts. Years after that early experiment, there are people in the department who no longer resemble their jowly driver's license photos, who live their lives differently. No one will ever know which of those people would have otherwise had a heart attack or a stroke or become diabetic. But the actuarial tables don't lie—some of those events have been forestalled or eliminated.

After a year of CrossFit in the Alexandria Fire Department, Thiel held a field day, literally. The field day announcement poster featured *300*-style Spartan warriors. In the converted truck-bay CrossFit box, intractable social schisms seemed to have melted. "There were people working out, doing this, who a year ago would not have talked to each other," Thiel says. "They had coalesced around CrossFit. We had a lot of cliques and a lot of factions and people who didn't get along. Now the CrossFit people have formed their own clique."

THE HOPPER

Trial by Lottery in the 2007 CrossFit Games

THE 2007 CROSSFIT GAMES WERE THE FIRST TIME CROSSFIT'S far-flung underground came together in force. On a desiccated California ranch, about 60 athletes and 150 spectators gathered to eat barbecue, drink beer, and throw down.

Dave Castro, a former Navy SEAL, had volunteered the place. He'd grown up there. His parents had raised animals, some horses and cattle. But mostly they ran a trucking business out of a hangar-size industrial barn. The flat section of the sixty-five-acre ranch was primarily a truck yard.

Not much of the ranch was flat, however. The Aromas hills were steep and numerous, and covered in scrub, poison oak, and trees. As a boy, Castro would hike, run, climb, and crawl around the hills until dark, sometimes after dark, playing G.I. Joe. As an imaginary ninja, he would stalk through the tall, dry grasses at night, silent and invincible on his do-or-die missions. The ranch's rolling hills were an epic stage for heroic sprints up, or scrambles down, to pretend battles. Peeking over the crest of a hill was the perfect vantage point for a grade-school recon scout. Navigating ravines, alert for bugs and snakes, any make-believe G.I. Joe knows the crack of a twig might signal an ambush. "Living there, and being part of the ranch, set the course of my life," Castro recalls. "Having the freedom to just run through the hills."

After school, it was a fairly straight shot to Special Forces, to Iraq and Afghanistan. More hills, ravines, gullies, more sprints, recon, night-stalking missions. And CrossFit. Having discovered that daily WODs kept them from getting winded on hike-in, find-the-target, hike-out mis-sions, a lot of SEALs had ditched marathon-length endurance train-ing for the intensity of box jumps, Olympic lifts, and heavily weighted sprints.

Stationed in Monterey for language training in 2005, Castro made a pilgrimage to CrossFit Santa Cruz. That day's WOD, a 15-minute se-ries of 1-minute sprints, alternating between metabolic misery (wall ball, box jump, rowing) and high-rep barbell movements, was aptly named "Fight Gone Bad." Glassman, noticing that Castro was active-duty mil-itary, told him to drop by anytime and train for free. A few months later, Castro started helping out at weekend CrossFit coaching seminars. He was, in the way of Navy SEALs, mission obsessed and neurotic about logistical details. He brought operational discipline to CrossFit's coach-ing certification staff, which consisted of a visionary intellectual with gladiators and warrior princesses in tow. Glassman ran CrossFit's Big Picture crusade. His firebreathers validated the concept and instilled general awe. Castro set up, packed down, and kept the trains running on time. "He went from a volunteer," Glassman says, "to 'Man, these certs go better when he's here,' to inde-fucking-spensible."[1]

By 2006, Castro had moved back to live on his parents' ranch, forty minutes from Monterey. In the years since his father's massive stroke, the Castro trucking business was in decline. Automotive detritus had accumulated into a small mountain of junked parts, oil, grease, and containers. Seemingly, nothing had been thrown away for years. The scrap hoard had a predictable effect on a sweat-the-details special oper-ator who remembered the place as a well-ordered home and workplace. He flew into a ruthless fit of clean-up and disposal, clearing thousands of pounds of garbage and gunk, and literally demolishing a disused trailer home where the trucking staff had once lived.

Sloping up and away from the industrial wreckage, the ranch's roll-ing hills had escaped relegation to junkyard status. The ravines were still steep and dry and beckoned for a breathless sprint, for old time's sake. The gigantic oak with overhanging branches was still a climbable fort. Buried in the terrain were the childhood memories of a grown-up G.I. Joe, a non-imaginary ninja.

The landscape was dormant in February when Greg Glassman came to visit, on his way out to Arizona. Glassman had always wanted to stage a CrossFit competition, a tournament open to all contenders. He'd just never had the time, or the right place to do it.

"Let's do it here," he said. "It'll be the Woodstock of fitness." It was a mission, and when you give a Navy SEAL a mission, the ball is in play. Castro shuttled back and forth from the Navy base in Coronado to Aromas, to make sure the ranch was cleaned up and presentable for the Games. Together they cooked up the structure of the event: a competition designed as the Ultimate Test of Functional Fitness. Anyone from anywhere could show up to compete, and the winner could lay claim to be the Fittest Man or Woman on Earth.

There would be three workouts. A 5K hill run with four steep ascents would test speed and endurance. A one-rep max strength test would measure pure weightlifting power. They were hoping to attract hotshot trail runners and local strongmen with cash prizes for winning individual events, which the specialists could collect only if they completed all three workouts. CrossFitters would outrun the best lifters and outlift the best runners and crush all specialists on a metcon. The idea was that this would force the endurance athletes and powerlifters to acknowledge the superiority of CrossFit. One can only imagine the sparks flying from all that eliteness if any hotshot trail runners or local strongmen had actually shown up.

The metcon was an archetypal CrossFit triplet, meant to whip athletes through a mixture of high-rep barbell and bodyweight movements and leave all finishers in a froth of sweat and metabolic agony. Just as important, this workout would invoke CrossFit's mystical and fearsome touchstone: the Unknown and Unknowable. No one, not even the event's organizers, would know the weighted element of the workout until minutes before it began.

At the last possible moment, Castro would reach into the Hopper—an improvised peanut roaster[2]—and pull out a colored ball. Green meant light variations of a movement. Blue meant heavy. Red was Coach's Choice—Glassman would get to pick the loaded weight of the movement. Yellow meant Glassman could pick both the weight and the movement. It was a mixture of fate and the whim of the CrossFit gods. Athletes favored by the Hopper's outcome would be fortunate. Athletes whose weaknesses were revealed by the Hopper would not be so fortunate. But the athletes who'd ruthlessly sought and driven out their weaknesses would be impervious to chance, and to the capriciousness of authority.

This is what makes the Hopper so compelling as a training tool, and why Glassman would constantly promote Hopper workouts as the Swiss Army knife in any coach's kit. The Hopper eliminates training bias, a coach's tendency to favor what he's good at, or what his athletes are good at. Imagine the Hopper, Glassman would tell coaches and athletes. Think about what you'd like to see come out of it—what you're good at. Now, think of what you'd *hate* to see come out of it. The task that's furthest from your comfort zone, that exposes your weakness. *That's* what you should throw yourself into, in your training. The thing you dread should be your first priority. Because if you're not willing to find the chink in your armor, the Hopper, the Unknown and Unknowable, the randomness of life, will find it for you.

CHRIS SPEALLER
A Lamborghini Among Diesels

ON THE FIRST MORNING OF THE 2007 CROSSFIT GAMES, IN THE truck barn, Dave Castro turns the handle of the Hopper and opens its door. Annie Sakamoto steps forward with her baby daughter, and cantilevers a pair of delectably pink and squishy arms into the barrel. A male voice rings across the room, "Something in green!" Oblivious to solicitation, the chubby hand chooses blue:[1] heavy push jerks.

A push jerk is the top half of an Olympic clean and jerk. The bar is already on your shoulders. You jump to transfer momentum from the legs to propel the barbell overhead, and quickly pull yourself under the bar to land in a partial squat, then rise to a standing position with arms straight overhead. With a heavily loaded bar, it requires a combination of strength in the legs and a flash of quick-twitch timing.

Push jerks also entail a triumph of muscle memory over survival instinct. When the bar is on its way up, powered by force from the legs, muscle memory from thousands of repetitions of this movement allows a trained athlete to quickly drop below the bar as it's rising. If you do this, the bar doesn't need as much force—it doesn't need to go as high—because you can catch it lower, in a squat, then use the large muscles in your legs to elevate the stack of torso, straight arms, and barbell all the way up. Legs are stronger than arms. So this movement pattern of quickly dipping under the bar, as it is rising, allows the human body to marshal its largest muscles for the effort, in the most efficient possible way.

The push jerk is a deeply counterintuitive and dangerous-feeling movement to learn. If there is something heavy that you've managed to jump above your head, the natural instinct is to keep your head above the heavy thing for as long as possible. You want to body-English the whole thing up, by moving yourself up, up, up, and then finish the push with your shoulders. That feels like the safe thing to do, because if the weight's too heavy, you can just drop it.

To pull yourself *down* and beneath a loaded bar that is momentarily weightless, but that you know will soon reach its apex and start falling again, seems semi-suicidal when you're learning to do it. It doesn't matter how well you understand the physics and mechanics, or mentally accept the fact that going down, while the bar moves up, allows the body to move more weight with less work. Survival instinct asserts itself when heavy objects are above your head. When your gut screams "Up!," the act of aggressively driving down and under the bar creates the same panicked trepidation as walking into a half-cracked building during an earthquake. It's hard to wrap your mind around. Some very strong people never do. Their personal records are limited by the load their shoulders will bear, to press out the weight, overhead. To master the movement, you have to repeat it correctly, starting light and using progressively heavier weight, until your muscles and nerves silence the conscious jangle of your mind.

Heavy push jerks, as determined by the Hopper and Annie Sakamoto's baby, means 135 pounds for men, 85 pounds for women, repeated 7 times, and 25 pull-ups. Five rounds of that, after a 1000-meter row, with a 20-minute cut-off.

There are eighteen rowing machines and forty-one guys, divided into three heats. The known all-stars among the men—the Fitzgerald brothers from Canada, and CrossFit's preeminent strongman, Josh Everett—are in the final heat. The second-to-last heat includes Freddy Camacho, a fixture on the NorCal CrossFit scene. Camacho owns a box on the blue-collar side of San Francisco Bay, and he's built like a bull. As he hauls into the final seconds of his row, Castro runs over to spur him on. "You're about to finish," he yells. "You're going to have the fastest time in the heat!"[2]

Someone taps Castro on the shoulder.

"Hey," says the judge who's been clocking another athlete during the event. "Chris Spealler, that guy over there, has been done for two or three minutes." Across a line of rowers, Castro sees a guy who weighs 129 pounds, which is less than the heavy push jerks most contenders can't even finish under the time cap.

Looking at Spealler, Castro instantly concludes that this is impossible. He sends the judge off to check that Spealler's rounds have been counted correctly. It is inconceivable that this tiny little guy could come out of nowhere, push-jerk his bodyweight thirty-five times, and finish ahead of guys who look like Freddy Camacho. But the count is correct. Somehow, Chris Spealler has managed to outperform guys who outweigh him by fifty pounds, on a heavy, high-rep barbell workout.

Chris Spealler has always been small, and he has always surprised people. He comes from a long line of insanely strong, tiny athletes. His dad was five feet five, a competitive gymnast, then a college football place-kicker at 125 pounds. Spealler's mom was a high school swimmer and a college field hockey and lacrosse player, a pint-size terror on the field. When Spealler was a baby, he wasn't even on the pediatrician's growth charts—the doctor had to draw extra lines on the lower end of the scale to track his height and weight. He was seven or eight years old before he made it onto the growth chart. "Chris, you made it onto the chart!" his mother chirped, elated to see her son in the fifth percentile.

She would have worried that something was wrong if Chris hadn't started tearing around the house on two legs at ten months, if he hadn't been so fast. He could move from anywhere to anywhere in a flash. He was strong. But the other boys were so much bigger that when he tried to play soccer, they'd just smash him in the scrum. By the time he was in high school, the boys were a head taller and thirty pounds heavier than he was, so football was out.

But there was one way to always compete against people his own size, even as a child, and that was wrestling. The first time his parents took him to youth wrestling practice at the local elementary school, he sat on the edge of the mat and watched, and saw that little kids only wrestled other little kids.

"I want to go every night," he told his parents when they got home, with a seriousness that belied his kindergarten age. "I want to do this." He was six years old when he wrestled in his first match. In junior high, he weighed 60 pounds, surrounded by kids who weighed twice that. But he never had to wrestle them. In high school, he wrestled as a 90-pound freshman, then at 103, 112, 119. He got concussions, sprained ankles, a broken arm. But he was relentless. He learned how to lever his weight, and other people's weight, under the grinding force of grappling holds and takedowns. Wrestling is basically contact gymnastics. It requires all the strength and body control of a gymnastic rings routine, with the added element of someone trying to pin you to the mat.

In the world's premier suffering sport, Chris Spealler learned how to suffer: how to be in pain, pinned to the ground, and still summon the strength to reverse positions. Suffering is a skill in wrestling, no less than the movements themselves. The ability to suffer is what allows wrestlers to tap what remains of their strength when they're exhausted, slick with sweat, forearms wrecked, back wrecked, and breathing hard against the anaerobic misery of a seven-minute struggle.

Spealler was a recruited walk-on, tapped for the team without a scholarship, at Lock Haven University in Pennsylvania, a Division I wrestling school. On Airdyne bike drills, when the coach challenged athletes to sustain maximum output with their arms and legs for as long as possible, Spealler maxed out higher for longer than wrestlers who outweighed him by seventy-five pounds. His conditioning was so good, the coach recalls, that "if a wrestling match didn't have a time limit, he would have won every match."[3]

There was one hitch: another wrestler, a three-time state champion with a scholarship, was in the same weight class, and the head coach was not going to bench a kid on scholarship to let Spealler compete. When the two bantam wrestlers squared off in a preseason match that customarily determined who would represent the university in each weight class, Spealler won. The result was negated. After Spealler held his own against nationally ranked wrestlers in competition and beat his rival repeatedly, the coaches simply declared that he didn't have enough experience. The kid with the full-ride scholarship had been promised the spot, and Spealler wasn't allowed to compete for the rest of the year.

There are a lot of hormones and heartbreak for an nineteen-year-old in this situation, and righteous indignation is so comforting: You can put a lifetime of work into becoming a Division I wrestler and want to be All-American, and prove you're the best, and in the end it's all politics. Why bother to work like a dog when the people in charge are just going to play favorites?

Instead, Spealler did what he'd done since fifth grade when a wrestling match turned nasty, when things were painful and not going well. He pushed himself through the sharp curtain of raw emotion, and mainlined his faith. On the other side of the mental noise and shock and fear of failure that makes you want to cry is a place where your heartbeat is still pounding, but more slowly. Adrenaline flows. But the fear is gone, because you know you are exactly where you are meant to be. The ordeal has a purpose, and all you need to achieve that purpose is utmost commitment to the next, decisive moment. Spiritual peace is not the opposite of physical force. Spiritual peace, in extremis, is a massive multiplier of physical force.

Faith is a competitive advantage. It eliminates psychic wobble, just as the tight integration of nerves and muscles eliminates physical wobble in CrossFit-trained firefighters, who can haul more weight faster with less oxygen. Faith eliminates inefficiencies. It is inefficient to stand around wishing an uncomfortable situation wouldn't suck so much. It is inefficient to lie on a mat wondering whether a guy is going dislocate your shoulder. The longer you stay there, the more psychic and physical energy goes to heat instead of work. If you believe that God put you in this moment for a reason, and your sole focus is driving up and forward to His purpose, the wobble drops out. God will pull you through the sharp curtain of raw emotion to the still place where all force can be applied to the point of a knife. Even if He doesn't exist.

Spealler figured, if God was keeping him from wrestling in the 125-

pound weight class, it might be because God intended for him to compete against bigger athletes—to be the small guy, up against big guys.
So, without gaining weight, he bumped up a weight class, and started
wrestling in the 133-pound class, and winning. Occasionally, when the
team's 141-pounder was unable to make weight, Spealler stepped up to
wrestle in the 141-pound weight class. Based on his performance on the
Airdyne, he could kick out as much power as heavier wrestlers, for longer. Being fully fueled and consistently hydrated was worth a few hit
points on game day, against wrestlers who were typically anorexic and
parched until just after weigh-in.

In his senior year, Spealler was one of the top twenty wrestlers in the
nation. In the 2002 Division I National Wrestling Championships, he
was two rounds away from becoming All-American, with no regrets.
After college, he moved to Park City, Utah, and became one of those
lean, good-looking twenty-somethings who repair rich people's gear in
mountain resort towns. He tuned bikes in the summer and skis in the
winter and coached wrestling at the local high school. He didn't have
much of a plan, until a Marine buddy, Eric Bova, introduced him to
CrossFit in October of 2006.[4]

Bova may as well have said, "Water, I'd like you to meet Fish. Fish,
Water." Within two weeks, Spealler had not just his first muscle-up, but
thirty muscle-ups in eight minutes and fifty seconds.[5] Two weeks later,
he smoked two of CrossFit's strongest athletes, Josh Everett and James
"O.P.T." (Optimum Performance Training) Fitzgerald on a workout
called "Linda," which is calibrated to the athlete's body weight: 1.5
bodyweight deadlifts, bodyweight bench press, and a 0.75 bodyweight
clean; 20 repetitions of each, then 9, then 8, laddering down to 1.
Spealler finished in 11:49.

Spealler is unrivaled in his ratio of strength to mass, and in his agility.
He is a Lamborghini among heavy-haul turbo-diesel pickups. On the
2007 CrossFit Games hill run, he seemed to fly, as if gravity weighed
more lightly on him than on the pack of larger and meatier competitors.
Until the final stretch, he drafted behind O.P.T., then flashed forward to
the finish line. On the Hopper, he was a marvel of precision timing and

efficient transfer of power from a ferocious engine to every moving part. This is what Lamborghinis are good at.

But when the task is to haul the maximum possible weight in a minimum amount of time, a Lamborghini has its limits. No matter how finely tuned it is, or how much the driver is willing to make it suffer, it's going to lose to a heavy-haul turbo-diesel pickup, and this is what happens in the final event of the 2007 CrossFit Games.

The strongman event, cooked up by powerlifting guru Mark Rippetoe, is called the CrossFit Total. Each athlete's score is the sum of the best of three attempts at back squat, strict press, and deadlift. Rippetoe's specifications for CrossFit Total's execution and judging standards hew to the established standards of USA Weightlifting (USAW), the governing body for the sport of weightlifting in the United States. These specifications dictate that the athlete must execute each lift on a raised platform, with three judges per platform and two volunteers to spot and change weights. Once the lift is deemed valid and complete from three different angles, the athlete gets a signal that it's okay to drop the weight. This rigorous judging protocol ensures that the results are sanctioned, incontestable, and boring as hell to watch.

On the first day of the Games, Castro and the CrossFit HQ staff calculate that if they run the CrossFit Total this way, it'll take from 8:00 a.m. until 9:00 p.m. to run every athlete through the sanctioned judging process. The results will be legitimate in the eyes of USAW. But does that really matter? This is the existential question: does anyone in Aromas, the athletes, the spectators, or the community online, give a rat's ass about USAW's opinion of what goes on here? If CrossFit borrows from other sports, does it have to adopt the competition rules and protocols of those other sports to be a legitimate sport itself? What if that drains away the thronging, berzerker joy of a dozen firebreathers gunning for PRs at the same time—the shared charge that makes one-rep max workouts such a compelling ritual in the box?

IT IS ALMOST INSTANTANEOUSLY DECIDED THAT ORTHODOXY doesn't matter so much. Hauling ass matters. Fun-to-watch matters. Standards are important, but points of performance from three different angles is complete overkill, and logistically impossible to boot. However, Rippetoe is going to be pissed, because he's been paid to design this event, whose rigorous judging standards are laid out in a lengthy and detailed memo.

It would be a breach of intersport diplomacy to engage a big name in one of CrossFit's major athletic components and then dismiss his contribution at the eleventh hour. So the top-ten men and women will do the CrossFit Total inside, in the USAW-sanctioned way. Everyone else will participate in what Castro calls "the ghetto CrossFit Total" out in the parking lot, with one judge per athlete and a raft of contenders going for max effort in one another's peripheral vision, amid the stomps and hollers of their friends and even their rivals. The CrossFit Games may be the only elite sporting event in which every athlete is also a coach. As competitors complete their efforts, they yell to their closest adversaries to push through the last reps, that they can do it, pick up the bar, you're almost there, you've got this, finish it.

The last athlete to finish a set of rounds for time usually has two or three top competitors gathered around him and the whole crowd cheering for him, louder than they do for the winner. People who don't do CrossFit, who watch the crowd going nuts at the Games for someone who's not going to win, while the victors crouch down to coach that last athlete across the finish, think it's Boy Scout courtesy, or some kind of trophy-for-ninth-place attaboy. The ritual of it sails right over them. But every CrossFitter sees, in that last athlete, his own whipsawed misery at the box. The last athlete has nothing left, and the noise of the crowd is to recognize the tenacity to go until there's nothing left. Every CrossFitter in the crowd tries to cultivate that quality in themselves. Struggle, not victory, brings that quality closest to the surface.

The winner is the winner. But the last athlete, if he finishes with nothing left, is the hero, just like Nicole Carroll in the "Nasty Girls" video. To really get a hero out of the Games, some athlete who's not winning has to go to failure. Someone who's suffering must refuse to give up and finish with nothing left, like the Greek courier at Marathon. This moment is more important than the winning finish. It is the crux of the event.

In 2007, Josh Everett is the firebreather who pushes himself to the point of failure. Everett, a Division III football player and track hurdler with two knee surgeries behind him, is the best weightlifter in the CrossFit pantheon. He has been surpassed in the Hopper and the hill run by lighter, faster athletes—Spealler, O.P.T., and another Canadian, Brett Marshall, who are tied for first, heading into the Total. Everett will not win. But everyone knows that he will pull a personal weightlifting record out of this last event, or fail in the attempt.

In the truck barn, Everett is the last of the top-ten athletes attempting the last lift of the CrossFit Total. As the volunteers stack plate after plate onto the bar, excitement rises in the room, until Everett is facing a 570-pound deadlift. He has never pulled up this much weight in his life. As Everett lowers himself to grip the knurled steel bar, everyone in the truck barn starts to scream. A stomping, shaking energy reverberates in the truck barn. Something is going on here, beyond a guy in a barn trying to nail a heavy lift. When Everett fails to pull the weight up from the ground, it doesn't feel like a letdown. For some reason, it feels like a great ending. This is the moment that goes down in CrossFit lore as the culmination of the event.

The podium winners, James "O.P.T." Fitzgerald for the men and Jolie Gentry for the women, each get a medal and five hundred bucks. But years later, people don't talk about the athleticism of the winners in Aromas in 2007. They talk about Everett and Spealler. As the purse grows, year after year, until the Games champions go home with a quarter million dollars, victory and veneration don't go together. Winners get the money. Heroes get the glory.

THE AMAZON AND THE ENGINEER

Rogue Gears Up

EVERY TIME SEVEN-YEAR-OLD CAITY MATTER MISSED A BASKET-ball shot, it was as if the universe had decided to spit in her eye and needed to be taught a lesson. She'd retrieve the ball, set her jaw, and with the next shot settle the grudge. It was this way with all sports—soccer, baseball (on the boys' team until high school), basketball, and, later, cross-country and track. She excelled, not just because she was tall and strong, but because she was the world's worst loser.[1] Anything could become a contest for time, quantity, or accuracy. Eating was competitive. Family board games escalated into psychic blood sport. Hungry Hungry Hippos, where marbles roll around a board and into the maws of frantically spring-triggered plastic hippos, was battle royal.

By the time she was in grade school, Caity was taking five hundred to a thousand basketball shots a day, outside her house. She moved through the arcs and angles of a perfect shot from different directions so many times that every neural and muscular glitch was wrung out of her body.

That's how you become the top-scoring three-point shooter in the United States[2] and a freshman starter at a Big Ten basketball school. As an Ohio State shooter, Caity was lighthearted with teammates. She'd make them laugh, to keep them loose in the middle of a hard game. But she was demonically focused in her own training. She'd dive for balls in practice. She broke her leg after seventeen games freshman year, broke her right foot and had knee surgery her sophomore year. Junior year, her fifteen-year-old brother died in a car accident. He was a younger, male version of herself: a starting quarterback and point guard on the high school team, even as a freshman. He was her rival and admirer, in the way of younger brothers.

She got the news in a hotel room in East Lansing, Michigan, the night before an away game against the Michigan State Spartans.[3] Ohio State's head coach told her the team would support whatever she wanted to do next. "If you want to play, or don't want to play. If you want to get in the car and have me drive you home, I'll drive you home right now," he said. "Whatever you decide is what we'll do."[4]

On Sunday morning, she knocked on the coach's door and asked to watch game film before facing the Spartans that afternoon. With her parents and a hundred Buckeyes in the stands, Caity took the team's first shot, a three-pointer that sailed over the court and swooshed though the basket. As the net snapped up, she leapt, punching the air with her fist, then pointed up to the vaulted ceiling of the arena and beyond, to recognize her brother.[5] As a luckless Spartan defender flailed to distract and deflect Caity's concentration and her aim, shot after shot flew from her hands to the target: twenty-three points, eighteen of them from the three-point line, four rebounds. With and around her, the tall, strong girls from Ohio played at an unprecedented level, for an upset win.

The last college game Caity played, as team captain her senior year, was to a sold-out stadium of 17,300 people cheering, singing the Ohio Buckeyes fight song, and chanting her name. She went pro, playing as a shooting guard for the Charlotte Sting for two seasons before breaking her left foot. This time the doctors drilled a pin into the bone.

The calculus of repetitive injury began to assert itself, in the way it does for all physically damaged professional athletes. On the give-up side of the equation is the weight of all the aches and creaks and scars. On the stay-and-fight side of the scale are livelihood considerations, an athlete's sense that she has not done what she set out to do, and well-founded or misplaced confidence that a banged-up body can recover to accomplish those things.

Caity loved playing ball for a living. "Every bit of it," she says. "Still miss it. Probably will until the I die."[6] But there was nothing left to accomplish with a left leg that had been sliced open five times and a matching set of busted feet. She wanted to walk with a normal gait after basketball and be active instead of stumbling around every morning trying to warm up. So she hung up her uniform and moved back to Ohio, to haunt the Buckeyes stadium and training facilities. She'd shoot hoops and occasionally garner a flash of recognition. She went to work as a strength and conditioning coach at Max Sports, an athletic rehab center and sports medicine clinic in Columbus.

Her boss at Max Sports was curious about CrossFit. Athletes were starting to talk about it, even though it seemed a bit crazy to maximize speed or volume or, God forbid, a combination of speed and volume, in Olympic weightlifting workouts. There was a place twenty minutes away, in Gahanna: Rogue Fitness. Rogue's owner, Bill Henniger, had been invited to come to Max Sports and talk about CrossFit and meet the trainers, but he wasn't interested. Go over to Rogue, Caity's boss told her. Check it out.

In January of 2008, the fallen star shooter pulled into the parking lot of Rogue Fitness. Her welcome was a frosty one. Bill Henniger knew where she worked, because her boss had been trying to get him to come over there. He strongly suspected she'd shown up to go to school on him, then go back and coach CrossFit at Max Sports. Sizing her up, he saw a tall, strong blonde, obviously an athlete in some former life. Basketball, maybe volleyball. But the WOD was a "Bear Complex," and unless this chick had done some serious weightlifting, it'd be pretty obvious she was a rank beginner in serious need of coaching. The ridiculousness of thinking she could pick up CrossFit, just like that, would be plainly apparent.

The "Bear Complex" is a fluid and unbroken chain of five weight-lifting movements that look easy when strong people perform it, even though their guts are in a blender the whole time.[7] In the first part of the complex, you grip a barbell on the ground, explosively jump it up, and slam your elbows forward to rack the bar on your shoulders (a power clean). With the bar racked on your shoulders, you do a deep front squat and rise back to a stand. A push press launches the bar from shoulders to overhead. You catch the bar on the back of your shoulders, behind your head, and ease on down into a back squat. After the back squat, you do another push press, then lower the bar to the ground. That's one rep. Seven reps is one round, during which you're allowed to rest anywhere, anytime, except with the bar on the ground. You can hang out with the bar on the back of your shoulders. Pass the time of day with the bar held straight overhead if you want. You just can't put the bar down, even to regrip, until the round is done.

The "Bear Complex" WOD is five rounds of seven reps, using progressively heavier weight from round to round. You can rest between rounds. Maximum weight goes on the whiteboard. There's no time component. It's a test of tenacity.

Henniger watched in shock as the blonde interloper annihilated the "Bear Complex." She beat all the women. She beat all the men. Getting the stink-eye from him may have sharpened her edge—it was an implicit challenge. In any case, it was the first time she'd felt a competitive charge since leaving the WNBA. And damn, the body still worked. And damn, it was fun to win.

"Where do I sign up?" she asked.

"On the website," Henniger shot back, "like everyone else."

Oh, she thought, *is that how we're going to play? I'll be back.* The next day, and almost every day after that, she crushed whatever workout Henniger had scrawled on the whiteboard. She was unapologetic about dominating the leaderboard. There wasn't any of the self-deprecation and excuses that women sometimes make when they win, to avoid compromising their femininity. Caity was a pro. She'd been paid to win. Unabashed desire to mop the floor with other people is a job requirement for professional athletes. She wasn't a bitch about it. She was outgoing and friendly. She could talk to anyone. But she had fire, and she was there to immolate any task that Rogue could dish out. She would own it, not vice versa.

Henniger had two options: He could continue to worry that Caity would go back to Max Sports and compete with him. Or he could hire her. The prospect of competing with this relentless Amazon became less palatable by the day. So he offered her a job. She coached during the week, and trained with Rogue's elite athletes, all guys, on Saturdays.

Hiring Caity freed Henniger up to focus on the gear he was selling to other CrossFit boxes. When he started Rogue out of his garage, Henniger had contacted all the niche manufacturers that CrossFitters were using to cobble together their training equipment. It was an expensive and time-consuming process to outfit even a small box this way. A Navy doctor, Ahmik Jones, was running a website that pulled everything a CrossFitter might want onto one page. But he was busy training Navy SEALs, working as a radiologist, and starting a CrossFit affiliate with his wife. Running an equipment e-commerce site was too much to handle. So he passed the baton to Henniger, and the website got reskinned as Rogue's online CrossFit trading post.

In late 2006, CrossFit was heating from a simmer to a slow boil, and a lot of people needed equipment. It doesn't take a genius to realize that selling picks and shovels during a gold rush is a good idea. But selling a bunch of iron gear—even on the web—requires something most gold rush hopefuls don't have: a knack for logistics and mechanized production. This was the trump card Bill Henniger had in his pocket. Because when he dreamed up the CrossFit über-dealership idea, he was working as an industrial engineer at General Motors' powertrain factory in Toledo. Mostly, that meant planning and deploying the layout and interplay of machines and people to manufacture transmissions. Eight thousand rear-wheel-drive transmissions a day for pickups and Camaros.

It was a shop floor MBA: how to work with steel, how to sweat the cost accounting and manage large groups of people. It was also a lesson in how snarled and sclerotic a manufacturing business can become when any new idea is subject to union work rules. On the factory floor, automated machine tools leached skill from highly repetitive tasks. As machines performed the movements, machinists were reduced to button pushers. Union work rules are a defensive reaction to loss of mastery on an automated production line: if it isn't skill that's keeping a machinist in his job, there'd better be some iron-clad rules about which kind of worker can stand in front of a million-dollar machine and press the green button.

"The union and management—they built this monster. It took a hundred years to build, and it'll take forever to undo."[8] In the same breath as Henniger acknowledges the value of his GM education, he deplores the decline of a twentieth-century industrial powerhouse. In the run-up to World War II, GM's people and machines could swiftly recombine and mobilize. Its factories could flex from cars to planes and tanks to win the war. In the generations that followed, the company lost its functional fitness. Bureaucratic and operational silos destroyed its ability to move in a coordinated way. It became the automotive equivalent of a health club franchise with overblown marketing and underwhelming results.

The layoffs came. For Henniger, it was a good time to get out. He took away all the knowledge of how to work with steel, and none of rules about how that has to happen. No rigid task specifications. No management bureaucracy. Rogue was born.

When he took over the website from Ahmik Jones, it was just an e-commerce front end. People placed orders that were relayed to a galaxy of vendors, who drop-shipped gear to the customers. Some vendors were prompt and reliable. Some were not. If orders arrived late, or in lousy condition, Rogue became the target of customer ire. So, to preserve his reputation, Henniger started warehousing items. When orders came in, products went out in Rogue boxes. The arrival of a Rogue box was a happy happy day in CrossFit Land.

In truth, Bill Henniger liked gear more than he liked sports. He wasn't a die-hard athlete. He wasn't even an avid sports fan. He liked programming WODs because designing CrossFit workouts allowed him to geek out on the mathematics of load and volume. In a well-designed WOD, and in a well-planned progression of WODs, constantly varied movements combine into a beautiful counterpoint of physical tasks and time domains: short sequences of power movements, medium-length AMRAPs (as many rounds as possible in a fixed amount of time), and long and breathless rounds-for-time compositions (in CrossFit, thirty minutes is considered an endurance event). For an industrial engineer, programming WODs was like formulating an ideal configuration of production machines on a transmission assembly line.

There was something about metal that just sang to him. He loved figuring out how to shape it and make things out of it. Shipping other people's barbells and bumper plates made him want to forge his own wares and make them better, indestructible and impervious to Cross-Fit's relentless brunt of force and load. In most weight rooms, equipment from companies like York can last a lifetime. But CrossFit is high volume, high repetition, high torque. Stuff gets jumped on. Stuff gets dropped. All that volume and intensity puts a lot of stress on equipment. It destroys barbells, dumbbells, kettle bells, anything with moving parts, anything with straps or stitches. Samsonite used to run ads showing their suitcases being thrown around by a gorilla, to make a point about how tough they were. A CrossFitter is the Samsonite gorilla of fitness.

Gymnastic rings were one of Henniger's pet peeves. When he was still running CrossFit WODs in a local park, rings were a pain to rig because the straps and buckles were so difficult to adjust. For gymnasts, who are all roughly the same height and train indoors, that doesn't matter so much. For a one-time setup, cheap buckles and straps from China are tolerable. But when you're hanging rings on a tree limb and your athletes range from small women to oversized men, you want bigger, easier-to-adjust buckles and straps.

On top of that, some of the popular rings were deformed in subtle ways that became annoying when people were trying to string together muscle-ups. And the texture was wrong: conventional gymnastics rings were too slick. That's not good when you're sprinting 400 meters and then doing all the muscle-ups you can squeeze into the remainder of three minutes, and you're sweating like a horse. The perfect CrossFit rings would be more grippy.

As visions of gymnastics rings danced in his head, Henniger saw a thread pop up on CrossFit.com's equipment discussion board: "Custom crossfit metal work in northern ohio."

"I would like to offer up my skills as a metal fabricator to any crossfitters that may want custom gear," wrote Ian Maclean, a metal shop fore-man working at his dad's retail display company in Cleveland. Ian had been fabricating hardware since he was a kid—his father gave him a pile of wood with instructions not to cut his fingers off. After working his day job, he went home and built custom furniture and hardware out of his garage shop. "Long story short, can build just about any crossfit gear you may need!" he continued. "Big nutty jungle gyms, pull up bars, wall ball targets, plyo boxes, custom bar racks, anything under the sun . . . if you need it i bet i can help out." He posted pictures of a ceiling-mounted pull-up bar and beautifully polished stainless steel ring grip.

"Not looking to make a living with this, just want to offer it up as a thank you sort of thing to others looking to be fit," he added. "Happy to work with any crossfitters within a days drive of cleveland. also would be more than happy to trade labor for training or gear that i can't build for myself."[9]

It was an irresistible appeal from exactly the right sort of person at ex-actly the right moment. Henniger rattled off a query to Maclean, with a sketch—a pair of gymnastic rings. Can you make this, Henniger asked? Yes, Maclean replied. He scrounged a metal bender from a Navy ship-yard and set to work.

Gymnastic rings are a simple geometric form, so it seems like it'd be easy to make them: take a metal tube, bend it in a circle, and join the ends together. But gymnastic rings are to metal fabrication what a roast chicken is to cuisine. Anyone can stick a chicken in the oven. But there's a surprisingly big difference between what most home cooks can do and what a master chef can do with the same basic idea. Between Henniger and Maclean, it took months to figure out the perfect gauge and diam-eter, surface grind, and textured powder coating that would hold chalk. A whole tasting menu of powder coatings failed to pass the Goldilocks test: When your exhausted body jumps to grab a set of rings so you can pull yourself over and and straighten your arms, which rings would tell your sweaty hands that *you have the effort in you*. Which rings said: *You are going to make it. Just hold on.*

When the perfect rings were bent and baked, Henniger got in touch with a friend's brother who'd just retired from the Army and was making tactical gear in Logan, Ohio. They solved the strap-and-buckle deficiencies with more-robust straps and hardware. Another set of annoyances, gone. All the not-quite-rightness was gone.

In the spring of 2007, Henniger put the rings up for sale on Rogue's website. Maclean loaded the first batch into his white van, like a baker on route to a wedding with some fondant masterpiece, and set out from Cleveland. All fifty rings were sold out by the time he got to Columbus. Fresh cardboard boxes were stamped on all four sides with the Rogue logo, a big stenciled *R*. The grippy rings and their thick straps and big buckles were carefully packed inside with a card describing how they were made and the care that had been taken to design them with Cross-Fit in mind. "I wanted people to feel, when they got the rings, that they were getting something special," Henniger says. "All we really did was listen to all the complaints and address all of them and make sure everything was built really robust. That's how we do it."

AS MANY ARTISANAL GYMNASTIC RINGS AS MACLEAN COULD hand-shape with a Navy shipyard bender were sold before he finished making them. After coming aboard as Rogue's fabricator-in-chief, Maclean built custom saws and drills specifically for ring production, so he could make the rings faster. Figuring out what tools to use next and how to keep up was the fun of it. When the shipyard bender proved woefully insufficient to meet demand, Henniger plowed profits from the rings into Rogue's first piece of high-end industrial equipment, a computerized numerical-controlled (CNC) bender. With rings rolling off the CNC like hot doughnuts ready for their glaze of powder coating, Henniger and Maclean could move on to a larger-scale design challenge: pull-up rigs.

At the time, there were stand-alone pull-up frames on the market. There was a rig that would support a barbell. But no one had built a pull-up rig that would allow a coach to give a cue and see ten people doing pull-ups simultaneously, with a sight line that would allow him to watch every person. So Henniger and Maclean designed, built, and patented a rig that came in six-foot sections, that was strong and stable enough to support troupes of CrossFitters jumping onto it and swinging from it like a pack of orangutans.

The next challenge was squat stands, to rack heavily loaded barbells at shoulder height. Existing squat stands had moving parts. When squat stands are raised and lowered for seven WODs and hundreds of barbell impacts a day, moving parts are a point of failure. The Rogue squat stand had no moving parts—just a couple of bomb-proof J-clamps with through-pins. "If you buy a squat stand from us," Henniger declares, "you will pass it from generation to generation."

It seems almost comical to describe a squat stand as an heirloom, but this is exactly how Henniger thinks about his products. "If you go into your grandfather's garage and pull out his tools, his hammer and his wrenches, it feels like they'll last forever. We've gotten away from that," he says, and the "we" is implicitly the system of outsourced manufacturing that produces cheap and annoying buckles and straps, and the planned obsolescence of the automotive and electronics industries, and maybe America in general. "I want to make things crazy over-engineered so they feel like they'll last forever. I want someone to open up the box and think, this is awesome. I never want to hear that someone thinks it's built just enough."

All of Rogue's gear was more expensive than other vendors' products, and it sold like hotcakes because it wouldn't break, because it was specifically designed for CrossFit. In the way it was made and even packed, there was a reverence for what it was designed to do. CrossFit's slogan, "Forging Elite Fitness," carried through to the forging of Rogue's elite equipment.

During the week, Henniger would build this indestructible gear, and on Saturdays Caity and Rogue's best male athletes would take it to town. Product feedback led to longer and more interesting conversations, and pretty soon Bill Henniger was breaking the two unwritten rules of CrossFit affiliates: don't date your employees, and don't coach your significant other.

As their relationship became more serious, the workouts Henniger programmed for Caity became more brutal: mixtures of Heroes and Girls, nasty hour-long WODs, and regular couplets and triplets with extra weight on the bar. Each day, Caity walked through the door, coolly reviewed the torture trial Bill had devised for her, and burned through the task. She had no idea that she was already a named competitor in the 2008 CrossFit Games.

One afternoon, Henniger tacked three sheets of paper to the whiteboard. Athlete registrations for Caity and two of the men. "I signed you up for this thing in California," he declared. "I'll pay for it. You're going."

It was late May. The Games were in July.

DARK HORSES
The 2008 CrossFit Games

IN THE SHORT SPACE OF A YEAR, AFTER THE FIRST CROSSFIT Games, CrossFit grows from a fringe fitness cult into a grassroots movement. It has a passionate following in the military and law enforcement, in the world of martial arts, and among former college athletes jonesing for a chance to compete again. So when CrossFit HQ sends out an open call for Games competitors in 2008, it isn't just a few dozen die-hards who sign up. It's three hundred athletes, with eight hundred spectators in tow.

Glassman's original idea was to have a festival environment where competitors could rotate between workout stations at will. "Greg's a genius," CrossFit Games director Dave Castro says diplomatically. "But sometimes his vision, in application, is almost impossible to create." As a SEAL team logistics guy, Castro quickly realizes there's no way a self-directed movable feast of CrossFit competition is ever going to work. If the Games have a snowball's chance in hell of moving three hundred athletes through multiple WODs in a single day, the whole thing has to be managed with military precision.

It's a given that the Games' physical gauntlet will vary across modal domains—speed, power, muscular endurance, and so on—to represent a true test of overall fitness. But unlike the full spectrum of CrossFit WODs, which range from three to forty minutes, every component event in the 2008 Games needs to be roughly the same duration, to prevent a traffic jam on the longest workout. Figuring out a format that exposes the chink in each athlete's armor, subject to Glassman's vision of competitors moving between stations and the sheer number of athletes involved, is a mind-wrecking multi-dimensional puzzle.

There is also the question of judging and movement standards, debated ad nauseam in the lead-up to the Games. Is CrossFit going to be judged like gymnastics, where technique matters and a movement with improper technique can be judged invalid? Or is CrossFit, like power-lifting, a sheer measure of output, regardless of whether form and technique are ideal or butt-ugly? Declaring CrossFit "the sport of fitness" doesn't clarify what sort of sport it is exactly.

To resolve this debate, Tony Budding, CrossFit's arbiter of stats-and-standards, publishes a precompetition article in the *CrossFit Journal*.[1] The purpose of technique, he explains, is to increase efficiency, power, and safety. Technique optimizes mechanics and minimizes injury. It doesn't have any value beyond that, except in sports in which points are awarded for style, and CrossFit isn't going to be one of those sports. Judging standards for the Games will be results based: Does the athlete complete a movement whose A-to-B work requirement is the same as for the other competitors'? If so, for scoring purposes, it doesn't matter if his technique is deplorable. That's between him and his chiropractor.

Having clarified this issue, CrossFit HQ still has to figure out a scoring system to determine the Fittest Man and Fittest Woman on Earth. Most of us take the point and penalty rules of competitive sports for granted, because the sports we watch have been around for generations. But all those scoring systems had to be devised by someone, then argued about, before they coalesced. Designing a scoring system for the Games is a particularly thorny problem, because the Games consist of multiple events that combine clock times, rep counts, and barbell weights.[2] Oh, and the structure of the competition changes every year, and may include some random element or last-minute on-the-spot shift in competitive requirements.

In the end, the logistical complexity of the event, and the statistical rat-hole of how to score victory, favor simplicity and time effectiveness at all costs. The Games are structured as a two-day event. On the first day of competition, Saturday, July 5, three WODs will run concurrently, from 9:00 a.m. to 8:00 p.m., with fifteen athletes starting a WOD at each station every twenty minutes. Each athlete will be guaranteed four hours of rest between WODs. Games organizers will somehow wrangle all of this onto a spreadsheet.

THERE ARE TWO BARBELL-BODYWEIGHT WORKOUTS ON SATUR-day. One is a more demanding version of "Fran," with chest-to-bar pull-ups instead of the standard chin-over-bar variety. The other WOD is five rounds of five deadlifts (275 pounds for men, 185 pounds for women) and ten burpees. Each has a time cut-off of twelve minutes. The third event is a 750-meter hill run over steep terrain, with a cut-off of twenty minutes.

The final event of the competition will take place on day two, Sun-day, July 6. In keeping with CrossFit's touchstone of the Unknown and Unknowable, the Sunday WOD will not be revealed until Saturday eve-ning, after the first day's final heats are completed. Every athlete's times for all four WODs, over the course of two days, will be totaled to com-pute overall rank. The fastest combined time wins. This quick-and-dirty scoring system gives rise to the overarching theme of the Games, "Every Second Counts."

As announcers shout "Three, two, one, GO!" every twenty minutes in three locations all day, the atmosphere of the event is one of con-trolled chaos and competitive uncertainty. In cumulative time trials like the Tour de France, it's easy for riders to know, after each stage, who's ahead and how much time they have to make up. But with CrossFit Games competitors scattered among three different events and starting in staged heats that run all day long, it's impossible for athletes to know where they stand against rivals across the field.

"Every Second Counts" is a paranoiac context for a parallel-track competition. Every athlete knows that every second of competitive performance, in any event, can make the difference between winning and losing overall. The amount of time it takes to pick up a barbell. An extra breath before jumping back onto the pull-up bar. Doing a set of five thrusters instead of stretching for seven. There is a heightened, moment-to-moment urgency in athletes' experience of each event, because it's so easy to imagine monstrously strong competitors, somewhere else, not resting. Every moment at less than full throttle is a gift to some rival just a hairbreadth behind.

It's the first time twenty-five-year-old Caity Matter has competed without a team, and the blur between athletes and the crowd is something she's never experienced. As a professional athlete, or even a college athlete, she'd travel to a game on the team bus, then hang out in the team locker room. When the team ran onto the court, it was obvious who the athletes were and who the spectators were. But in this crowd, everyone is an athlete—the friends and family look ripped and ready to throw down. Competitors mingle in the crowd between events. The only sure way to distinguish competitors from noncompetitors is to look at their arms and see who has a number scrawled in black Magic Marker.

Caity's first workout is chest-to-bar "Fran," alongside last year's female champion, Jolie Gentry. Jolie, in her SWAT team shades, looks like a *Sports Illustrated* swimsuit model trained to kill people. She pounds out chest-to-bar pull-ups in a gray sports bra, black tights, and a perfect French manicure,[3] and finishes the WOD in 5:43, more than a minute ahead of Caity. Tanya Wagner, a Pennsylvania PE teacher and former Division I soccer goalie, finishes in 5:55. On the deadlift/burpee WOD, where the barbells are more than 120 pounds heavier than "Fran" weight, Caity plays to her comparative advantage—power and muscular endurance—and beats Tanya by seventeen seconds and Jolie by almost half a minute.

The rolling curves and hollows of Aromas, covered in golden grass, look so idyllic—until you have to sprint across them. The run, two brutally vertical loops around an unforgiving hill, is Caity's last event, and she's dreading it. As she barrels up and down the course, she is haunted by the specters of past injury: a three-inch pin in her foot and a torn

ACL. On the downhill scrambles, her quads are shot. But muscular fatigue pales in comparison with the fear that on some misplaced footfall, her knee might unravel. It is an evil place to be.

As she arcs round a downhill bend, hoping her joints don't explode, Bill catches sight of her. Caity's arms are flapping at her sides. She looks tired. She isn't as fast as Jolie or Tanya, but she's in the hunt. "Don't give up, Caity!" he yells. "Don't you give up on me! Come on!" As Caity pulls ahead of a competitor, he screams, "THAT'S WHAT WE TRAIN FOR, CAITY! Go! Don't quit now! Go! Go! Go! Go! Go!"[4]

Meanwhile, in the men's competition, Chris Spealler has put on 4 pounds of muscle since his 129-pound CrossFit Games debut. He is still dwarfed by his competitors, which makes quite an impression as he beats them. On the deadlift burpee WOD, cranking out twenty-five 275-pound deadlifts and fifty burpees, Spealler finishes first in his heat. The men's WOD is fun to watch—an alternating spectacle of manly deadlifts and burpees, which have a bunch of ripped shirtless guys diving into push-ups, then jumping up and clapping their hands above their heads. No one looks tough doing that.

Spealler finishes with the fastest chest-to-bar "Fran" time of 3:01, almost half a minute ahead of 185-pound CrossFit strongman Josh Everett, who is favored to win the Games. Once again, Spealler is managing to move his body (and "Fran's" relatively light 95-pound thrusters) in what seems like half gravity, or fast forward. On the hill run, he tears ahead of a dozen shirtless competitors. A hulking athlete no one recognizes makes a valiant charge in the beginning but quickly falls behind. One by one, so do the others. On the second loop, everyone but Spealler is making an obvious weary effort. Arms are pumping. Torsos zig-zag up the trail. Heads bob from side to side. Some athletes stop, leaning on their legs to walk uphill and resuming speed on the downhill. Others barely maintain their footing on the way down. Last year's champion, O.P.T., leans back, managing his descent.

Ahead of him, Spealler moves smoothly through the dried grass. He makes speed look easy, the way his feet find the right place to land and his muscles spring and flex forward over the terrain. He outpaces O.P.T.

by twelve seconds. The side of beef who came charging out of the gate finishes twenty-four seconds later. Across the finish line, all of them lie sacked out on their backs, panting on the grass. The final trial of the day is done.

At the end of the afternoon, all athletes assemble to hear Dave Castro announce the final event. "As a test of everyone's mental fortitude, we're going to go ahead and do 'Fran' again with the same requirements," he declares. There is a chorus of nervous laughter. "Nah, I'm just kidding. Tomorrow's workout is going to involve one simple move: clean and jerk." Thirty of them, for time.

"Not just any clean and jerk," he continues. "Squat clean and jerk." Instead of just jumping a bar from the ground to shoulders, the athletes will have to jump it up to their shoulders, sink down into a full squat, then rise to a standing position before driving the bar from shoulder to overhead. If an athlete isn't fast enough and strong enough to catch the bar in a squat before rising to a stand, he can jump the bar up to his shoulders, then, in a separate movement, do a full-depth front squat. This is much more work, because the bar has to move all the way up before it starts moving back down. But it's a less intense way to accomplish the work. At the top of the clean, before the squat, there's a chance to breathe, although standing with a loaded bar on your shoulders is no one's idea of rest. Once an athlete has the bar in the bottom of a full squat, he can get it overhead however he wants, as long as his feet are next to each other and his arms are straight up at the top.

An athlete raises his hand and asks if it's permissible to launch the bar overhead with a thruster—to explode from the bottom of a squat to launch the bar straight overhead in one propulsive movement. Castro is highly amused by the idea. "From the squat clean, you can go into a thruster with 155 pounds, if you like, for thirty times. Go ahead and try that, Jacob. I'll be watching you tomorrow. Straight into a thruster, 95 pounds is easy; 155 pounds is a little harder."

The weight, 155 pounds for men, 100 pounds for women, is a last-minute decision. The original Sunday morning workout was going to be a benchmark Girl WOD called "Grace": thirty clean and jerks with 135 pounds for men, 95 pounds for women. But Castro has been watching the competitors and sees how strong they are. The day's workouts have been, in CrossFit terms, relatively high speed, lightweight. So, after conferring with Glassman and Budding, Castro intensifies the final WOD by requiring the squat and ratcheting up the load.

Castro knows this will kill Spealler, who leads Josh Everett and the rest of the pack by over a minute. There is no way a 133-pound guy can finish "Grace's" evil sister at the same rate as a 185-pound powerhouse like Everett. Castro knows that by deciding at the last minute to bump up the weight, he has denied victory to Chris Spealler. It is now Everett's race to lose. And this is something every Games athlete should remember: The CrossFit gods are making all of this stuff up as they go along. They want to see how much wattage they can pull out of the fittest human beings on earth. They are not malicious. But they are curious, and perhaps even greedy for energetic outlay. As the cadre of Games athletes get stronger, the trials become more taxing. The field goals are never fixed.

The time structure of the final event is geared for drama. The top-twenty men and the top-twenty women are each assigned a starting time based on their cumulative time on Saturday's events. The athlete with the lowest combined time will start first. The next nineteen athletes will start after the precise time interval that separates their combined time from the combined time of the leader. If the leader is thirty seconds ahead of second place and a minute ahead of third place at end of day one, he starts the final event first. The athlete in second place starts thirty seconds after the leader, and the third-place athlete starts thirty seconds after that. Thus in the final event, there's no need to cross-check with yesterday's results to determine the winner. The first athlete to finish the final WOD is the champion. The staggered start, with leaders jumping out of the gate ahead of lower-ranked competitors, makes the last heat a winner-take-all sprint to the finish line.

Caity Matter is in fourth place overall. There are eighty-three seconds between her and first place. But as Tanya Wagner and Jolie Gentry enter the fray ahead of her, Caity knows something that they do not. A hundred pounds on the bar, which Dave Castro thinks is such a daunting challenge, is light compared with the brutalizing WODs Bill has been programming for her at Rogue. She hasn't touched a bar weighing less than 115 pounds in months. She's been throwing around 125-pound bars for thirty to forty minutes at a time. Clean and jerk is her favorite lift. "Grace" is her favorite workout. It's a sub-four-minute effort. This is going to be fun.

The most Tanya Wagner has ever clean-and-jerked is 95 pounds. Everyone is looking at her like she's going to win, but she doesn't even know if she can finish the WOD. As she grinds through it and fatigue sets in, Nicole Carroll is watching. She knows the face of how-the-hell-do-I-finish-this, and she threads her way through spectators and athletes, to where Tanya is struggling to maintain her pace, to spur her on. "You can do it," she yells. "You've got it."

In a fog of oxygen debt, lactic acid, and the noise of the crowd, Tanya doesn't perceive anything in the middle distance. So it seems as though Nicole Carroll has appeared out of nowhere. *Nicole Carroll, from the "Nasty Girls" video*, is yelling at her to keep going. Tanya is so starstruck by the apparition that she resolves to finish, if only to avoid disappointing the woman whose epic muscle-up battle inspired her to do CrossFit in the first place. "I'm going to do this," she tells herself. "I'm going to get through this one. It's going to be all right."

Tanya puts her hands on the bar, gathers the tension in her body, and sends a 100-pound barbell rising on the clean, falling as she sinks into a squat, and flying overhead to complete each rep. It is a series of complex movements that harnesses dozens of muscles, the heart and lungs that fuel them, and the nerves that send electricity coursing through the whole human machine. Seeing this WOD performed by an elite athlete at the limit of her strength is like watching lightning strike the same spot thirty times. The awe-inspiring moment is the split second each bolt leaves the cloud.

As Tanya battles to maintain her lead, Caity Matter is gunning for her, and gaining on her. Caity knows that, as long as she doesn't take her hands off the bar, she can win. It's like the "Bear Complex," the first time she showed up at Rogue. Just don't drop it, don't let go. Bill is yelling his head off, "Don't drop the bar! Don't drop the bar!" His voice breaks into the hoarse and desperate cry that comes only when someone you love is about to win. "Dig in! Come on, Caity, turn it on! Go go go go! Finish it! Come on, Caity, go go go! Two left! Two left, Caity, go Caity go!" Caity's judge calls a no-rep on her second-to-last squat, for insufficient depth. "One more!" Bill screams. "One more!!! Yeaahhhhhh!!!!"[5] She misses the last rep after Bill's Kermit-the-Frog yelp and has to marshal one last rep. Bill keeps screaming until his voice is in shreds.

Across the arena, Tanya has finished her final lift, and Dave Castro is announcing "Tanya Wagner is the champion of the 2008 CrossFit Games!" Because Caity wasn't one of the first starts, and is flanked by lower-ranking athletes in a corner of the arena, no one has been watching her. Everyone, including the master of ceremonies, has been watching the woman they expected to win: Tanya.

"Hey!" Bill rasps, waving his hands to get Castro's attention. "Hey!" Caity's judge runs over to tell Dave Castro that, in fact, Tanya Wagner is not the champion of the 2008 CrossFit Games. Startled, Castro makes a rapid retraction and declares Caity the winner. As she steps under the rope dividing the arena from the crowd, someone hands her a beer. Her legs are aching for an ice bath.

Finally, it is time for the men's last heat, the fox hunt where Chris Spealler will be set loose, and then a minute later, a pack of larger animals will be released to run him down. After Spealler, the next nine competitors are close, within a thirty-second range. It will be a powerful pack, and Everett is expected to be the first one to roll over Spealler en route to the podium. Everett is such a sure favorite that CrossFit's media team has been interviewing him for months for a documentary about the Games, and their cameraman hovers around him like a horsefly.

Spealler gathers his thoughts before the countdown. Asked what he's hoping for, he's unflustered. "I'm hoping that maybe these guys tire out a little bit," he says before insulating himself with his trademark earphones and shades.[6] At the signal to begin, he leans down to a barbell that weighs more than he does, and jumps it up to a clean. The judge calls a no-rep on his first attempt, because Spealler doesn't lock out his hips to full extension. When you're lifting more than body weight, no-reps from a judge can be more demoralizing than failed reps, because you thought you had it, before it's declared that your energy has been wasted. Spealler finishes his sixth rep at forty-one seconds, his seventh at fifty seconds. He is on his eighth rep when Josh Everett hurtles out of the gate. As Spealler finishes his eleventh rep, Dave Castro announces that Everett is seven reps into the WOD. By the time Spealler can muster another squat clean, Everett has a dozen.

THIRTEEN REPS FOR SPEALLER, CASTRO ANNOUNCES. THIRTEEN reps for Josh Everett. They are tied at a pace that Chris Spealler cannot possibly match. By his fourteenth rep, Spealler has been overtaken by Everett, at nineteen reps. Everett is fired up by the power of his own momentum. "This is it," he thinks. "I'm the CrossFit Games champion."

Spealler fails on his eighteenth rep. He can't get under the bar, and it drops. He's wrecked. Remarkably, he is still ahead of O.P.T, who fails on rep seventeen. Even Everett begins to fail, three reps short of the finish, then again at rep twenty-nine. He drops the bar and pauses for a moment. Castro shouts, "One more rep!" Everett leans down, puts his hands on the bar, and cleans it to his shoulders. The camera is on him. The crowd is cheering. Everett's bar begins moving from shoulder to overhead. This is the crowning moment.

And then, Castro's voice, strangely distant, carries across the arena. The twenty-two-year-old meathead who tried to charge up the hill, the guy who looks like some kind of Muscle Beach bodybuilding specimen, has just finished his thirtieth rep. There is no camera on him, because he started so far behind the pack. But the whole time, he's been doing what Dave Castro laughed off as an impossibility in the athlete briefing—squat clean thrusters with 155 pounds—to churn through the WOD more than a minute faster than anyone else. Castro grabs his hand, raises it up, and shouts, "Jason Khalipa is the champion of the 2008 CrossFit Games!"

The same question occurs to everyone simultaneously: Who the hell is Jason Khalipa? Glassman is delighted. "I expected a dark horse," he says. "You don't have to be famous to do well at this. You have to have a medicine ball, some rings, some weight, and you can get really, really good in your garage and come out on Game Day and be the best in the world. It doesn't get any more egalitarian than that. It's perfect."

A CLYDESDALE
LEARNS TO RACE

KHALIPA HAD COME OUT OF NOWHERE TO WIN THE 2008 CROSS-
Fit Games. Moments after he won, and for weeks thereafter, all anyone
wanted to know was how he'd done it. How long had he been doing
CrossFit? Had he formerly been a Division I athlete? Where was the
underground CrossFit bat cave where he'd been secretly training?

Facing this volley of inquiry, the Mysterious Champion sheepishly
lowered his head. He had a confession to make: He had been doing
CrossFit for a year, and thought it was the greatest thing ever. But before
he saw the light . . . he had been working out . . . working in membership sales, actually . . . at a globo-gym.

Globo-gym is CrossFit's derisive epithet for conventional health
and fitness clubs. The term comes from the 2004 movie *Dodgeball*,
starring Ben Stiller as the villainous bleached-blond, mustachioed
owner of a slick fitness club filled with expensive machines, steroidal
bodybuilders, and blonde gym bunnies in spandex. Stiller's gleam-
ing globo-gym was such an exquisite parody of the fitness industry's
cosmetic ideals that the fictional gym quickly rippled across Cross-
Fit's boards and blogs as the symbol of everything that CrossFit was
not. The warped body culture of exercises done purely for cosmetic
effect—bicep curls and crunches. The narcissistic flex of isolated muscle groups on resistance machines. The mindless grind of cardio. A
fat (but superficial) society's abandonment of functional fitness and

primal vigor. All of these things could be neatly encapsulated in the word *globo-gym*.

Globo-gym was, and remains, CrossFit's code-word shorthand for The Way Things Are Is Wrong. It's a loaded phrase, like "factory food" or "the 1%" or "the mainstream media," that defines a culturally dominant Them, and by opposition, a scrappy, righteous Us.

So for the CrossFit elite, having Greg Glassman's anointed "Fittest Man on Earth" ruefully recall alternating days of chest-tricep and legs-and-shoulder sets was like hearing a recovering alcoholic's tales of week-long benders and bottles hidden around the house. Khalipa's recovering globo-gym bodybuilder story, which becomes funnier and more self-deprecating every time he tells it, is a Born Again story that follows the same contours of degeneracy, revelation, and redemption as any religious testimony.

Here's how a Born Again story goes: Life wasn't working for me, or felt meaningless. Details of sin, carousing, infidelity, and such are laid out with brio. Then a friend opened a conversation about faith or took me to church. There's always a humbling moment: I realized how wrong and inadequate I was (the more outward success someone has in life, the more humbling and effective this moment is). But that was okay—there was a way to be better. I was welcomed into a community of faith. It changed my life and my identity, and I never looked back. I'm grateful for it, and I try to spread the Word.

When CrossFitters meet for the first time, the opening conversational gambit is "How did you find CrossFit?" It's an invitation to testimony. It almost always goes something like this: My gym or running routine wasn't working for me. I was overweight, my knees hurt, I was bored. Then a friend pointed me to the CrossFit main site, or brought me to their box. I did my first WOD and ended up gasping on the floor (the fitter someone looks and feels going into it, the more humbling and effective this experience is). But that was okay—all these superstrong people start the same way. We're all in it together—the sense of community is awesome. I kept at it, and I've gotten so much stronger (the person lists milestone workouts and personal records). It's changed my life and the way I think about myself. I've gotten my sister into it, and she's lost twenty-five pounds.

People embellish this story with their own personal details and flourishes, and that's what makes it fun to hear and exchange. Storytelling has fallen out of memory as an everyday mode of social exchange. But people like telling stories. We evolved to share stories as a way of belonging. It feels good. And CrossFit provides a wealth of milestones along the path that everyone travels: First WOD, the first few puny benchmarks, the first time you get a pull-up, or a handstand pushup, or a muscle-up. First Hero WOD. The first time you rope a friend or relative into trying it.

Khalipa's is the story of a reluctant convert. After playing high school football and throwing shot put in Northern California, he stayed close to home and studied for a business degree in Santa Clara. All through high school and college, he worked, and worked out, at a globo-gym in Milpitas. All he wanted was to someday own his own gym. So he sold memberships at the desk.

He did all the standard globo-gym exercises. He got big, doing three sets of eight to twelve reps, the tried-and-true formula for maximizing muscle mass. But it was monotonous. "You get tired of bicep curling fifty pounds," he says. "Then maybe next time you try fifty-five pounds. It's just stupid." He tried Muy Thai and started to develop some athleticism doing pad work with a partner and sparring. He enjoyed the intensity of it. But what he now describes as "heavy globo-gym bicep bullshit"[1] was his fitness bread and butter.

In December 2006, his friend Austin Begiebing, a trainer at the Milpitas gym, started getting on Khalipa's case to try CrossFit. Austin had been rabidly consuming articles and videos on the CrossFit main site since his own conversion experience earlier in the year. Austin had heard about CrossFit back in 2002, when his mother came across the website while searching for nutrition information. But he was already a trainer and wasn't interested in yet another fitness trend that would end up fizzling away. "As much as I turned my back on CrossFit, it kept resurfacing in different ways at least once a month for years," he explains on his CrossFit coach's profile, veering into a variation of the Born Again story known as God-was-always-there-waiting-for-me-to-come-around.[2] "Looking back, it is so obvious I was meant to do this."

Eventually, sheer boredom with standard gym workouts drove Austin to a local box. After his first WOD, he lay on the floor wondering how it was possible for a fifteen-minute workout to do this to him. He was hooked, and binge-read materials on the CrossFit main site. Fired up by Glassman's "Foundations" manifesto and determined to meet the man himself, Austin flew to Santa Cruz for a CrossFit certification seminar. "It was a life-changing experience in many ways. Since then I have been on a never-ending quest to improve my knowledge as a CrossFit coach and share it with others."

His evangelization started with Khalipa, whom he eventually dragged to the same CrossFit box where he'd started, to try it. Khalipa's first workout was "Fran." For a guy with massive bodybuilder thighs, the thrusters were no problem. But he couldn't do a pull-up. Because all his exercises had been isolation movements, his nervous system wasn't wired up to move his whole body through space using many muscles at once, in coordinated succession. A lat pull-down, plus a row, plus a bicep curl does not equal a pull-up. Pull-ups knit all those muscles together into a whole-body movement that also includes the trunk and hips. It requires a level of brain-body and muscle group integration that isolation exercises cannot achieve.

On top of that, Khalipa's strength-to-mass ratio was abysmal, because he'd been lifting weights to maximize muscle mass, not strength. The reason bodybuilders hew to the formula of three sets of eight-to-ten reps is that this rep scheme builds muscle volume (in the clinical parlance, it "maximizes hypertrophy"). If the goal is to bulge on a podium, this is the ideal rep scheme. It optimizes muscle-man aesthetics.

The bodybuilding rep scheme builds bulk and definition. But bulk and definition are not the same as power or endurance. Powerlifters and Olympic weightlifters train for maximum effort with one to three reps per set. Athletes looking to build muscular endurance rep out sets of fifteen to twenty. Eight to ten is for show ponies.

Khalipa was a show pony. He was so massive from the bodybuilding that it was impossible for him to haul his bulk up and over the bar. When most people show up to a CrossFit box and can't do pull-ups, they clove-hitch a thick rubber band over the bar, and lodge their heels into the bottom loop to give themselves a spring on the way up. Khalipa wasn't even on the band. He did jumping pull-ups: stand on a box, grab the bar and jump, using your arms to provide a bit of pulling assistance to your legs. Jumping pull-ups are what new moms, grannies, and clinically obese people are given to do with a pat on the shoulder and an encouraging word ("Don't worry—you'll get there! You're doing great!").

Doing jumping pull-ups, it's almost impossible to achieve the intensity of a CrossFit WOD, even "Fran." Khalipa finished and felt good. He hadn't been laid low. So the revelation would have to wait. Over the next couple of months, Austin cherry-picked some WODs off the CrossFit main site, exercises he thought Khalipa would enjoy. But it took some time for the mentality of isolation exercises to dissipate. The habit of moving methodically from movement to movement over the course of an hour wouldn't allow Khalipa to truly push himself to the level of intensity that CrossFit WODs are designed to achieve. It was just he and Austin in the same environment where they'd been parked on a bench doing hamstring extensions. There was a clock, but there was no sense of urgency, no "3-2-1-GO!" and the pounding of a pack on the run.

But even as a very bulky lone wolf, after ten or fifteen WODs Khalipa began to realize that these were the toughest workouts he'd ever done. He saw that he was becoming more athletic. What if, he wondered, I could apply some CrossFit intensity to my old-school weightlifting routine?

He went over to the bench press and loaded the barbell with 135 pounds. "I'm going to rep this out a hundred times," he thought, "and see how long it takes me." The next time he tried it, he had a time to beat. Every time, the set got faster and more intense. As the guys in the weight room realized what he was doing, they tried it. And of course, this became a competitive event. And now, there was a reason to really go for it. As Khalipa shoved the bar up and away a hundred times, his

body and mind flooded with a distinctive CrossFit cocktail of adrenaline, fatigue, determination, and a sprinter's consciousness that every
second counts. A hundred and forty seconds, in the end, was all it took.

"Oh," he thought, gasping and glowing. "I *like* this." It clicked.

From then on, he and Austin did CrossFit workouts from the main
site, and eventually convinced their boss at the Milpitas globo-gym to let
them convert a racquetball court into an 800-square-foot CrossFit mini-
box. They'd work out there, recruiting intrigued passers-by gawking
through the glass. Over the months that followed, Khalipa felt himself
becoming stronger and faster. His body began to become more efficient.
His mind was dialing into the intensity, the red-zone push that didn't
happen anywhere else in the gym. After the 2007 CrossFit Games, he
started watching O.P.T.'s workout times online, and he put the champion in his sights. A year of CrossFit workouts turned him from a show
pony into a racehorse—an unusually large, bulgy sort of racehorse, but
a snorting champion all the same.

After hitting the flat-out intensity of workouts that blurred "strength"
and "cardio" into a single sweaty smear, Khalipa would go back to his
job selling globo-gym memberships. He'd been selling gym memberships since high school. He was good at it. He loved sales and had visions
of selling memberships to his own gym someday. At the same time, he
knew that the people buying his gym memberships were never going
to achieve the results they wanted on cardio and muscle isolation machines. "It was a dilemma," he admits. "Obviously, I wanted a pay-
check. And I was working on commission. But I didn't really believe in
the product."

There are more than fifty million gym members in the United States,
and most of them aren't fit. Most of them don't even work out regularly.
This isn't a glitch in the health club business model. It's fundamental to
how modern fitness facilities make money.

GLOBO-GYM
The Spandex Juice-Bar Business Model

THE GRANDDADDY OF THE MODERN GLOBO-GYM WAS A CLUB
called Vic Tanny's, which opened in Los Angeles in 1947, just as California became a spawning ground for cultural trends. Before World War
II, there had been three types of gyms:[1] There were private member-only clubs like the New York Athletic Association and the Olympic
Club of San Francisco, where business executives went to swim and play
squash. There were YMCAs, which offered a full array of gymnastic
equipment, dumbbells, pools, and sports courts to middle- and working-class youngsters in the spirit of health and wholesomeness.

Lastly, there were bodybuilding gyms owned by strongmen. Sig
Klein's Studio of Physical Culture, in midtown Manhattan, was a shrine
of strength training that nursed the bodybuilding movement in its infancy. Sig himself was known to press 299 pounds overhead with one
arm. In Philadelphia, Hermann's Gym and John Fritshe's Gym became
clanking capitols of hard-core weightlifting. Across the Susquehanna
River in York, Pennsylvania, Bob Hoffman's York Barbell Club was
home to some of the greatest bodybuilders and weightlifters of the era,
and Hoffman's York Barbell Company was synonymous with the grimace and grunt of serious muscle men. Muscle gyms were vulcan armories of steel and iron. They were suffused with sweat and testosterone
and filled with working-class guys who looked like comic book characters. Although warm hearts beat in the barrel chests of the proprietors,

these dungeons of strength training seemed forbidding to men with unimpressive biceps, or to women of any sort.

Vic Tanny's was different. It was geared for middle-class consumers in the postwar suburbs. The facilities were brightly lit and tricked out in carpet and chrome. In addition to gym equipment favored by men, there were pools and saunas to attract women looking for spa amenities. And mirrors. Lots of mirrors. You could look in almost any direction at Vic Tanny's and see your own reflection in a wall of mirror. Tanny's pioneered the modern health club's architectural impetus to stare at yourself in the mirror during exercise. Curl the bicep. Look at the bicep in the mirror straight ahead. Put down the dumbbell and notice how the bicep looks larger than it did in its precurl state. Scrutinize the whole shoulder/chest/ab situation and move to the next mirror-facing workout station. This was one of Vic Tanny's major innovations.

The other major Tanny's innovation was the hard sell and contractual lock-in that's become a ubiquitous feature of major gym chains. Salesmen had daily membership quotas to hook new prospects into contracts ranging from six months to "permanent" seven-year contracts. Many of these salesmen worked strictly on commission and were aware that if they outsold their manager, the next day they'd be the new manager. If their ex-boss outsold them the day after that, they'd be back in the sales pool. Vic Tanny himself sent out a mimeographed set of instructions for calling prospects on the phone. "If you fail to get an appointment," he concluded, "take a gun out of the desk and shoot yourself."

By 1960, Vic Tanny's had grown to eighty-four health clubs across America and a million gym memberships. Sales volume was king, and pressure and intimidation were part of the job. A Cook County Vic Tanny's salesman went to trial for false imprisonment after a girl claimed he locked her in his office for an hour while trying to persuade her to sign up. At the same gym, a blind man was conned into signing a lifetime membership contract he thought was a free membership application. New York State authorities received so many complaints from Vic Tanny's members that the state attorney general's office made the chain sign a fair practices code that prohibited deceitful, fraudulent, or misleading claims in its sales process.

Nobody remembers Vic Tanny's anymore, even though it was the largest chain of health clubs in America. But in 1963, when Tanny's Glengarry Glen Ross management finally imploded the company, the clubs he didn't shutter were bought by a former Tanny's employee, Don Wildman, who'd taken his high-pressure sales training and started a new gym chain, Health and Tennis Corporation, which continued to attract regulatory attention for its opaque membership agreements and strong-arm sales tactics. Despite its reputation, the chain expanded aggressively. In 1983, it changed its name to Bally Health and Tennis and became the largest health and fitness club operator in the world.

In 1994, Bally paid to settle Federal Trade Commission charges of illegal billing, cancellation refund, and debt collection practices.[2] In 2004, it was still being hounded by the New York State Attorney General's Office for the same reasons.[3] In 2010, the Texas attorney general announced the company had mailed more than eleven thousand fake past-due notices to former members, urging them to immediately pay nonexistent late fees that would fraudulently roll into new membership contracts.[4]

Bally Total Fitness is Vic Tanny's. And not because the ghost of Vic Tanny, who died of heart failure in Tampa at age seventy-three, is still rattling around the locker rooms. Globo-gym contempt for membership didn't persist and proliferate across the industry because salesmen were troglodytes, or had supervisors with minimal ethics who were themselves terrified by ruthless regional managers. High-volume health clubs—facilities that sell year-long memberships to use cardio machines and weight circuits—have a financial model that succeeds when members pay but don't actually exercise.

In the globo-gym business model, the best-case scenario is to maximize membership while minimizing members' use of the gym itself. The gym's billing system is going to extract money from members' bank accounts every month, regardless of whether they work out. Contracts allow the gym to do this for at least a year, often multiple years. At the same time, the gym gets crowded during prime morning and evening hours. If more than a fraction of members actually show up, the facility becomes unacceptably crowded. Waits at the cardio machines become long enough to require sign-up sheets. Sniping ensues, and cardio-machine queue altercations require manager attention. Classes get full, and the people in them get possessive about their spots. Water bottles become territorial markers. It gets ugly.

So the art of marketing a globo-gym is to maximize the group of members who don't use the gym but aren't motivated to cancel their memberships. In January, you recruit new members, people who've made weight loss resolutions but aren't actually going to change their habits. You take steps to alleviate crowding in January and February as those new members (and existing members racked by guilt) hit the floor. By March, member attendance has fallen off—Gold's Gym has statistically identified February 7 as the "Fitness Cliff," when the daily check-ins take a steep drop, a mere thirty-eight days after January 1.[5]

But people who signed up in January are now captive subscribers who are legally committed to monthly bank debits for the rest of the year. If it's legal in the state, you build auto-renew clauses into contracts that extend membership for an additional year unless a member explicitly cancels within a certain period of time. Inertia is the most powerful force in the universe. Even when people are still overweight after a year of cardio machines and crunches, or don't even find time to use the gym, it's hard to make a change. It's especially hard when the available alternatives look just like what you're already doing. Except that some of them are closer to your house or work, and some of them are cheaper.

In recent years, globo-gym members have realized that the machines are exactly the same, regardless of how much the gym charges. If the main benefit people get is a sense of virtue for using the machines, then it doesn't make sense to pay sixty dollars a month when you could pay twenty dollars for access to the same apparatus within the same radius of your home or office. Economic doldrums, financial crises, and a shaky job market mean that more people are looking to trim their monthly expenses.

The result is the rise of so-called high-volume/low-price (HVLP) clubs: 15,000- to 25,000-square-foot warehouses of cardio and weight circuit machines with no classes, no trainers, just a manager at the desk. Some of them don't even have a manager—they are twenty-four-hour keycard access facilities with no staff on the premises. For this, you pay less than twenty dollars a month, even as low as ten dollars a month. In the United States, and across Europe and Australia, HVLP clubs are leading a globo-gym race to the bottom.

It's good for the companies that make the machines, because it converts both the supply and the demand side of fitness into an industrial assembly line exercise: the facility owner obtains capital to lease a large-scale facility and fill it with machines. Members' interaction with the facility is entirely mediated by machines, via the web, electronic funds transfers, and soon their pedometers and heart rate monitors and other Quantified Self gadgetry. Using radio-frequency identification (RFID) access cards, they key themselves into the facility and operate the machines as directed. Management pays for the continued maintenance and occasional replacement of the machines, and the accounting department makes sure that leasing and depreciation schedules are optimized for the bottom line.

The machines require a lot of up-front capital and floor space. But they are less expensive and more predictable than employees. They're good at maintaining a Goldilocks level of member indifference: still paying (because it's so cheap), but not excited to show up. Trainers and instructors, especially good ones, screw up this equilibrium. Groups of people start to attend their classes regularly, and the classes get crowded. Gym use goes up, which in the Bizarro world of the fitness club business model isn't always a good thing. When trainers realize that members love the class experience more than the machines, they demand more money or they move, taking clients with them. Machines don't play pied piper with the membership. They have no social contract. They enable a business model that scales beautifully. Row upon row of self-serve machines in a self-serve facility, fully industrialized fitness, cleansed of the inefficiency and nuisance of human interaction.

The old-school globo-gym, with its chrome and mirrors and airhead instructors, may be easy to deride. But it's also under siege. On the low end, it's being squeezed by HVLP machine-circuit warehouses that charge a fraction of the globo-gym price for access to identical equipment.[6]

On the high end, members willing to pay a premium are starting to realize that globo-gym programming doesn't achieve all that much in the way of results. "The membership portion of the business that we've been so dependent on in the last fifty, sixty years is starting to evolve," says Thomas Plummer, who runs the National Fitness Business Alliance, an industry trade association. "The consumer is starting to, in significant numbers, gravitate toward a results-driven environment and away from a do-it-yourself fitness environment. That's going to spell bad news for some of these old-style chains."[7]

People who care about outcomes, versus giving themselves a gold star for gym attendance, are gravitating to fitness activities that double down on human expertise and social interaction. That means coaches, trainers, groups, and sports activities that feel like fun, even an adventure, rather than a chore or a mindless calorie grind.

The irony is that, as cardio machines have evolved to make exercise more comfortable (the modern elliptical machine is a moderate-intensity Barcalounger), "fun" turns out to be the opposite of comfort. Fun is what gets your blood racing and makes you a little nervous. It messes up your hair and may leave your clothes permanently stained. And it all but requires a friend or strangers who, by the end of it, are friends. In the last five years, the biggest boom in running hasn't been marathons or triathlons or traditional 10Ks. It's mud races—obstacle-studded runs, often on summertime ski slopes, that friends tackle on a lark (or a dare).

Obstacle races started as military-themed variations of ultra-endurance events like the Camp Pendleton Mud Run. A British variation on this theme, the Tough Guy Challenge, originally included a 40-foot crawl through flooded tunnels and long mud slithers with machine-gun blanks fired overhead.[8] Ultra-endurance obstacle events like the 48-hour Spartan Death Race still warn (on the website www

.YouMayDie.com) that 90% of participants will not complete the course, knowing that this kind of admonishment is catnip to the hard-core elite who ultimately sign up. Every summer, two hundred maniacs in the Vermont woods tackle the course, where they may be asked to chop wood for two hours, crawl through mud under barbed wire, or memorize Bible verses in order to progress to the next obstacle.

But this is a sideshow. The real action in mud racing is in kinder, gentler versions of the same weekend hell. The Spartan Sprint, run by the same outfit as the Spartan Death Race, has more participants than the Boston Marathon, the New York Marathon, the London Marathon, and the Chicago Marathon combined. Held in dozens of locations across the English-speaking world (apparently, there is something Anglo-Saxon about running headlong through the mud), the Spartan Sprint is a three mile run with fifteen obstacles: rope climbs, tunnel crawls, jumping over (or into) a mud pit, leaping over flames. Although the flame leap isn't that challenging, pictures of it make excellent social media postings. In keeping with the Spartan theme, there's a spear throw into a hay bale. If the spear doesn't stick into the hay, the penalty is thirty burpees. People running Spartan Sprints already know how to do burpees. Most of them do CrossFit. "99.9% of all people who try this event will finish," assures the event's web page, "and 100% will have their thirst for mud fully satisfied!"[9]

The three top male and top female finishers of a Spartan Sprint receive a free entry into the Super Spartan race of their choice. The Super Spartan is 8 miles instead of 3 miles, with 20 obstacles. Top Super Spartan finishers get free admission to a Spartan Beast race, which is 12 miles and 25 obstacles. People who run the Sprint, the Super, and the Beast get a Spartan Trifecta patch, and Spartan Beast champions automatically qualify for the Death Race. It's like scouting, with a dash of *Hunger Games*, live music, and delectable outdoor-festival food.

There are half a dozen large, sponsored, well-organized outfits that stage mud races around the world. Warrior Dash started in 2009 with 2,000 participants. By 2012, it was running 700,000 people through dozens of 5K obstacle races a year—15,000 to 25,000 people per weekend, November through August. Tough Mudder, a ten- to twelve-mile event whose signature obstacle is a finish-line curtain of live electrical wires, has run almost 1 million people through a gauntlet of mud swims; fire trenches; rows of gymnastic rings four to six feet apart suspended above ice water pools; sprints with fire hoses battering participants from both sides; and other tests of strength, agility, grip strength, and pain tolerance.[10]

Mud races are sporting events. But they are being run for completely different reasons than marathons and triathlons or 5K and 10K road races. Finish time is completely beside the point. What's important is the dramatic intensity and social bonding of the event, the laugh-about-it-later, we're-in-it-togetherness of the suck.

Marathons and triathlons are certainly rites of passage. But there's a serious and solitary quality to them. Even as thousands of athletes crash forward from the starting line, they're setting out alone, together. It's everyone for himself, putting one foot in front of the other until it's over. The story you can tell is that you completed the event in a certain amount of time. No one cares how long you trained for it, or how much your knee or ankle hurt at mile twelve, or what it felt like to "hit the wall." Fast or slow, it's predictable. There's no drama.

Obstacle races are campfire tales. Did you cut yourself crawling under the barbed wire? Did you get zapped by the 10,000-volt live electrical wire? Tough Mudder's twelve-foot sloping wall, emblazoned in giant letters, NO QUIT IN HERE, absolutely requires a running start, accelerating to a flat-out sprint, a leaping scramble up, and a hand at the top to help you over. The topography of the course guarantees moments of action-movie heroism and a satisfying buddy adventure about how you all got through it, and whose crazy idea it was in the first place.

If marathons, triathlons, and road races are the weekend fitness event of the Me Generation, obstacle races are how socially meshed millennials challenge their bodies. These events are designed for small groups to tackle as coordinated teams or larger packs. Races like Muddy Buddy explicitly require you to have a partner for team-based challenges every mile or so.[11] Tough Mudder flatly states that people can't complete the course alone. Not just because it's physically impossible, but because "you'll need teammates to pick you up when your spirits dip. To get over 12 foot walls and through underground mud tunnels, you'll need teammates to give you a boost and a push. Tough Mudders are team players who make sure no one gets left behind."[12]

Who runs obstacle races? CrossFitters,[13] and the people they're trying to recruit into CrossFit. Because if the friend powers through discomfort and intensity and ends up grinning, exhausted and sore, covered in mud, and posting to Facebook about it, well, why not try that again, without the mud, on a weekday? Walk through the door of a CrossFit box for an introductory class, and what do you see on the desk? Flyers, for an obstacle race.

What most people don't realize when they pick up that flyer or fill out a waiver or sign the membership agreement that authorizes monthly debits to their bank accounts—the same motions you go through at a globo-gym desk—is that the business model of a CrossFit box is completely different from that of the globo-gym. It makes its money differently. CrossFit headquarters doesn't make money the same way as a globo-gym's corporate headquarters. And that affects everything.

GLOBO-GYMS ARE FRANCHISES. EVERY REVENUE STREAM, FROM membership subscriptions to personal training fees and smoothie sales, is split between the local gym operator and corporate headquarters. Gym corporations, most of which are owned by private equity funds, have a business imperative to maximize the money flowing back from all those local gyms to headquarters, to maximize shareholder value or dividends to limited partners. In any franchise business, there are three ways to do this. The first is to open more franchises. The second is to increase the amount of money coming into the franchises, by advertising or making the facilities more attractive. The third is to slice the pie differently, so that headquarters expands its share of the take or reduces its share of the costs. Every franchise in the world is under pressure to increase its profitability in all these ways. There are benefits that flow from centralized management and hierarchy. All the computer, billing, and human resource (HR) systems are standardized. The logos are already done. The trade-off for these benefits is that no one who works at the gym, from the owner to the trainers, gets to decide much of anything. Pricing, hours of operation, staffing policies, gear for sale behind the desk are informed, if not determined, by headquarters. And every dollar that flows into the joint is subject to a franchise royalty.

CrossFit doesn't work that way. It's not a franchise. All CrossFit HQ requires from CrossFit gym owners is a coaching certificate—to make sure they understand the movements and methods—and an affiliate fee to use the CrossFit name. The methods are open source—trainers can use CrossFit methods to run a gym and charge people. They just can't call the place a CrossFit gym unless they license the trademark. Once they do that, the minute they've set up a web page and paid the affiliate fee, CrossFit HQ lists the box as an affiliate on its website. It's official.

This setup began with the first affiliate, run by Dave Werner, a former Navy SEAL who'd been doing CrossFit in his garage. Werner wanted to open a gym and train people to do CrossFit in Seattle. So he called Greg Glassman in Santa Cruz. "We want to affiliate," said Werner.

"That's awesome," replied Glassman. "What's an affiliate?" So Werner explained his idea to open a CrossFit box, like the one in Santa Cruz. Glassman thought this was a fantastic idea. "Let's do it!" But, Werner asked, what about using the CrossFit name? Didn't Glassman want to charge him for that?

"Yeah," Glassman replied. "Like, five hundred dollars a year. You've got yourself a deal." Werner's box, the first CrossFit affiliate, opened as CrossFit North in 2002. At the same time, TJ Cooper in the Jacksonville, Florida, sheriff's office was running a box for his fellow cops, and he wanted to make his CrossFit business legit.

No problem, Glassman told him. "It costs five hundred dollars every year. But I'll waive your fees, because you're one of the early ones." The Jacksonville box became CrossFit East. Because the first two affiliates named themselves after compass points, Glassman jokes, "I thought, this is incredible. There's probably going to be five someday: north, south, east, west, and us. We'll be headquarters."[14] But he knew that CrossFit's online discussion boards would light up with this notion of becoming an affiliate. The brethren, scattered across the country but connected on the web, were passionate. They were primed to pounce on the idea of replicating what Glassman had built in Santa Cruz, as long as it was cheap enough, and hewed to the garage do-it-yourself ethos, and left them free and autonomous.

Every affiliate from the first to the current crop, more than seven thousand in total, has the same arrangement. The affiliate fee has gone up over the years, to three thousand dollars. But everyone is grandfathered into whatever affiliate fees they started paying. The guys who started paying five hundred dollars a year in 2002 are still paying five hundred dollars a year, and any income over that amount belongs to the box—there are no franchise royalties.

The kind of space that's perfect for CrossFit is industrial. An empty warehouse with a concrete floor and twenty-foot ceilings is ideal. Compared with leasing space in a big-box strip mall or a shopping center, it's dirt cheap. Cheap space, plus cheap equipment, plus a small affiliate fee and no franchise expense means the cost of entry to open a CrossFit box is orders of magnitude lower than the stand-up cost of a conventional health club.

It doesn't require seven figures of net worth. A prospective Planet Fitness franchisee needs to prove he's worth $1.3 million, with $400,000 in liquid cash available. It can take anywhere from $700,000 to $1.7 million to open the doors.[15] Young trainers, taking home less than half of what a health club charges their clients, don't have that kind of money. CrossFit gives them an alternative to fitness sharecropping at the globo-gym.

From 2001 to 2011, according to the US Labor Department, the number of personal trainers increased by 44% to 231,500. That's about 70,000 new trainers. During that same period, CrossFit certified 40,000 trainers (most, though not all, in the United States), bringing the total to 50,000 by the end of 2012. So more than half of this dramatic surge of personal trainers in the US fitness industry is just from CrossFit. It's not more bimbos and himbos at Bally's. It's twenty-seven-year-olds flying the Jolly Roger, rigging pull-up bars, and hoisting climbing ropes over steel rebar in a warehouse in some industrial park.

Glassman had been one of those young guys. He had no experience running a franchise operation, and no interest in it. He only grudgingly attended to the operational mundanities of his own business. Contrarian by nature, he detested being told what to do or how to do it. The only thing worse than being told what to do was having to manage other people and their operational mundanities. So Glassman decided the whole affiliate thing was going to be hands-off, and that he'd only offer terms a younger version of himself would have taken. CrossFit's affiliate model is the Golden Rule, applied by a renegade who can't work for anyone.

Affiliates don't have to get permission or approval from headquarters for any aspect of their business, from hours of operation, pricing, and staffing levels to workout programming and the obscenity quotient on wall posters and T-shirts (or whether T-shirts are even required). If affiliates want to give military discounts, they can. If they want to assign burpee penalties to members who arrive late or fail to sign in, that's their call. They are tribal leaders, entrepreneurs, pirate captains, accountable only to the athletes who choose to train with them.

"I'm a libertarian by birth," Glassman says. "We have a system in place. I think it's just free market unfettered capitalism that is creating these affiliates, and their fidelity to the original is just amazing. . . . Their instincts are free market instincts. They're natural instincts. The unfettered have a deep appreciation of being unfettered, even if they are not able to express it."[16]

CrossFit HQ protects a culture that embraces competitive fitness. It's a cult of excellence. The cultural imperative for affiliates can be boiled down to four words: make your pack strong. If you pursue excellence and make your pack stronger, you will thrive. If you need support, reach out to the community. Band together. It's a strategy for resilience.

The clearest case in point for this strategy is CrossFit's organizing principle for liability insurance. In 2008, a Virginia affiliate was sued by a member who got rhabdo. The box owner had liability insurance. But the insurance company lawyers didn't know anything about CrossFit. They could Google "CrossFit" and "dangerous" and see dozens of blog screeds about this "controversial" fitness movement. So they weren't inclined to defend it. They just wanted to limit the potential damage. So they settled.

It was a nightmare scenario: if every time some out-of-shape CrossFit newbie torqued his back and hired an ambulance chaser to sue, and an insurance company settled instead of mounting a vigorous defense, a trickle of precedents would snowball into an avalanche of liability. Because any legal claim against an individual CrossFit box would also compromise the CrossFit brand, HQ could have required affiliates to purchase comprehensive liability insurance through headquarters and made a profit on the underwriting, while giving affiliates a sweetheart deal on premiums.

Instead, it set up a co-op. Members of the co-op—the policyholders themselves—set the premiums. If there's money left over after any claims are paid, the profit gets distributed as dividends. CrossFit HQ doesn't own the insurance company or profit from it. The members buy into it and own it. Affiliates don't have to buy their insurance from the co-op, although it's the easiest and cheapest option. Local insurance agents, when they hear descriptions of what goes on in a CrossFit box, tend to categorize the enterprise as Crazy People Doing Dangerous Things and set rates accordingly.

But if they buy into the co-op and pay premiums set by their peers, affiliates know they'll get an insurance policy written without loopholes and exclusions that allow insurers to renege on coverage for, say, training on homemade equipment. Trainers know that if it comes down to a court trial, they'll be defended by lawyers who do CrossFit. And the expert witnesses on the stand will be doctors and exercise PhD professors who also hit three WODs a week. The defense will be well organized and intensely committed. The community protects its own.

CrossFit HQ's insistence on minimizing its own role to essential functions—a corporate theory of limited government—includes an absolute refusal to regulate competition between the affiliates themselves. If a new affiliate wants to open three blocks away from an existing affiliate, there's no territorial exclusivity (standard among franchises) to prevent that from happening. It's uncomfortable for established boxes when a new affiliate opens a mile up the road. And when CrossFit boxes began to proliferate in earnest, there was a lot of online pot banging by veteran affiliates clamoring for "quality control" measures that would serve as a gating mechanism for affiliates run by less-experienced coaches.

In response, CrossFit HQ's famously pugnacious Russell Berger posted an article to the *CrossFit Journal*.[17] "It is human nature to want someone with power to step in and fix your problems," he wrote. "The truth, however, is that intervention rarely comes without a price. 'Thou shalt not directly compete with a veteran affiliate' may sound like a good notion, but telling someone they can't act in their own best interest is futile, and inevitably leads to more problems.

"Territorial protection, rating systems, and stricter requirements for affiliation might appear to help your affiliate in the short term, but they would eventually hurt everyone involved, including you. It might allow you to monopolize a certain amount of high-intensity functional training in your area, but until CrossFit HQ starts deploying tactical units to arrest people for doing thrusters at local gyms, your 'protected' affiliate would just be an endorsement of mediocrity. Without competition, you have no incentive to improve your product. This complacency would eventually dull the constantly alive, open-source revolution that is CrossFit. And when that happens, it will hurt CrossFit—and that would hurt us all."

CrossFit HQ's libertarian philosophy is consistent: excellence is the only source of sustainable advantage. Trainers are leaders. If they're good leaders, their people will stay. The relationships between coaches and athletes, and between the athletes themselves, will keep a group rooted. If a box owner is not a good leader—if his coaching or programming is lacking, or the box isn't socially cohesive—he should view competition as a spur to improve. If he doesn't want to step up his game, he shouldn't be surprised when a better leader builds a larger, stronger tribe in the same hunting ground.

Ben Bergeron, who runs CrossFit New England,[18] delivers a compelling sermon on coaching acumen as the test and evidence of leadership, published as a *CrossFit Journal* essay, "The Deeper Side of Coaching." "The essence of CrossFit coaching is to get our clients to move better," he begins.[19] "Good coaches can see faults and have the tools, knowledge and ability to correct these faults. If you can get your athletes to consistently move better, you are a considered a 'good coach.'

"But what then makes a 'great coach'?"

Great coaches, he says, connect with their athletes by being intensely aware and attuned to the person in front of them. Not just the fine details of movement—whether knees are tracking over the feet, or shoulders are in the right position—but what the athlete is thinking and feeling. "Is your athlete absorbing the message or is he lost?" Bergeron asks. "Is he motivated by competition or turned off by it? Does he like the spotlight or the shadows? Does he learn visually or verbally? Is he in a good mood today? Is his mind somewhere else? Is he moving faster or slower than usual? Are you making a true connection with your athlete? What is his goal? Not everyone is training to get a better 'Fran' time."

Any great trainer brings focused attention and awareness to his work, inside or outside a CrossFit box. But because affiliates are running their own businesses, Bergeron argues, they are responsible for setting an example in their personal character and conduct. His favorite case in point is gossip: a bunch of people hanging around after class and talking lightheartedly about someone who isn't around. If a coach joins that conversation, he's basically telling the gang that when they're out of earshot, he'll gossip about them too. "Conversely, if you opt not to join in that gossip but, on the flip side, defend that person when they're not present, what you're saying to those people that are present is, when you're not here, I'm going to defend you.

"One of the most visible displays of integrity is being loyal to those who are not present," he concludes. "You always lead with integrity.

People will follow your lead. That's where the community starts."[20] The community bonds of a CrossFit gym are most obvious in its congregational activities: the charity events and the celebration of birthdays and holidays, the happy hours and competition teams and the way dozens of people show up to cheer those teams. But on a day-to-day level, in quiet, subtle ways, the trust and respect of athletes is earned by coaches who lead by example, in ways that transcend the correct form for an overhead squat.

It is hard to imagine a globo-gym trainer designing a workout routine that drums out blowhards and narcissists. But this is what Bergeron explicitly promises to do, on CrossFit New England's home page: "There are no egos, no room for bad attitudes. Those type of people just don't last here."[21] The site also asks prospective members to check whether the class they can attend still has open slots, because the gym is close to capacity. It is unheard-of for a globo-gym to create speed bumps to a membership sale because peak times are crowded. That's something for a member to find out later, after committing to a year of payments. It probably won't affect members anyway, because they're statistically unlikely to show up on a regular basis.

But a CrossFit box doesn't make money by charging low fees to thousands of members who don't show up. It makes money by charging a premium to a couple of hundred people who attend religiously. If a conventional gym is a kind of fitness feedlot, herding members into tightly packed rows of cardio machines, a CrossFit box is grazing organic free-range livestock. It's a smaller-scale enterprise. With one class running at a time, there are usually about twenty people working out at any given time. Most boxes run seven or eight classes a day: three or four in the morning, three after work, and one lunchtime session. There are a few warehouse megaboxes running multiple classes at once, but most boxes top out at two hundred to three hundred members making full use of 5,000 square feet.

AS ANY SHOPPER KNOWS, FREE-RANGE ORGANIC MEAT IS A more expensive proposition. CrossFit memberships are typically $150 to $200 a month. That's pricey compared with the monthly fees of a machine-based fitness club. It might be ten times what you'd pay to access a high-volume/low-price twenty-four-hour keycard facility. But a CrossFitter who hits four WODs a week is getting sixteen training sessions a month. He's not getting 100% of a trainer's attention, but he's getting enough instruction, cueing, and coaching to build skill from session to session and to set personal records month over month. Compared with paying a globo-gym personal trainer $50 to $75 an hour, it's a good value, and the results justify the cost. CrossFitters with three to six months under their belts are measurably stronger and faster. They can do things that, when they started, seemed impossible. They look better, but in the end, this is not what motivates them.

What keeps them going, and makes it almost impossible to go back to a globo-gym, is a change in their identity: they become athletes. If they were never athletes, they are on a team, with a coach, for the first time. If they played sports in high school or college, they get to experience the competition and banter and sweat and smell of the old weight room. The sense of belonging that happens in tournaments and on road trips comes from having ridiculous amounts of energy to squander, and burning that energy to compete as a group. Most athletes, after school, think that feeling is like first love and a full hairline, lost forever. Until they find it again, in some converted auto body workshop. Along with their genetic endowment for sports, they bring a deep and abiding gratitude with them into the box. It's given them back their varsity letter.

The small group size of a CrossFit gym is part of what makes its social fabric so strong. Even though it's an artifact of how CrossFit trainers use physical space, the carrying capacity of a CrossFit box happens to match the tribal size of Pleistocene hunter-gatherers whose tribes typically numbered between 110 and 230.[22] A daily shared struggle to survive, in groups of this size, defined the human experience for tens of thousands of years. Like the ritual of a Hero WOD, it is a buried genetic memory.

Joining the sprint and clang of a WOD is physically difficult. But it is socially easy, because everybody from elite firebreathers to journeyman and novice CrossFitters has tacitly agreed to test their limits. Firebreathers load up the bars as prescribed. Beginners scale down and modify the movements, enough to make them achievable but still all-consuming. As long as there's nothing left to burn when the WOD is over, everyone feels like they're a part of it. The strongest person may have lifted the equivalent weight of three cars, and the weakest may have hauled the weight of three refrigerators. But the stronger person isn't more central to the experience or the group. If the weaker person is pushing harder than the strong person, in some ways the weaker athlete has more status.

The only way to feel not included in a WOD is to slack. Because athletes scale the workouts in different ways, performing at a sub capacity level isn't obvious. No one would ever be called out for dogging the workout (although a coach might ask, after class, if everything is okay). It just creates a gnawing sense of free ridership.

When a veteran encourages a beginner, it's an acknowledgment that exhaustion is a common denominator. Elite athletes, flat on their backs, are no less exhausted than rank beginners. Elite athletes are probably even more exhausted because they've learned how to tolerate a higher level of discomfort. Sometimes beginners, building muscle memory with lighter weights, are quicker to recover, while the strongest athletes seem to suffer the most.

In this respect, CrossFit is the exact opposite of what kids experience in PE class. Weaker, starting-out athletes—the kids who would have been picked last—are cheered by stronger athletes who would have lapped them on the track. The last two or three athletes to finish, a mix of heavily loaded high performers and newcomers laboring on a downscaled last round, hear "Last set!" and "You got this!" from their peers on the sidelines.

It's counterintuitive, but one of the big reasons beginners drop out of CrossFit is a perfectionist streak: being coached or boosted means you're not doing everything perfectly (in front of people!), and this can be mortifying to a certain sort of person. Social perfectionists either bow out, or stay and accept the cultural norm that people at all levels struggle. Being able to appreciate, or at least tolerate, a holler of support is part of the equation. Finish-line esprit de corps varies from box to box and from country to country. Gregarious coaches foster gregarious boxes. But any box is more gregarious than a globo-gym—so much so that CrossFitters moving to a new city will find a box they like and look for housing within a radius of the box. It's the fastest way for a transplant to establish a new local set of friends.

Viewed through a business lens, the rampant proliferation of CrossFit boxes looks like a new market or product category, driven by a huge number of small businesses. But if you think of affiliates as social groups, CrossFit's big bang looks like an explosion of voluntary associations, the kind whose demise Robert Putnam mourned in *Bowling Alone*. CrossFit boxes have a strong sense of tribal identity. When a CrossFitter visits a box in another city, he's introduced by name and home affiliate: "This is Matt from LoCo CrossFit in Leesburg, Virginia." And when Matt, wearing the LoCo team shirt, hears "3-2-1-GO!," he feels pressure to perform, to represent his Leesburg homeboys. No one dropping into an Equinox from an LA Fitness has ever experienced that.

Communities, especially face-to-face communities of a couple of hundred people, have a much higher long-term survival rate than new businesses. In the United States, a start-up business providing services has less than a 50/50 chance of celebrating its fifth year in operation.[23] The five-year survival rate for CrossFit boxes, from 2008 to 2012, ranges from 95% to 98%, depending on how the statistic is calculated.[24] And those were some pretty rough, belt-tightening years.

A month before half the US mortgage market tumbled into federal receivership, Jason Khalipa opened his first CrossFit gym, NorCal CrossFit, in Santa Clara. It was 1,200 square feet. There were six months left on the lease, and he vowed to outgrow the space before the lease was up. The son of a Syrian Christian who emigrated from Iran during the 1979 Islamic Revolution, he had what a lot of immigrants' children thirst for: his own business. He spent all day at the box. He slept there.

Six months later, as the Dow Jones Industrial Average continued to free-fall, Khalipa moved a hundred CrossFit NorCal members to a 3,000-square-foot space with eighteen months on the lease. When that lease was up, he moved twice as many members into 8,000 square feet. He opened another box in Mountain View, and two in San Jose. The promotional knack that had made him a star salesman at the globo-gym was in full effect. But now he had a product he believed in. In Silicon Valley parlance, he was eating his own dog food. And if new members didn't like it, they were free to walk any time. No contracts.

The idea of forcing people to pay for something they don't want is repugnant to Khalipa, as it would be to any affiliate. The whole phenomenon is philosophically consistent, from an individual athlete's performance to an affiliate's business practices. It's based on freedom and accountability: Freedom to scale the workout, and the accountability of scores on the whiteboard. Autonomy from the micromanaging franchise corporations, and accountability to members who can cancel their memberships at will. Those members are not bound by a legal contract. But they are bound by a social contract. It's the one that Amundson defined back in Santa Cruz: listen, acquire skill, use judgment, encourage others, put your name and results on the board, work on your weaknesses.

The world is full of heavy things to carry and distance to cover. Cheap industrial space becomes training ground, a gathering place, a playground. Barbells, pulled straight up the center line of the body, shave shins en route from the floor. Calluses rip. A newcomer tries jumping on the box instead of stepping up onto it. Three or four people yell "Get it! Get it! Get it!" as a guy locks out his first muscle-up. The place is suffused with the unmistakable smell of a CrossFit box: a mixture of plywood, chalk powder, rubber matting, and the asphalt/ beef-jerky tang of bumper plates. A heavy brass ship's bell, the kind you can hear a block away, is mounted on the wall. Anytime someone hits a personal record, the bell clangs. It is a world away from the globo-gym filled with cardio machines, televisions, and no-show members captive to their contracts.

"People walk in here and they ask, 'Where are the machines?'" says Khalipa.

"*We* are the machines."

CAVEMAN KOSHER
Post-WOD Potlucks and the Paleo Diet

AFTER A YEAR AND A HALF IN THE BLUE ROOM, JERRY HILL KNEW it was time to find another space. The jujitsu studio had been an inexpensive way to get started, but running down stairs to sprint outside, taking shoes off to protect the mats, and not being able to drop weights was a drag. The owner was accommodating. But the dojo was someone else's space, and someone else's space would never feel like home. There is something about having your own four walls that beckons young adults and couples and garage start-ups. It makes them feel like their efforts are legitimate, that they've come into their own.

In mid-2008, Jerry had just enough athletes to justify the lease of a dedicated space a couple of miles away. The place had been a car wash, and a vestigial driveway at the entrance sloped down toward double doors. Regrading the front of the space with concrete would be idiotically expensive. So this would be the spot for squat racks, rowers, and other gear that wouldn't roll down the slope.

When Jerry posted a Facebook request for help getting the pull-up rig assembled and anchored, Dan Wilson was the first to volunteer. "Have muscles, will provide support," Wilson replied. "No real tool skills though!" If there was a Marine who needed help migrating CrossFit equipment to a new facility, as the Pendleton Marines had done, Wilson was the self-appointed go-to guy. Semper Fi.

As it turned out, Greg Glassman was in town to give a speech at the

Naval War College, where Wilson was getting his master's degree. Tagging along with Wilson the next day, Glassman stopped in to check out the Blue Room, which was in many ways a carbon copy of his original martial-arts sublease, back in the day. Same blue mats, same compromises, taking shoes off and not being able to drop weights. He checked out the new space, with its bare concrete floors and fresh paint. The pride and excitement in Jerry's eyes was the same as his own chest-thumping sense of ownership on Research Drive. With a box of their own, the Santa Cruz CrossFitters had thrown themselves into Olympic lifts and out-the-door sprints and become firebreathers. The Blue Room gang at CrossFit Oldtown would be no different.

On January 20, 2009, the new space was ready to move into. All Jerry needed was the muscle to carry about 3,000 pounds of bars, bumper plates, and other gear down two flights of stairs, load it into vehicles, and unload it on the other side. It was a perfect testament to functional fitness. "I need your help," he posted to Facebook. "The WOD on Sunday is moving day! No class but plenty of lifting—whattya think we have been doing so much strength work for? Let's meet at 0900 in the Blue Room and move the entire contents to CFOT v.2.0."

On Sunday morning, a Ford 350 hauling a forty-foot flatbed trailer pulled up to the jujitsu studio. The driver, Pete Stramese, was a crew coach at T. C. Williams High School in Alexandria, and he was hauling the trailer that carried fiberglass racing shells to rowing events. In less than fifteen minutes, 3,000 pounds of equipment was hustled down two flights of stairs and loaded onto the rowing trailer. In short order, it was all unloaded through CrossFit Oldtown's double doors on Royal Street. It is difficult to imagine the members of a globo-gym showing up on a weekend to help the franchise owner move cardio and Cybex machines, even if they were strong and coordinated enough to do so.

One long wall of the new box had been been painted a deep primary blue, to match the color of the old jujitsu mats. Like newlyweds, the gang was elated at the sight of mundane fixtures that were special because they were "our own." Our *own* rubber floor matting, just waiting to have fully loaded barbells thunderously dropped on it. Our *own* cubbies, bathrooms, water fountains. "It finally feels like we're a family. We have a home," said one of the gang. "We do," another replied on her blog, "and a beautiful, spacious one, with lots of toys, at that."[1]

ALMOST IMMEDIATELY, CROSSFIT OLDTOWN ESTABLISHED A monthly potluck social gathering. On the first Friday of the month, everybody got to choose their own workout: a Hero or a Girl, a one-rep max or some self-determined benchmark. Then they'd go home and change, or shower at the box, for a 7:00 p.m. party in street clothes. Accustomed to seeing their fellow CrossFitters in the exhausted flop sweat of post-WOD cool-down, Oldtowners were surprised to see how well their peers cleaned up. Very few people had seen Harold Doran wear a shirt for more than five minutes, ever

Tables were unfolded. Bowls and plates of food were laid out to cover them. But the food in these bowls and plates bore scant resemblance to the edibles at most congregational potlucks. No pizza, pasta casseroles, sandwiches, puff-pastry canapés, chips, pretzels, or crackers alongside the cheese. No cake or candy, sweetened beverages or juice. Instead, there was meat: giant aluminum trays of barbecued pulled pork and sliced flank steak. Platters of fresh vegetables and fruit with nut butter dips. And bacon. Lots and lots of bacon. Bacon-wrapped asparagus. Bacon-wrapped shrimp. Bacon bits mixed into the yolks of deviled eggs. Stumped for a crowd-pleasing recipe, CrossFitters reach for bacon like 1950s American housewives reached for mayonnaise.

In a mainstream food culture that equates "light" with "healthy," CrossFit's diet culture bucks conventional wisdom with heretical amounts of fat. There are lots of nuts, egg yolks, coconut milk, and avocados. For people who eat dairy products, skim is replaced with more high-octane grades of milk, butter, and heavy cream. The consumption of animal fat at CrossFit gatherings is gleeful and unstinting. As a popular T-shirt proclaims, "Meat Is Murder. Tasty, Tasty Murder."

As with their dedication to "constantly varied functional movement, executed at high intensity" in a way that's "measurable, observable, repeatable," CrossFitters' rejection of refined carbohydrates has a strong empirical rationale. Their personal experiences provide firsthand evidence that dropping sugar and starch eliminates body fat, regardless of how much they eat. But there's also a substantial body of scientific evidence to support their firsthand conclusions.

The physiological mechanism for this counterintuitive insight, exhaustively documented by science writer Gary Taubes,[2] is as follows: Refined carbohydrates quickly raise blood sugar (glucose) levels, which triggers the pancreas to release the hormone insulin. Insulin causes the tissues of the body to absorb blood sugar, and a spike in blood sugar elevates insulin until the sugar is absorbed and glucose levels drop. People whose blood sugar levels are always high, because they're constantly eating refined carbohydrates, also have elevated levels of insulin. Over time, tissues bathed in chronically high levels of insulin lose their sensitivity to the hormone. As insulin sensitivity drops, blood sugar levels climb even higher, which triggers the pancreas to produce even more insulin. The cycle viciously repeats. If unabated, the result is what we now call Type 2 diabetes.

But insulin doesn't just regulate sugar. It also regulates the absorption of fatty acids, which the body also uses for fuel, into fat cells for storage. When carbohydrate-boosted insulin levels are high, fat cells grab more fatty acids out of the blood and convert them into stored fat that accumulates under our skin and around our organs. Essentially, the high insulin level is telling the fat cells, "There's a lot of sugar floating around. If the cells burn fatty acids instead of sugar, we'll never clear this glucose backlog, so get those fats out of circulation, into storage, and keep 'em there until the sugar gets chewed up. When that happens, we'll be ready to take some fat out of storage. You'll know we're ready for that when insulin drops. Don't call us; we'll call you."

If a carbohydrate-rich diet keeps insulin levels high, the fat never gets released, *even when blood sugar is low*, because elevated insulin is telling the fat cells to hold on to fatty acids like grim death. The result, Taubes argues—and this is the controversial part—is an obese person who feels ravenously hungry but is actually starving on a cellular level, even though her body is cloaked in fat. Because of carbohydrate-driven insulin elevation, her fat cells keep grabbing the fatty acids out of her blood and depriving her body of their availability as fuel. If she tries to cut calories without cutting carbohydrates to lower her insulin level, the cellular starvation gets more severe and triggers the typical symptoms of semi-starvation: a lower metabolic rate, which makes her move less and generate less heat, and a semi-starving person's fixation on and obsessive thoughts of food.

Cut carbs, and these phenomena abate, even if the total number of calories goes up. In controlled experiments, when carbohydrates are eliminated, people don't feel hungry even when their caloric intake is significantly reduced, and don't put on weight even when their caloric intake is jacked up. When they eat more, their metabolism goes up. They get hotter, and they move around more. Conversely, subjects on a high-carbohydrate diet constantly feel hungry, even when their intake goes up by thousands of calories a day. When their caloric intake is cut, their metabolism slows down. They move around less, and feel cold. They lose some weight, but when food intake goes back to normal, their weight shoots back up to normal and sometimes higher, as post-famine gorging pushes insulin levels to unprecedented heights.

With an avalanche of research citations and a capsule course in endocrinology and biochemistry, Taubes argues persuasively that refined carbs, not fats, are the root of all metabolic evil. The conventional wisdom of "calories in, calories out" and "a calorie is a calorie" is, in H. L. Mencken's words, "clear, simple, and wrong." And the public health establishment's promotion of a low-fat, high-carbohydrate diet has made the obesity epidemic worse. In short, the middle aisles of the grocery store, including the boxes marked "high fiber," "heart healthy," and "organic," are making us simultaneously fat, hungry, and sick.

Taubes's thesis dovetails perfectly with the Paleo Diet favored by CrossFitters. The core tenet of the Paleo Diet is that the human digestive system evolved before agriculture, and so it is fundamentally geared for the diet of a Paleolithic hunter-gatherer. As *Homo sapiens* shifted from hunting and gathering to agriculture, our genes stayed essentially the same. Therefore, the argument goes, the modern diet is fundamentally inappropriate for the biology of our bodies, which truly thrive only on the nutritional template of the Stone Age. Basically, it all went south ten thousand years ago. The prescription is to approximate the diet of our caveman forebears, to the extent possible, and eat lots of vegetables and meat while eliminating new-fangled Neolithic dairy and grains. Industrial foodstuffs—refined sugar and high-fructose corn syrup, lunch meats, and anything that's been a slurry at any point in its production—are the fourth horseman of the Apocalypse.

The key characteristic the Paleo Diet is its overwhelming emphasis not on what to consume, but on what to reject. In this sense, it is like any religious dietary code and draws on the same narrative: In the beginning, we existed in a state of innocent perfection, ideally adapted to our hunter-gatherer environment. And then we tasted sin, in the form of cultivated wheat and beans and vegetables that were bred to be more appetizing than the roots and leaves we'd been gathering from the wild. And all that sinful, toxic gluten, lectin, and other plant proteins banished us from our state of grace. Poisoned and corrupted, we live in a fallen world. We can never return to our Edenic past, because nothing available to the modern shopper, even the grass-raised meat and organic vegetables, bears the slightest resemblance to what Paleolithic human beings actually ate. But by rejecting abominable foods, we can purify ourselves.

It may be true. But it's also Leviticus. The Old Testament litany of unclean foods that forms the basis of kosher law is also the book that lays out the rules for ritual sacrifice. It's not a coincidence that Paleo dieters describe their favored fare as "clean food" and the transition to the Paleo Diet as "getting clean."[3]

But this is why it works. Religious dietary taboos are a lot more effective at getting people to restrict their eating behavior than the sternest warnings of medical authorities. If a public health agency or a medical journal or even your own doctor tells you to change your diet, it's easy to rationalize ways to ignore their advice. "Everything in moderation"

or "I just want to enjoy my life" is all it takes to dismiss nutritional guidance from the experts, even if you believe they have your best interests
at heart.

For someone following an unconventional diet on their own, the
social cost of bucking mainstream eating habits—the squints from coworkers as sandwich bread is discarded, the passive aggression of the
menopausal office food-pusher when her brownies are declined—can
only be weighed against a lonely sense of "sticking to it." But for people
observing tribal dietary customs like keeping kosher or halal or CrossFit
Paleo, the social cost is more than offset by a sense of kinship that grows
stronger every time they peel off the bread, toss the bag of chips, ignore
the cookie plate.

When you choose not to eat the corrupt and unclean foods of the
Outsiders, you reaffirm your tribal membership, even if members of
the tribe are not around to witness it. The more rooted you feel in your
tribal identity, the easier it is to routinely make nonconformist choices,
even if nutritional nonconformity has a social cost. It's not an individual
consumer decision. It's an act of social allegiance.

For most people in the globo-gym supermarket world, food choices
are individual consumer decisions, and have been for generations. But
choices about what to eat and not to eat have drawn bright lines around
social groups for thousands of years. It's not a coincidence that the Paleo
Diet became popular as CrossFit affiliates exploded in number. CrossFit
boxes are the tribal bond that makes the diet stick.[4]

CRUCIBLE
The 2009 CrossFit Games

IN 2009, THE CROSSFIT GAMES GO GLOBAL. WHAT STARTED AS an informal throw-down at a California ranch now has regional qualifiers in the United States and Canada, Europe, Asia, Africa, Australia, South America, and online, where far-flung athletes post videos of their qualifying WODs. Rogue Fitness is providing all the gear as the Games official equipment sponsor. Jason Khalipa and Caity Matter are competing as Rogue-sponsored athletes—the first CrossFit athletes to garner any sort of endorsement.

At the Mid-Atlantic regionals in Virginia Beach, Jerry Hill is a volunteer judge. On the 21-15-9 squat snatch pull-up WOD, he's counting reps for an Air Force wife named Nicole Gordon. Like many military wives, Nicole found CrossFit through her husband's warrior-fitness grapevine. She was home in Virginia Beach, five months pregnant and chasing a toddler around, when her husband, Jeremy, came home from Korea for a visit. He was raving about CrossFit and thought it'd be a perfect way for Nicole to stay in shape after the baby arrived. "You won't have to drag both kids to the YMCA—you could do it here at home! I'll send you the workouts from Korea!"

As soon as Nicole was medically cleared for exercise, she and Jeremy started trading CrossFit WOD results back and forth from Korea. As the weeks and months passed, Nicole became stronger and leaner— but also fiercer, more confident. Something about the ritual intensity of CrossFit training was pulling her toward the Dark Place, as she calls it: the psychic trench where a person looks for strength when the body seems to have nothing left. There is a reserve cache of power buried in this place. But it is spiritually difficult and painful to reach in and dig that power out.

For a woman whose life revolves around supporting others—the husband, the kids, keeping the house and everything going single-handedly—the Dark Place is where all the emotional habits of a good wife, sister, mother, neighbor, and gal-pal are incinerated. No one else matters. There's no compassion. It is the ruthless headspace of a cornered animal.

"It's kind of an indescribable place. I know what it takes to go there. But I don't do that very often," she says. "I just reserve it for special times, because, emotionally, I cry when I come out of that. It taps into something very deep, and it makes me even cry thinking about it. There's something very deep about those times in your life that took every ounce of effort in your being. It's an extreme emotional trial, even more than an extreme physical trial. You have to be emotionally ready to push your body and mind to an extreme limit, when your body is telling you no, being willing to say yes.

"In the Dark Place, it is all you. It is all a battle against yourself. It is almost like everybody else disappears," she says. "None of that talking-yourself-through-it happens in that Dark Place. You just go. And afterward, the emotion of that experience just overwhelms you."[1]

At the 2009 Mid-Atlantic regionals, Nicole is in the Dark Place. As she staggers under her last set of lifts, Jerry is transfixed by the intensity of her effort. He has never seen anything like it. On her last pull-up, he notices her chin doesn't quite make it over the bar, and he calls a no-rep, knowing the worst thing an athlete can hear from a judge at the end of a WOD is that she's not actually done. Nicole scrambles back to the bar, gives her hips one last explosive swing to propel herself over the bar, and collapses on the ground.

She is on the floor, and her heart is pounding. Heat is radiating from her exhausted body as her husband Jeremy, tattooed and shirtless from his own competition round, breaks through a crowd of spectators to kneel beside her. He covers her with his arm, cradles her sweaty head, and nuzzles her sweaty neck. "I love you," he says. "You made it."

Jerry steps back, shocked and fascinated. *I don't want to judge this anymore,* he decides about competition, which makes regular CrossFit training look like a globo-gym workout. *I want to do this—or coach people to do this.*

Nicole ends up taking second to Christy Phillips, a nursing student, and both travel to Aromas for the CrossFit Games' last year at the ranch. Because the field has been winnowed at the regional level, there are half as many individual competitors as at the 2008 Games, and five times as many fans in the stands. Four thousand CrossFitters have assembled to watch their strongest peers vie for the titles of Fittest Man and Fittest Woman on Earth.

For Glassman, this competition is a means of inquiry. It's part of his ongoing experiment: if you release an inherently variable and modifiable open-source training method into a population of athletes, and each of them puts their own spin on it, what works? Stage a competition that pushes genetically gifted, highly trained athletes to the limits of their capabilities and find out.

A large barn houses the athletes' warm-up area and medic station. Above the door is a banner trumpeting CrossFit's manifest destiny: "The strength and value of CrossFit lies entirely within our dominance of other athletes," it announces with Glassman's characteristic combination of militance and Barnum. "This is a truth divined through competition, not debate."

"You're standing in the world's proving grounds for elite fitness," Glassman declares. "The men and women competing here today have a legitimate claim to the title of fittest men and women on earth, by the same rights and logic that Lakers, the Steelers, the Penguins, and the Phillies are the best basketball team, the best football team, the best ice hockey team, and the best baseball team on earth. Let the Games begin."

The theme of this year's games is "The Unknown and the Unknowable," and the athletes have been promised that no one has done any of the workouts that make up the Games, or even performed many of the movements in competition.[2] The first day's WODs are announced the night before the event, and there is an element of uncertainty, even fear, as returning champions find the ground has shifted under their feet. As CrossFit has absorbed more and more elite athletes, the Games' competitive pool has gotten bigger and deeper. The WODs have gotten harder and heavier. The event itself seems to have morphed into a survival challenge, not just a test of strength and speed. Many of CrossFit's well-known names find themselves failing amid a new crop of champions from overseas.

Greg Amundson, CrossFit Santa Cruz's original firebreather, fails to even qualify. Despite a personal invitation from Glassman to join the athletes in Aromas, Amundson decides that showing up to compete as the founder's favored son wouldn't be an honorable way to go. It would tarnish the purity of the Games, and his own self-respect, not to earn his place in the arena like everybody else. He won't go unless he can win a legitimate spot in the Last Chance Qualifier, an opportunity for athletes from all regions to give it one last shot at Aromas.

In the Last Chance Qualifier, staged online, three WODs are announced in the morning and must be performed, and video uploaded, within twenty-four hours. One of the WODs includes jump rope doubleunders. Simply defined, a double-under is jumping once while whipping a jump rope under your feet twice. It's not the most taxing movement in the CrossFit repertoire. But it takes skill and timing. There's a knack to double-unders that requires trial, error, and practice before a person finally "gets it" and can string them together.

Double-unders are the only Zen element of CrossFit, one of the few instances in which it's possible to do better by not trying quite as hard. The unfocused focus of double-unders is about timing under fatigue. Nerves have to trigger movement along different axes at different rates: wrists rotate while ankles and calves flex vertically at half the speed. The task is to keep the body locked into the counter-

point of wrist and leg movements while the aerobic demands of the
movement flood the brain with noise: the rapid, irregular rhythm of
breathing and a spiking heart rate. Two variable meters of heart and
lungs boom over the double metronome you're trying to maintain
with your hands and feet. It's "pat your head and rub your tummy"
on a unicycle in gale-force winds—as much a neurological exercise as
a cardiovascular one.

The morning of the Last Chance Qualifier, Amundson's wife is up
early to check the WODs online. She wakes him up. "Honey, do you
know how to do a double-under?" Amundson tries to remember the
last time he's even held a rope in his hands. All these years that he's
been preaching "constantly varied movements," Amundson hasn't
exactly followed the CrossFit main site's prescriptions. He's been
cherry-picking the stuff he's good at—fast heavy lifts and strenuous
gymnastic movements—and getting incredibly good at them, while
not bothering with less macho stuff like double-unders. But it's jump
rope, he figures. How hard could it be for someone with a sub-three-
minute "Fran" time?

Amundson, his wife, and his friend Paul Szoldra, an active-duty
Marine, drive out to CrossFit Camp Pendleton, storied home of the
original Santa Cruz equipment. There is a special magic in this place,
as if all the early firebreathers' physical force was cast into the apparatus that absorbed their energy. The first Girl WODs were con-
cocted with these racks, rings, medicine balls, and boxes. The gear's
heavy use by young, tough Marines has only amplified and deepened
its provenance and aura. This is where Amundson wants to make his
competitive stand.

The first WOD is "Jackie": a 1000-meter row, 50 thrusters with 45
pounds, and 30 pull-ups. It's right in Amundson's wheelhouse, and he
nails it in 5:55. In the rest interval between the first and second WOD,
he tries to learn double-unders, only to discover that he can't do them.
After trawling the web for instructional videos, he finds a helpful set
of step-by-step progressions and cues by Jon Gilson, the owner of a
speed-rope company that manufactures high-end double-under ropes,

the niche-iest of niche items for CrossFitters. By the time Amundson is ready to tackle the next WOD, he can string ten double-unders together. He spends the next two hours practicing double-unders before he has to perform them in the final WOD.

With a "Three, two, one, GO!," the WOD begins, and Amundson gets ten consecutive double-unders before tripping on the rope. Trying to hold on to the mojo, he picks up the rope and attempts to clear his mind. To his utter shock, he whips through thirty-three double-unders in a row. Based on his performance in previous WODs, a ticket to the Games is within reach. This is doable.

On rep forty-four, Amundson misses, and things begin to unravel. He spends the next mortifying minute in a series of failed start-overs, and at one point is unable to execute a single successful jump. His brain and body are crossing signals. The knack is gone, only to flicker back into existence for the last seven reps of his first set.

After his fumbling sequence of double-unders, Amundson grinds through his second set of ten 275-pound deadlifts. He wades through the next set of double-unders by alternating single-under and double-under jumps. He finishes, wrecked, in seven minutes and twenty seconds. On a second attempt before dawn the next morning, just under the time cutoff for uploading video, his time is ten seconds slower. The original firebreather has been humbled by a jump rope.[3]

But Amundson is not the only elite athlete to fall by the wayside. In Aromas, the first workout is a brutal 7-kilometer trail run with five seriously steep ascents and descents. A creek bed cuts along a middle stretch of the course. "Don't go down there," warns Dave Castro, the Games ringmaster and athletic programmer, whose parents' ranch this is. "There's lots of poison oak down there."

An escalating ladder of heavy deadlifts begins in ninety minutes. So athletes who finish the trail run in thirty minutes will have sixty minutes to recover. Athletes who take an hour will have only thirty minutes to rest. Slower athletes must start the second workout first, so they have less time to recover, and begin the next leg at a disadvantage. The reward for finishing first or early isn't just rank. It's rest.

It's brutal, the way that survival in the wild is brutal: when the pack moves, slower animals (or people) get less rest and become more vulnerable. In a real-world survival scenario, the difference between good leaders and bad leaders is that good leaders gauge the fatigue of the group's weakest members and set the pace accordingly. Bad leaders let the strongest members of the group set the pace, then berate stragglers who run out of steam or get injured. But this event is not about keeping a group alive. It's a test of individuals, and how to separate strong individuals from an even stronger pack.

As the race begins, morning light shines through dried grasses along the road. Dust from the runners' feet begins to rise. By the time they reach the top of the first hill, athletes are walking with hands on their thighs. These are not endurance athletes who train for steep runs in dry heat. They're sprinters used to gunning down 100 or 400 meters, or doing a flat mile to benchmark their speed.

In the lead are Russell Berger, Chris Spealler, and Mikko Salo, a Finnish firefighter whose bony Scandinavian face bears a striking resemblance to Viggo Mortensen's. For someone who lives 370 miles from the Arctic Circle, Mikko seems surprisingly at ease in the desert scrub. Spealler, five feet five ("on a tall day") with his hair buzzed off, is a lean 139 pounds, shirtless and agile. With his trademark headphones, sunglasses, and mountain-trained lungs, he seems insulated from the toll this event is taking on sea-level athletes from California and the East Coast.

Jason Khalipa, last year's champion, is in thirty-fifth place at the bottom of the first steep slope. He is, at heart, a weightlifter, 205 pounds of muscle packed onto a five feet nine frame, and he's having a tough time hauling all that meat uphill. His female counterpart, Caity Matter, last year's champion, isn't faring much better as she slogs toward a finish in sixty-fourth place.

The steepest hill, halfway through the course, puts competitors on their hands and knees on the way up, and has many of them sliding on the way back down. Loping up the slope on his hands and feet, like some kind of desert cat, Spealler is in first place.

Tanya Wagner, the Pennsylvania PE teacher and Division I college goalie who came in second in last year's Games, is seeing asses right in front of her face, all the way up the hill. As she descends, she hears gravel falling down from the feet of people just above her and prays, "Dear God, please don't let them slip. They'll wipe me out," as she slides down, grasping and holding on to weeds to keep the slide from turning into a tumble.

Spealler is peeling into the final descent in first place, with Mikko on his heels. Mikko is four inches taller and twenty-five pounds heavier. As he closes the distance between himself and Spealler in the lead, Mikko looks like a predator in the final, fatal moments of a chase. As the hill turns back into flat road, they both veer left, and Mikko charges forward to capture the lead. Spealler stares at this stranger from God-knows-where, who looks like Aragorn from *Lord of the Rings*, and figures, why not let this guy pick the pace, as long as it's not too fast: stay tight, leave something in the tank, and gun it in the end.

As they head into the final stretch, Spealler realizes Mikko is trying to tell him something. He pulls his headphones aside.

"What's that?" he says.

"You still have strength," Mikko asks in a thick Finnish accent. "Energy?"

"Yeah, a little bit. You're Mikko, right?" Spealler extends his hand.

"Yes, I'm Mikko," the Finn replies, and shakes Spealler's hand.

"Nice to meet you, Mikko."

Spealler pulls his headphones back on and tucks back in to draft behind his opponent. Mikko speeds up, and Spealler stays with him until they both spot the tent that marks the finish. Hoping his new friend from the frozen north doesn't have much left, Spealler hits the accelerator and barrels into the finish.[4] The lightest and fastest of the CrossFit brethren hurtles over the line in first place, by a second and a half. It is the only victory he will taste at the Games.

Mikko, unlike many of his competitors, refuses to hit the ground after this or any workout. He explains that he read once, in an article, that when animals surrender, they lie on their backs. From then on, he de-

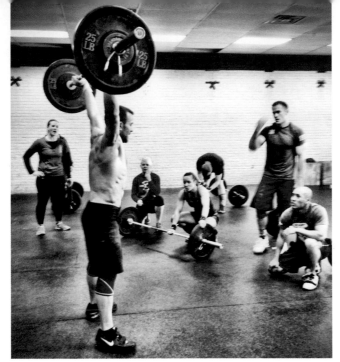

CrossFit Oldtown gathers around their firebreather coach as he burns through a qualifying workout for the 2013 Games. *Photo by Catherine McNally*

Caity Matter, former pro basketball player and Bill Henniger's future wife, crushes the clean and jerk finale of the 2008 CrossFit Games. *Used with permission of CrossFit, Inc.*

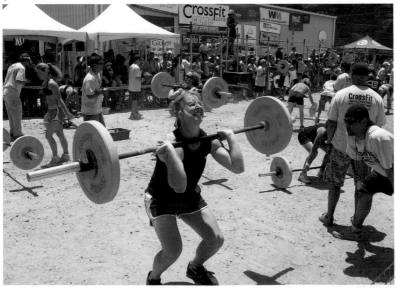

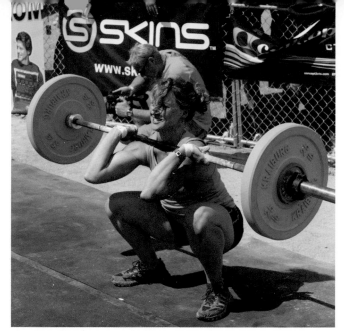

Tanya Wagner grimaces through 15 thrusters in the 2009 CrossFit Games' final chipper. Tanya won the Games in its last year at the Castro ranch. *Used with permission of CrossFit, Inc.*

Nicole Gordon throwing wall balls at the 2009 Games shortly after nailing her finger with a sledgehammer. *Used with permission of CrossFit, Inc.*

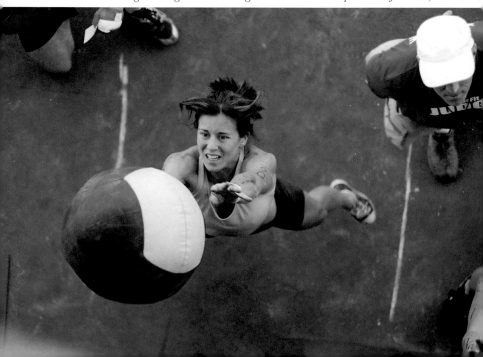

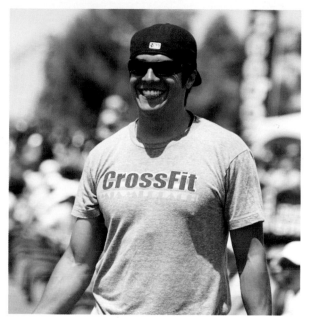

Dave Castro, former Navy SEAL and director of the CrossFit Games. *Used with permission of CrossFit, Inc.*

Greg Glassman, CrossFit's inimitable founder.
Used with permission of CrossFit, Inc.

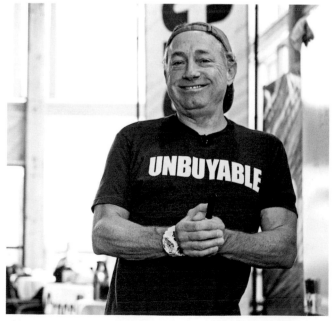

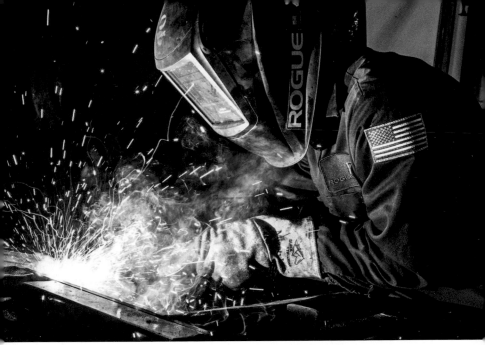

Sparks fly off a steel rig at Rogue, CrossFit's armorer of choice. *Photo by John Cropper for Rogue*

Harvard's Hemenway Gymnasium, shown here in the 1880s, carried the banner for functional fitness. Its director, Dudley Allen Sargent, also invented the pulley machines that ruled gym floors for the next 130 years. *Courtesy of Oldtimestrongman.com*

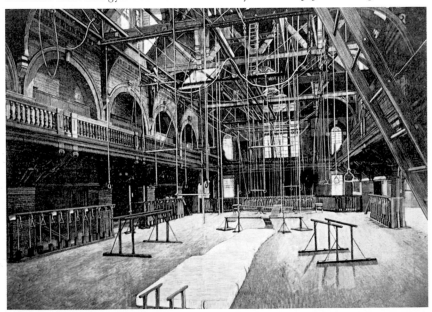

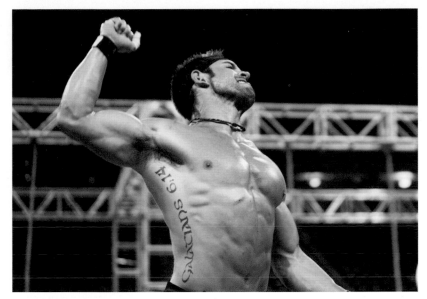

Rich Froning, three-time CrossFit Games champion, celebrates victory in 2011
and makes Galatians 6:14 the most re-Tweeted biblical tattoo in history.
Used with permission of CrossFit, Inc.

Chris Spealler, 142 pounds, pushing a 385-pound sled (with his head) in the
2011 Games—one of many superhuman feats of fortitude that make Spealler a
legend in the CrossFit community. *Used with permission of CrossFit, Inc.*

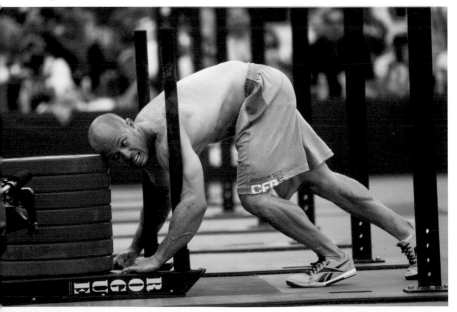

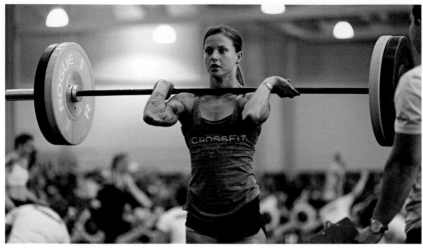

Christmas Abbott, oblivious to the crowd at the 2013 Mid-Atlantic Regionals. *Used with permission of CrossFit, Inc.*

Jerry Hill, wearing Wolverine sideburns for luck, pulls a one-rep-max clean and jerk in the 2013 Masters competition. *Used with permission of CrossFit, Inc.*

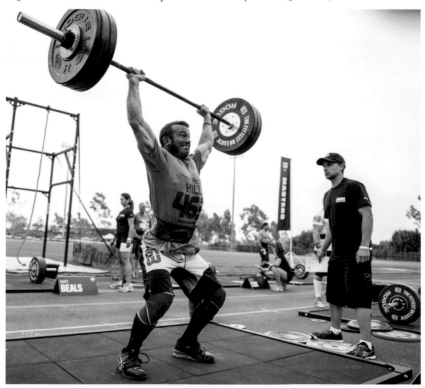

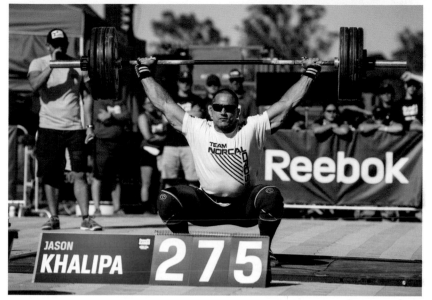

Jason Khalipa, CrossFit's Clydesdale, eases into a 275-pound overhead squat. All day long, baby. *Used with permission of CrossFit, Inc.*

Laura Novotny channels the thrill of post-WOD victory at the 2012 Team Superfit competition. © *Christopher Nolan—MetCon Photos LLC*

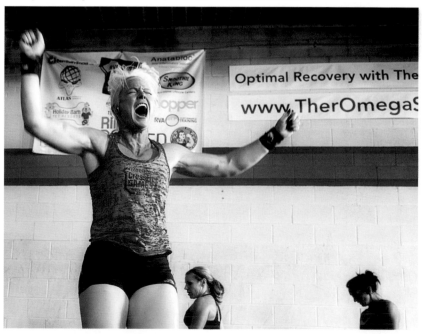

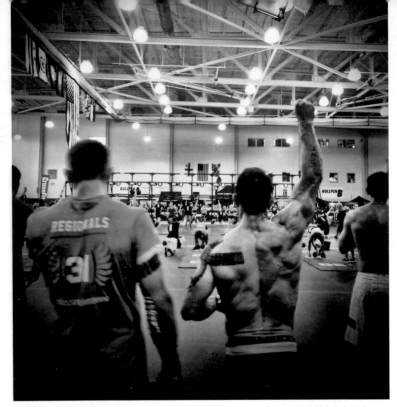

Jerry Hill cheers on the CrossFit Oldtown team at the 2013 Mid-Atlantic Regionals. *Photo by Catherine McNally*

Greg Amundson, celebrating a latter-day athletic victory. *Photo by Mike Hennick*

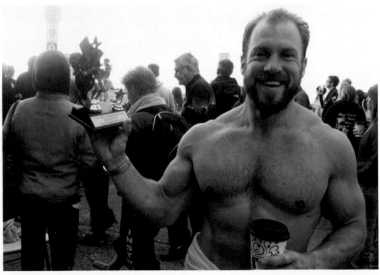

cided he would never lie on his back after a WOD. It was a sign of weakness and surrender. He would never show submission to a workout, even though hitting the deck after a CrossFit workout is an orgasm of relief. Not lying down is Mikko's way of proving he has conquered the workout, not the other way around. It is the purifying ritual of a true ascetic, and entirely consistent with a culture in which people beat themselves with birch branches in the sauna.[5]

Jason Khalipa collapses in the final stretch of the run. Within earshot of the finish line, he is on his belly, dry heaving and groaning on the ground. His calves are cramping, and his whole body feels like it's going to explode. He's never experienced this kind of pain in his life. Two medics rush over to him and ask what's going on.

"I think I'm going to die," he replies.

A medic surveys the big slab of athlete he has to get off the ground, hopefully with some assistance from said athlete. "We're going to pick you up," he says. "We want you to give us a hand. We're going to get you back to medical, stick you in a dunk tank, and hose you off, got it?"

It does not look as if getting up is on Jason Khalipa's agenda. "Want to wait one?" the medic asks. "Okay, I'm going to give you about thirty seconds. I don't want to see you lying on this hot-assed fucking asphalt."

Khalipa groans at a faster rate, "I have poison oak all over me. I can't breathe." The medics are pouring water over his broad back and promising to clean him up and telling him to take slow, deep breaths. A thought flits through his head, as he realizes they want to put him in an ice bath. "Could you take off my iPod please?" The medics roll him over and pull a blue nano on its cord out of his shorts pocket. They ask him if he wants to keep going.

"Fuck, yeah, I'm going to keep going." True to his word, he does get up to lumber through the remainder of the course, finishing seventy-second in 54:35, leaving just 35 minutes to recover before the deadlifts.[6]

James "O.P.T." (Optimum Performance Training) Fitzgerald, winner of the 2007 CrossFit Games, finishes sixth and heads for the physical therapy bench in the barn. As a former champion, he got to skip the regional qualifier and go straight to the Games. But his past victory has not kept his calves from cramping on the hills, and he is grimacing in pain, knowing there's more pain to come.

The next event is the deadlift ladder, with one lift, starting at 315 pounds for men and 185 pounds for women, executed by each athlete every 30 seconds, escalating by 10 pounds at each lift. Athletes move from bar to bar until they fail, and are ranked according to their heaviest successful lifts.

The men's ladder tops out at 505 pounds, even though a few competitors have recorded one-rep maximums of 550 or 600 pounds. But those personal records were set in different conditions, when the athletes were fresh, with 3 to 5 minutes of rest between attempts. CrossFit HQ figures that after humping around the hills for 7 kilometers, the most these guys are going to be able to lift is 75% to 80% of their one-rep max.[7] The strongmen, who were also the slowest on the run, have had barely half an hour to recover.

The rotation signal sounds, relentlessly, every 30 seconds. There is no time to think. Just "Three, two, one, GO!" and the noise of the crowd. Put your hands on the bar, get tension in your hamstrings, go. Drop the bar, move, put your hands on the next bar. Go.

Tanya Wagner's mind is blank. She can't process, in the usual human way, what is going on. There is no internal dialogue. Her body is moving with no conscious control, just muscle memory and animal instinct. Time collapses as her body moves itself from bar to bar, lifting and dropping, *boom, boom, boom,* one after the other. When it's over, she regains awareness and thinks, *holy crap, I just lifted a lot of stuff.* But she doesn't know what the numbers are until the judge tells her the last lift was 325, 25 pounds over her previous PR.

Sixteen men max out the ladder in a tie for first place. Five athletes, including Graham Holmberg, who works out a few miles from Rogue's Ohio foundry, and Jason Khalipa, who passed out on the run, set new personal records for deadlifts on their way up the ladder. Khalipa is five to ten years younger than competitors who trounced him on the run, and he is testament to the regenerative advantage of being twenty-three. Endurance isn't his strong suit. But he can recover faster than anyone.

And the adrenaline of competition has juiced his performance, even after the ordeal of the hill run. Game Day is when personal records happen—this is one of the big reasons CrossFitters compete, even in local throw-downs. When you're up against competitors, and the clock is running in front of spectators, your body performs better than it does in training. Everything is heightened. It's go time.

Mikko gets the 505-pound bar to midthigh but can't lock out his hips. He finishes a point behind the sixteen men tied for first in WOD #2. Spealler, at 139 pounds, is as disadvantaged on the deadlift ladder as he was golden on the run. He maxes out at 375 pounds, in seventy-first place in this power event.

Spealler makes up ground on the next WOD, a 170-meter sprint up-hill with a 70-pound sandbag in an unexpected desert rain. In Spealler's heat, the leaders are Khalipa and an even bigger athlete, Brandon Philips. Both are a head taller than Spealler and outweigh him by sixty to eighty pounds. With half his body weight slung over his shoulder, Spealler slips through the narrow space between the heavyweights and tears ahead up the hill. He finishes just ahead of Khalipa, as both tackle their sandbags over the finish line and lie panting on their bellies in the damp dust. Spealler, gasping for air on his hands and knees, reaches up to shake hands with Khalipa, who kneels with his head on the ground.

Spealler finishes two-tenths of a second ahead of Mikko on this event. Mikko's fellow Scandinavian, Sveinbjorn Sveinbjornsson from Iceland, finishes first in the sandbag sprint. Sveinbjorn's fellow Icelander, Annie Thorisdottir, just nineteen years old, finishes first among the women in this event by draping a 35-pound sandbag around her neck like a gym towel and booking it up the hill without even using her hands to stabilize the weight. As a gymnast in Iceland, she qualified for the national team at age fifteen, and she's no stranger to tournament pressure. But competing in a series of new and surprising physical tasks is a completely alien experience.

For Annie and Sveinbjorn, this competition is something of a lark. Neither had even tried CrossFit when they decided to enter the European regional qualifier for the Games. Over the last six weeks, they've been picking it up as they've gone along. There are still movements the Icelanders haven't mastered. But they completely dominate all other nations at running uphill with sandbags.

After the sandbag sprint, Caity Matter, the 2008 women's champion, succumbs to heat exhaustion and takes herself out of contention entirely. Like Fitzgerald, she took advantage of her automatic qualification for the Games and skipped regionals. Between planning her wedding to Bill Henniger, scheduled a month after the Games, and the knowledge that her place at Aromas was assured, she let her training slip. But it's a bad year to arrive in Aromas in less than optimum condition—the physical demands have been heavily ratcheted up, and recovery periods have been ratcheted down. The competitors are stronger. The champions' pre-qualification for the Games is an honor. But as O.P.T., Caity Matter, and Jason Khalipa have discovered, it is also a trap.

The fourth event of the day is consistent with the Games theme of the Unknown and Unknowable: each contestant must row 500 meters, then pound a four-foot iron stake into compacted sand with a sledgehammer, then row another 500 meters for time. Before the stakes are firmly planted in the ground, they have to be held in place. This turns out to be a risky proposition for several athletes.

On a series of sledge drives, Nicole Gordon nails her finger and yells the least ladylike expletive before pounding her stake the rest of the way into the sand. The handle of her rower is smeared with blood as a nearby medic snaps on a pair of latex gloves. The second she finishes the row, the medics descend, and Nicole turns back into her regular self. As alcohol splashes over her hand, she screams and cries like a little girl. She is led, whimpering, into the barn and rushed to the hospital to x-ray her finger.[8] Annie Thorisdottir, a fair-haired Valkyrie with hammer in hand, finishes twenty seconds behind the winning time.

The men's sledgehammer victory goes, unsurprisingly, to a onetime construction worker, Tommy Hackenbruck. After playing middle linebacker for the University of Utah, but before discovering CrossFit, Tommy was swinging a hammer six days a week for three years, framing houses. His hammer technique puts him in a tie for first place overall.

As the sun sinks, the day's last trial begins. It is a couplet—in Cross-Fit terminology, an alternation of two exercises for multiple rounds, in this case three rounds of thirty wall balls and thirty squat snatches. To execute a squat snatch, you jump a barbell from the ground to overhead, straighten your arms, and sink, with straight arms holding the bar overhead, into a deep squat with hips below the knee. This is the quick part. At the bottom of the squat, with straight arms holding a weighted bar overhead, you still have to get back up to a full standing position with arms still extended straight up in a V. Rocket launches from Cape Canaveral seem to require less propulsion when the fuel is lit.

The target for the men's twenty-pound wall ball shots is the competition banner, ten feet above the ground across the length of the barn. At the beginning of each set, each man is poised below a single word and has to hit that word, ten feet in the air, with a twenty-pound ball, then catch that ball in a full squat before jumping up to launch the ball again. Mikko stands under the word *competition*. Tommy Hackenbruck's word is *dominance*. James "O.P.T." Fitzgerald's is *events*. Jason Khalipa has the word *this* to target, a perfect mantra for the second-to-second misery of a wall ball workout: "this . . . this . . . this . . . this . . . just this." He crushes the workout, finishing thirty-eight seconds ahead of Tommy Hackenbruck, who's in first place overall.

Chris Spealler, currently in thirty-second place after the deadlift ladder torpedoed his overall rank, tilts his face upward and throws a wall ball toward the sky. It hits the word *within*, and gravity does its thing to drive the ball down. He accepts the force, bends his knees, and springs up to launch the ball upwards before it descends to shove him back down.

Tanya Wagner peeks through the curtain that divides the athletes inside the barn from the men chucking wall balls against the building's exterior. Behind her, athletes are preparing themselves for the couplet. She hears the chatter: it's just wall balls and squat snatches—the weight on the bar is seventy-five pounds. Seventy-five pounds is light, less than most of these athletes warm up with on a regular day. Everyone's done these movements. After wild cards like the run and weird-assed random things like the sledgehammer stake event, this is a break from the Unknown and Unknowable. It's known and knowable. The consensus in the barn is, *it'll be fine—just pace it out.*

Tanya takes stock of her body. Because her legs were so tired from the run, her form fell apart on her last two deadlifts, and now her lower back is smoked. She's watching the men's first round, thinking: *Thirty. That's a crapload when it's wall balls and the number doesn't go down from round to round.* Josh Everett, one of the best Olympic lifters in the CrossFit pantheon, is struggling to do single repetitions with this supposedly trivial amount of weight.

Then she looks at her husband's face. Josh Wagner is right next to Everett, and he can't string together wall balls to save his life. Tanya has trained with Josh nearly every day they've been together. She knows him better than anyone, and knows the ratio between his capabilities and hers. She knows he never breaks a series of wall balls, and now he is laboring to do them one by one. Josh's eyes are glazed, and he's hurting. She sees and feels this, the way any wife looks past the tough-guy mask on her husband's face and just knows.

It dawns on her that this task that seems so simple and mundane is going to be a lot harder than it looks. She walks back to the athletes crowded around the screen who are telling each other it's all going to be okay. "This is not okay," she says. "This is not going to be okay." But she can't convince them, because the movements are so familiar and the weight is so light, that this is going to be the most grueling trial they've faced at the Games.

But she goes into the couplet knowing it's going to knock her, and everyone else, flat on their ass. She knows not to go out too fast or too hard, because she's not sure how her back is going to hold up. Every time she brings the bar, just forty-five pounds, below her knees, it cranks the muscles along her lumbar spine into frayed ropes of pain. "Just get me through this," she says to herself and to God. "Just get me through this. I need it to be over." Now that she's at the wall, Josh is in the frame of the barn door watching her. He knows how much it's taking out of her, because he's just been through it himself.

"It's your last round!" he yells. "Get through it. Last round. Keep breathing."

It hurts, and seems to go on forever, and then it's over. Tanya finishes sixth for the WOD, still in first place overall and two full minutes ahead of Annie Thorisdottir. Like her fellow Norseman, Mikko, Thorisdottir doesn't crash onto her back after the agony of wall balls. She crouches on her hands and knees. A flash of aggression in her eyes gives her a strange dignity in this last moment. She's like a cat that's been caught on a kitchen table. Her face says, "I know I'm not supposed to be here, and that you've seen me and I have to move. But just so you know, I'm still in charge."

Fifteen women fail to complete the WOD before the twenty-minute time cap—a DNF (Did Not Finish) result that gets them automatically cut from the rest of the competition. One of the women to DNF is Nicole Gordon, back from the hospital. Her finger isn't broken, and she's got some relief from the Vicodin they gave her in the emergency room. But the force of gravity on fourteen pounds for ten feet falls hard into Nicole's bandaged hand and drives through her back and legs, round after round. She finishes her last thirty wall balls, leaving the final set of lifts unfinished when the buzzer sounds.

The sun is down, and exhausted athletes can eat, drink, and sleep. Of the 144 athletes who started the day, all but 1 progressed from the hill run to the deadlifts. Seventeen more finished the deadlift ladder and bowed out before the sandbag sprint that put Caity Matter out of contention. After the sledge strike, 19 more of the fittest athletes on the planet decided they'd had enough. Twenty-seven DNF'd on the wall ball workout. Of the 78 that finished before the time cutoff, only 32, 16 men and 16 women, will be allowed to compete on day two.

On Sunday morning, the sidelined competitors have become spectators who watch the last three events with a mixture of regret and relief. The surviving 32 are steeling themselves for the day. Khalipa's calf is messed up, and his back is feeling sore. Tommy Hackenbruck was too excited to sleep through the night and hasn't recovered as well as he could have. Mikko seems chipper when asked if he got enough rest. "Sleeping like baby," he answers.

The first WOD of the morning is an Olympic lifting event—sort of. Contestants have ten minutes to do their heaviest single lift, ground to overhead with arms locked out in a V. In Olympic lifting parlance, the movement is called a snatch (Tanya, as a school PE teacher, is used to snickers around the room when she introduces the term). But in the official universe of US Olympic lifting, there are a lot of formal rules about what the bar and the athlete can or cannot do on the way from the ground to the final lockout. For instance, in a USA Weightlifting tournament, an athlete cannot throw the bar up, lock out his arms, fall to his knees, then stagger up to standing and count that as a successful lift. Not so in CrossFit—as long as the athlete doesn't rest the bar on any part of his body on the way up, and his arms are fully extended overhead at the end, the lift can be as ugly and desperate as sin. Just get it done.

"For what CrossFit stands for," remarks Mike Bergener, CrossFit's Olympic lifting guru, "it's great." Bergener is the father of an Olympic weightlifter, and he's coached national teams to Olympic standards. But sometimes in the real world, he observes, you've just got to get something heavy over your head. "In the military environment, the firefighting environment, the policing environment, and even the mother at home trying to lift something up, I think it's absolutely right on."[9]

Neither the male nor the female winner of the snatch event ends up in the overall top ten. Josh Everett, CrossFit's fabled Olympic lifter, is conspicuous by his absence after failing to make the top sixteen on Saturday. But the power athletes, Jeff Leonard and Tamara Holmes, demonstrate their dominance on a test of maximum effort. Attention has been paid. Khalipa pulls a second-place showing on the event, clawing his way up the leaderboard to eleventh place overall. Tanya also pulls second in this event, putting distance between herself and Annie Thorisdottir, whose final lift is twenty pounds lighter.

The end—the real end of the Games—is in sight. Tommy Hackenbruck has barely held on to first place. Mikko Salo, the indefatigable Finn, is just one point behind him, and Tommy knows it will be tough to beat Mikko in the final WOD. "I can feel him breathing down my neck," he says, with a mixture of foreboding and admiration. "He's a great athlete."

There is just one more task: the chipper, a single-round workout in which athletes have to finish a full set of one movement before moving on to the next movement. Some people interpret the term for this kind of workout in a positive light—just "chip away" at the WOD until it's done. Others see a clearer analogy in the progress of a log moving in one direction through a wood chipper and coming out as mulch on the other side. This chipper is a gauntlet of ten movements, starting with barbell cleans (155 pounds for the men, 100 for the women) and ending with a 25-meter stretch of walking lunges while holding a barbell plate (45 pounds for men, 25 pounds for women) with straight arms overhead.

By far the most daunting aspect of this workout is a set of ten muscle-ups.

Annie Thorisdottir has never done a muscle-up in her life. Nicole Carroll, who struggled through muscle-ups in the "Nasty Girls" video, is now CrossFit's director of training. She shows the Icelanders how to do muscle-ups the morning of the final event. Mentally, they understand what needs to happen on the rings. But understanding the split-second physics of what needs to happen and being able to actually do it are two different things.

In the barn, Tanya continues the conversation with God she's been having all weekend. "Dear Lord, I don't know what you want for me right now, but please just give me strength," she prays. "I don't know where you want me to place, or what you want me to do, but just give me the strength to get through it." At this point, she is relying on faith to fill the void between the sense that she has nothing left and the massive effort she's expected to summon for this final event. She finishes her prayer knowing that whatever God intends for her will happen in the arena in a few minutes. But she still doesn't know how she's going to do all ten muscle-ups.

As the women line up to enter the arena, Tanya looks at Jolie Gentry next to her in line. A California-gorgeous SWAT team offi-cer who won the Games in 2007, Jolie is a woman at ease behind the sniper sight of a high-powered rifle. A smile has been playing around the edges of her mouth all weekend, the way a smile plays around the edges of Bruce Willis's mouth during a *Die Hard* movie. She seems to relish this whole ordeal in a bring-it-on, action-movie kind of way. If Jolie were in Tanya's position, she'd be firing up the afterburners to win. She's a champion, and she recognizes the next champion. "You got this," Jolie says.

Tanya, a PE teacher in pigtails, doesn't feel like a champion. Desperately, she admits that she's a nervous wreck, that she's never done ten muscle-ups in a row, that's she's afraid she'll fail to get through them and choke out there in front of everyone. "How do I do this?" she asks.

Jolie drops her smile for a moment and fixes her brown eyes on Tanya's baby blues. "Dive through," she says. "Just fucking dive through."

It's time. The women take their places in front of 100-pound bars that have to be jumped up from ground to shoulders fifteen times. The same high-nutrient diet that fuels their muscles with protein and fat makes their skin beautiful, their hair lustrous. The same genetics that made them Division I college athletes also gives their faces near-perfect symmetry. Their bodies are lithe, strong, and tanned, except for Annie, who almost glows with Icelandic pallor in the California sun.

Tanya Wagner and Annie Thorisdottir, dressed almost identically in lime-green tank tops and black shorts, finish their box jumps and arrive at adjacent sets of rings. They could face each other. But they both turn away, to tackle the challenge in a more solitary mental space.

The Icelandic blonde takes a deliberate sip of water and stands there, under the rings, breathing hard. The American blonde chalks up, as if getting the right amount of chalk on her hands is the secret to success. Having dispensed with their preparatory rituals, the two blondes square their shoulders, back to back.

Tanya takes the rings, swings, and fails, stuck in the chicken-wings position. She tries again, fails, and drops to the ground. On her third attempt, she punches through and pushes herself up, arms straight above the rings. Annie is a flailing knot of legs and elbows splaying up and down and sideways, to no avail.

Tanya gets a second muscle-up, and a third. This is real now. It's happening.

Annie Thorisdottir gathers herself again and grabs the rings. She swings up, furiously kicking her legs like a prisoner at the gallows, pitches herself over the rings and pushes herself up. As she straightens her arms, the crowd cheers, the way any crowd of CrossFitters cheers a first muscle-up, except there are thousands of them. So the shared pride is heightened, amplified, when someone passes this milestone in the heat of competition.

Tanya gets her fifth muscle-up, then fails three times in a row. She can still win the Games, even though she's not ahead in this event. All she has to do now is not choke on the muscle-ups. She completes her sixth rep, then fails expensively on number seven. Her arms, almost straight, have just given out. It's not faith that's lacking now—it's strength. She fails again, and again.

Nicole Carroll has lived this moment. She doesn't want to see Tanya fail on the rings, the way she struggled from failure to failure in the "Nasty Girls" video, and get left behind. She runs to where Tanya is struggling and gets in her face, cheering, coaching, screaming a different outcome into existence. Tanya pulls herself up and over, four more times.

Having achieved her first muscle-up, Annie Thorisdottir is determined to get through all ten. But whatever she had the first time, in terms of strength and sheer will, is gone. Flailing like a fish on a line, her efforts become increasingly desperate and uncoordinated, until finally Dave Castro intervenes. "Annie," he says quietly, "no more attempts. It's getting dangerous. You're going to hurt yourself. One more and that's it, all right?" She nods, and throws herself at the sky one more time before falling defeated to the ground.[10]

As Tanya grinds through the remainder of the workout, she doesn't know where she is supposed to be going, and moves toward the wrong station. Her obsession with the muscle-ups has blotted out the memory of what she heard about the workout after "muscle-ups." She moves between stations like an amnesiac, shepherded by her judge.

In the final minute of overhead plate lunges, she is almost overtaken by Lindsey Smith, a tall Division I athlete who played three sports in college and semi-professional soccer afterward. Lindsey's inspiration to start CrossFit was a video of Tanya on the CrossFit website, and now she's poised to overtake her role model.

As Tanya maintains a two-second lead over Lindsey at the finish line, Josh Wagner is yelling from the sidelines, "C'mon, keep moving! Just like the garage, babe. C'mon!" She comes in seventh on the chipper, but she's held on to her overall lead. Tanya's legs are shaking, and her face is flushed. She is promptly directed to the medic station to rehydrate and recover.

Christy Phillips and Lindsey Smith, rivals just minutes before, sneak into the medic station like fans getting backstage at a concert. They hug Tanya and congratulate her. As they relive each other's highlights, the excruciating final WOD is chalked up as "fun." They laugh with a lightness of heart that belies the weight they've had to carry.

While the women are celebrating, Dave Castro is looking for James "O.P.T." Fitzgerald, who should be getting ready to start the chipper. "James Fitzgerald?" he asks a volunteer outside the barn, who tells him that Fitzgerald is out.[11]

"He's out?" Castro says, sounding shocked. "He's not out of the competition, is he?"

"He's injured," answers the volunteer. "He's broken down."

"O.P.T.? What happened to him?" Castro asks, heading into the barn, where a volunteer massage therapist has set up a physical therapy station.

O.P.T. is lying facedown on a padded table. All day, he has been coming back here to get the kinks kneaded out, and no matter what the massage therapists do, muscle cramps all over his body are getting worse. Now he can barely move without seizing up in pain.

Castro goes to the head of the table and crouches down. "James," he says, grabbing Fitzgerald's wrist. O.P.T.'s face is a spasm of pain. Castro steadies Fitzgerald's shaking shoulder with one hand as this champion, the athlete Castro declared the Fittest Man on Earth, weeps on the table.

"We're proud of you, all right?" Castro tells him. "Hold your head high. You did great. You have a lot to be proud of."

After seeing his first champion broken on the rack of this two-day Quest for the Fittest, Castro walks from the shade of the barn into the glare of the arena to announce the final heat. At the starting signal, seven competitors dive into the chipper. Tommy Hackenbruck, in first place, charges into the lead, and now it is his turn to be stalked and over-taken by Mikko Salo. But unlike Spealler, Tommy has no way to draft behind Mikko until the final stretch. It's just each man, in his own lane, hacking away at a mountain of work.

On the muscle-ups, Tommy and Mikko hang from the rings, facing away from each other as Tanya and Annie did. Tommy is two reps ahead, and every time he gets a muscle-up, Castro announces that Mikko has one more. After Tommy finishes his thirteenth muscle-up of fifteen, one of his compatriots yells from the sidelines, "You can do any-thing for two reps, Tommy. Go!" Mikko closes the gap between them to just one rep.

By the time Tommy has churned through dumbbell presses and most of his double-unders, Mikko and Khalipa are both attacking his lead. Khalipa is the first to throw aside the rope and grab a 135-pound barbell for a set of fifteen thrusters—"Fran" weight plus 40 pounds. On the pull-up rig, the massive V of Khalipa's back unfolds like the wings of a *Transformers* robot as he churns through thirty pull-ups. As Jason, then Tommy, dives into a set of thirty burpees, Mikko has left them behind.

Next rep, thinks Mikko. *Next rep, next rep. The end will be coming.*

In the final minute, each man holds a 45-pound plate overhead for a 100-meter plate lunge. With each step, their back knees touch the ground, then move up and lunge forward into the next step. As the ath-letes' shoulders go from fatigue to failure, the weights are dropped, sec-onds lost, until each athlete leans over, grabs the plate, hoists it up, and lunges forward for as long as he can before dropping the weight again. Khalipa, living down his collapse on the hill run, takes a 10-meter lead over Tommy and holds on to it like grim death.

Third across the finish line, having relinquished the championship, Tommy collapses onto the ground to lie down, at last, and fill his lungs with oxygen. "Mikko," he yells after he's caught his breath. "Mikko, help me up, man." Mikko gives him a hand and slaps him on the back. As they leave the arena, Tommy holds Mikko's arm aloft,[12] paying respect to the guy who knocked him off the top of the podium—the only male athlete whose back never touched the dust.

At the awards ceremony, Mikko and Tanya are each given a golden sledgehammer and five thousand dollars for being the Fittest Man and Fittest Woman on Earth. The Spirit of the Games Award, given to the athlete who embodies CrossFit's competitive ethos, goes to Khalipa, whose final rank is seventh overall. Jolie Gentry, seventh place among the women, is declared the Games' winningest law enforcement or military officer. She gleefully accepts a Viking Tactics gift certificate for the Smith & Wesson pistol of her choice, knowing she had to beat a male Marine to get it. For bragging rights, out-competing a Marine for a weapon is right up there with winning the Games.

Tanya has nightmares for weeks after the Games. In these nightmares, she's still in first place, but somehow, after the chipper, it's not over. There's another event, something else they're fetching her to line up for, that she has to pray for the strength to get through. That sense of the bottom dropping out, of giving it all in the finish and then being shocked to discover she's not done, jolts her awake wondering, "Did that really happen? Is it over? Okay, it's over. Tell yourself it's over. It's done."[13]

The 2009 CrossFit Games were, to use the phrase Donald Rumsfeld employed to describe the fall of Baghdad, a catastrophic success. In the aftermath, a few things were evident. The first was that if the CrossFit Games were going to be a legitimate sports championship, not some kind of fringe survival event, the competitors had to be treated like professional athletes, not Roman gladiators. That meant giving them a reasonable amount of time and space to recover between events. Shelter, ice baths, physical therapists. Facilities. It couldn't be tents and a barn anymore.

It was also clear that, regardless of conditions, these athletes would do whatever they were asked to do in competition, whether they'd trained for it or not, to the point of breaking, and past the point of breaking. It was clear that the energetic tribute of CrossFit's elite would bind the community. It would test the limits of human capability. And it would at least momentarily satisfy Greg Glassman's curiosity.

A GOOD CULT

NICOLE GORDON SPOTTED CHRISTMAS ABBOTT AT THE COACH'S Prep Course, and then a few months later when Christmas was first tapped for an internship on the Level 1 staff. CrossFit's thousand-dollar "Level 1" certification is the entry-level credential that allows trainers to become CrossFit affiliates. It's a weekend firehose of CrossFit 101, group WODs, and a standardized test. After passing the test, certified trainers can take the Coach's Prep Course, which is a master class on the art of coaching: how to spot and correct faults in the way people move and set up to move, how to cue corrections that boost performance, how to program and effectively manage group workouts.

CrossFit courses like Coach's Prep and a bevy of specialty seminars provide a cornucopia of continuing education options for certified CrossFit trainers: Olympic lifting, endurance, and gymnastics, as well as courses tailored for football coaches and law enforcement agencies. Kelly Starrett, a kayaker and physical therapist, teaches a mobility course on how to tune up creaky or injured knees, hips, and shoulders so they can move the way they're supposed to, function better, and not get hurt. Starrett (aka "K*Star") is the patron saint of aging athletes with old sports injuries and muscle-bound beasts who are lacking in the suppleness department. He combines a ballet master's attention to the subtle arcs and angles with a litany of stretches and techniques to therapeutically torture your muscles and tendons with a lacrosse ball.

Most CrossFit certification seminars cost six hundred bucks and require attendees to possess the entry-level CrossFit Level 1 certificate.

One of the reasons it's easy for CrossFit HQ to maintain its libertarian purity with regard to affiliate competition is that the company's financial bread and butter is certification courses. Midway through 2013, Greg Glassman estimated that CrossFit Inc. would clear fifty million dollars on certs by the end of the year,[1] with only 140 seminar trainers, who are contractors. Monday through Friday, most of the Level 1 staff are box owners. Weekends, they hit the road to train the trainers. Some CrossFit affiliates host certs at their boxes and get a share of the revenue. In lieu of their hosting fee, they can sponsor certifications for a handful of friends or prospective employees.

It's an incredibly profitable business, and it's exploding. On any given weekend, there are between twelve and twenty Level 1 CrossFit certifications running on six continents. Most certs have a sixty-person limit and sell out. These are just the entry-level certification seminars, not the specialty courses. And 40% of Level 1 seminar attendees aren't even planning to use the credential in a professional capacity, to train other athletes or open a box.[2] They're just regular CrossFitters who want to level up.

This is puzzling, considering the wealth of information and media that CrossFit HQ makes available online. There are literally thousands of free articles and videos delving into every aspect of the CrossFit training methodology, dissecting all the common errors and faults of a squat, power clean, or pull-up and ways to correct them, emphasizing the underlying importance of nutrition, or laying out the building blocks of workout programming. All the CrossFit WODs are available open source online. Literally every topic that's covered in this thousand-dollar certification seminar is easily accessible on CrossFit.com in greater breadth and depth, and this isn't a secret. So why do people who don't actually need this certificate as a professional credential spend a cool grand and a weekend on a face-to-face seminar?

Partly, it's for the badge. Recreational CrossFitters with Level 1 certs don't open new CrossFit boxes, although they might daydream about it. But they have earned their stripes as fully fledged members of the CrossFit training cadre. It's kind of a fitness bar mitzvah—they've demonstrated they have enough knowledge to take full responsibility for their own training. They're fairly well equipped to course-correct themselves without having to ask a trainer what they're doing wrong. Some boxes give a discount to certified trainers because they're less likely to need constant attention and more likely to be competitors. They may not be coaching and correcting, but they provide a good reference point for other athletes to mirror.

When we see someone execute a movement, there are specific neurons in the brain that allow us to match and synchronize our movements with theirs. Even if we're just watching people move, the mirror neurons in our brain fire as if we were doing the same movements. The mirroring circuitry of our brain allows us to project ourselves into other people's actions, and also into their emotions (people unconsciously mirror one another's facial expressions during tales of woe). When the person we're watching catches the pass or crosses the finishing line, we feel like we have caught the ball, that we have broken the tape, that we have won. The connection is so strong that we irrationally sense we can influence the outcome on a sports field by leaning hard in the direction we want a player to veer. This circuitry for mapping ourselves onto another person's movements is the most basic, ancient wiring for interpersonal connection—the kind that babies have with their mothers. It's how we evolved to learn.[3]

Sometimes no amount of verbal coaching will help as much as seeing someone in front of you get it right. Mirror neurons fire up. You move at the same time. You map from joint to joint, how the hips extend, how the elbows turn. If more people are executing Olympic lifts correctly, beginners will imitate correct executions of the movement, not the faulty efforts of other beginners.

Recreational CrossFitters with coaching certifications are easy hires, because they're already a member of the tribe at their box. As boxes grow, they hire from within—it's almost unheard-of for coaches to be hired off the street, no matter how many certifications they have. It's more common for an athlete who's been training at the box for a while, who gets along with everyone, to go for her Level 1 cert and start coaching at the box where she's been working out for years.

As a credential, the CrossFit Level 1 is also a kind of secret Cross-

Fit handshake. It goes on the bottom of people's résumés. To non-CrossFitters in HR, this just looks like another hobby. But if the person handling that résumé happens to be a CrossFitter, the applicant will probably get an interview. A candidate with a CrossFit coaching credential won't get hired, necessarily. But the badge carries more weight than a school tie, because it reliably indicates that someone is able to work outside their comfort zone. There's a whole set of assumptions you can make about certified CrossFit trainers: They know how to buckle down and focus on results. They're not allergic to accountability. And they're extremely unlikely to harbor any kind of chronic disease.

So the badge matters to some people. Others go for the experience. At a Level 1 seminar, odds are the person scrawling on the whiteboard, or leading a WOD, got their coaching certification at a seminar Greg Glassman ran with Greg Amundson, Annie Sakamoto, and Nicole Carroll. For CrossFitters, the Level 1 is like a ballet master class with one of Balanchine's ballerinas, or a guitar tutorial with a session musician who played with rock legends, or the Manning football dynasty's offensive skills camp.[4] It's not just about picking up skills. It's the chance to experience and absorb the original lightning-in-a-bottle that made the virtuosos great in the first place.

The main thing that's changed in a decade is the confrontational undertone that used to give seminar WODs the quality of gladiatorial combat. In the old days, when attendees were DEA agents or Army Special Forces operators, Glassman needed Greg Amundson and the girls to dominate their competitors, because their competitors were alpha males who needed to be taught a lesson before they'd accept the validity of the training method. The WODs delivered a serious physical beatdown. The results humbled people and commanded respect. In places like Russia, CrossFit seminars still work this way. CrossFit HQ has to send unbeatable beasts to lead the seminars, because strong-like-bull attendees won't accept the training principles until they're decisively defeated in competition.

But in most of the world, Level 1 certs are kinder and gentler because 99% of the people who go to them are already drinking the Kool-Aid.

They are so excited to be around CrossFit veterans and Games athletes who run the seminars that when Level 1 trainers run "Fran" as a benchmark WOD, every attendee hits a personal record. So the dogfighting of yore has given way to a shiny, happy fanboy experience. Glassman's pugnacious irreverence and contemptuous dismissal of every other training method on earth has given way to a more ecumenical tone. It's less of "Whatever you're doing that's not CrossFit is idiotic and here are the reasons why" and more "Oh, you do something outside of CrossFit? You know what'll make you *more awesome* at it? CrossFit, and here's why."

Level 1 staff are selected for their empathy, not just their expertise and athletic prowess. Like box members who take on coaching responsibilities, they're the ones who know how to set a good example and can invest as much energy in other people's improvement as in their own performance. They're people like Nicole Gordon, who, when she's not going to the Dark Place in competition, just wants to be everybody's mom.

"Nana Gordon is what I've had a couple of girls call me," she says. "Always making sure that everyone is 'Are you taken care of, baby? What do you need?' Hopefully everybody will feel safe with me. Safe is such an odd term to use, but their needs will be met. They will be taken care of. I like to figure out what's going to make it work for them, and when it clicks, that's awesome. There's a little happy dance that happens. I don't give up on people. I want them to know that, no matter what, I'm going to be working to find what they need."

She asks questions, and she's genuinely interested in the answers. Why are people there? What are they looking to get out of it? When did they get into CrossFit? What has changed since they started? "Within three minutes," Gordon says, "I could find out so much about somebody's life. And that connection could make somebody's entire weekend, because they feel like someone's listening.

"There's a way to deliver information: You can stand up there and give a lecture, or you can make them feel like they're a part of the lecture, like their lives are in the lecture. Not that we're actors, but we're giving a performance. Do they feel like they're being drawn in and a part of it and almost know what's going to come next, but maybe not, and be excited to hear it, with lectures, movements, just hanging out and talking, with their workout? You have to give them something to remember forever. If you're not on and doing that, you haven't done a very good job."

Nicole Gordon will teach you how to squat with your torso upright, knees flared out, butt below the knees. She'll make it seem like a life-changing experience and, simultaneously, as if someone is making you a peanut-butter-and-jelly sandwich with the crusts cut off. She is incredibly passionate about this air squat interaction. They all are. Before the seminar, the Level 1 seminar staff huddle in a moment of personal gratitude that they have the opportunity to teach air squats to future Cross-Fit trainers and, by so doing, change people's lives.

This isn't as kooky as it sounds. Better movement does improve people's lives. Making measurable improvements, a sense of progress, reinforces the idea that incremental effort will yield dividends. CrossFit in general inures people to escalating levels of physical and psychic discomfort, and builds strength of will. It spills over.

When Christmas was tapped as an intern for the Level 1 seminar staff in late 2010, Nicole Gordon and another military-wife-turned-CrossFit-coach, Sara Wilkinson, were there to keep a hawk-eye on her. The Level 1 internship is CrossFit's Top Gun School. People in it are supposed to be excellent to start with, and then get taken to task by people who are even more excellent before they can join the ranks. So Nicole and Sara were on the lookout for any minor fault or flaw in Christmas's coaching or interpersonal skills.

They both intended to play the schoolmarm "you think you've got what it takes?" role. But like everyone, they were dazzled and seduced by Christmas's luminous smile and how she seems like a trained assassin, but also a Mouseketeer. In some very deep ways, they recognized that they were alike. Nicole had been to the Games. Christmas was on a Games competition team. She knows what it's like to go to the Dark Place. Women who've been there recognize one another. There's something in the way they carry themselves.

They tend to have tattoos. In addition to her full-sleeve sword-wielding woodland goddess, Christmas has a life-size pistol tattooed on her right thigh and hip, right where she'd holster a real weapon. Sara's got a full-sleeve Buddha surrounded by flowers on her left arm, and a Chinese guardian lion on her bicep. Nicole has a spray of cherry blossoms that unfurls from her back, across her right shoulder blade and onto her arm. It's delicate, even girly, but it covers some real estate. "[In CrossFit] there's this idea of sexy but don't-mess-with-me at that same time" she explains. "These [are] girls that are wearing cutesy hot pink, but they're badass."

Until a few years ago, Nicole Gordon did a good job of keeping up with her high school friends, because she's that girl who remembers birthdays and sends Christmas cards and calls to say, "Hey sweetie, how are you?" The last time she got together with a bunch of them, they looked at her body, and it didn't match theirs anymore. Nicole is not big—intense CrossFit training builds gymnast/sprinters, not jacked-up bodybuilders. On the other hand, the definition in Nicole's arms and legs make it clear that she's an athlete, not just another suburban mom.

"Why all the tattoos?" asked her old classmates. "That's so not you. Why all the muscles?" These were women who'd taken one another through big life changes, from junior high to getting married and having kids. They'd celebrated everything from prom to baby showers, and maintained long-distance connections for more than a decade. They just hadn't seen Nicole's body in a while. She tried to tell them about starting CrossFit. "I've heard of it," said one. "But that looks hard. Why would you do that?"

Men get a lot of flack for ogling women's bodies. But when it comes to aesthetic standards, women are the enforcers. Women are the ones who look at another woman's body and make negative remarks to her face, or communicate disapproval with a furrowed gaze or the curl of a lip. Women's bodies reflect a social order that's largely upheld by other women. By decorating her athlete's body with tattoos that drew attention to her strength, Nicole had run afoul of the standards and violated the social order, even though she was still Miss Congeniality. The questions were rhetorical—none of her high school friends wanted to know what motivated her, or what she was getting out of it. They were just making her aware that she'd stepped out of bounds.

She looked at her friends and for the first time thought, *You're weak. You can't handle yourself. You have to have someone do shit for you. Don't get me wrong, I love chivalry, but all you do is* yoga. *All you can do is stretch and bend. How does that get you through life?* She imagined these women in forty years, being skinny and brittle, breaking and languishing and being frail. She thought of her own mother, who'd done aerobics and dieted herself into bird-like slenderness in her thirties, who is now pushing sixty and overweight and loses her balance and falls and worries about chipping her teeth. These were the women telling Nicole she was becoming less feminine, as if fracturing a hip was the height of femininity.

"Until then," she says, "I didn't realize how different I was becoming, and how proud I was of the difference. I felt, in that moment, closer to the CrossFit women that I was used to being around. We had a stronger connection than I had understood up until that point." When she sees another female CrossFit athlete, coach or competitor, she feels that they understand each other. "There is a thread that runs through us."

CrossFitters joke that they're part of a cult. John Wellbourn, a former NFL offensive lineman, now runs CrossFit Football, a CrossFit variant tailored to the physical demands of football, for high school, college, and pro players. "In college," he mused in a CrossFit-produced documentary, "in one of my classes we defined what a cult was. The number one was: special diet. CrossFit promotes a diet, the Zone. They have a terminology that only people within the cult understand. If you were to say to somebody 'What's your Fran time?' on the street, he doesn't understand. But if you tell it to a CrossFitter, he knows exactly what you're talking about. Special clothing: I see these CrossFitters, their biggest thing is to go get T-shirts from other CrossFit gyms and wear them proudly. Meeting places: your CrossFit gym, that's your community. A lot of CrossFitters tend to only associate with other CrossFitters. Now, is it a good cult? It's a fitness cult—it's making you better. Is it a cult? Yeah, it is."[5]

Even Greg Glassman asks this question. "So many people say it's a cult—at some point you've gotta ask yourself, *is* it a cult?" He shrugs. "Maybe it is a cult, where people get really fit and support each other."[6] This is probably the biggest counterpoint to the characterization of CrossFit as a cult in the negative sense: Cults don't generally instigate discussion about whether they're cults. They're low on inquiry. They're opaque. CrossFit is pretty transparent. Unless you're trying to suss out next year's Games workouts, it's a fairly open book.

None of this mitigates the social torque that happens when CrossFit devotees gravitate away from their high school friends and toward their box-based communities. As they weave into their kettle-bell-swinging social groups, and try to drag in as many friends and relatives as they can, they're engaged in the same social migration that happens with any radical change in health habits. Smokers who quit want everyone in their family to quit. People who've given up drinking don't like hanging out in bars. When obese people lose 20% of their body weight, sometimes they find that they have to make new friends, because their old friends pressure them to reprise unhealthy eating habits. They are shifting position on the map of like-attracts-like. That's not without its moments of social awkwardness.

Guys hitting personal records on WODs want to impress other guys who understand what the hell they're talking about. Women who like to pull heavy weight over their heads find it easier to hang out with other women who don't think Olympic weightlifting is a deviant behavior. Every time someone pulls a friend or relative into the craziness, it gets a little easier. Families become fitter. Moms swap recipes for Paleo desserts while their grade-schoolers learn to snatch wooden dowels with perfect form. It's a lifestyle, promulgated by the Level 1 laity.

It's a good cult.

FAITH AND THE FINISH LINE

2011 WAS THE YEAR THE CROSSFIT GAMES WENT VIRAL. IN JUST a few years, the competitive field had grown from dozens to hundreds to thousands. In 2009, the Games staged seventeen regional qualifiers around the world, as well as the "Last Chance" online qualifier. In 2010, regionals had to be subdivided into thirty-three preliminary sectional competitions, with sectional winners moving on to regional events.

Competitions have participation limits. Facilities are only so big, and there are only so many heats you can run for men, women, and teams in the course of a weekend. For CrossFit HQ, the growth had become unmanageable. It was logistically absurd to organize an ever-expanding pyramid of local qualifiers. That would have involved hierarchy and centralized control, both anathema to the corporate culture. So in keeping with CrossFit's original open-source approach, HQ transformed the first phase of the Games into a massively distributed serial competition called the Open.

During the Open's five-week season, a new workout is announced early in the week. Athletes around the world have until Sunday afternoon to either go to an affiliate and have their performance judged, or to post a video of their performance online. All results are submitted online, validated by the affiliates or volunteer video judges, and sifted into global and regional leader boards. The top thirty males, females, and teams in each region progress to the regional qualifier. The top three males, females, and teams from each regional competition go on to the Games.

The Open does two things. The first thing is, it cheaply and effectively increases the accessibility of qualifying competition. Anyone with an Internet connection and a video-capable smartphone can sign up, even if there's no affiliate for hundreds of miles. If the Fittest Man on Earth is holed up in some hinterland, as long as he can find an Internet-connected computer, the competition can find him.

The second thing the Open does is create a competitive season for regular Joes and Jills. The Open workouts are deliberately designed to be accessible to beginning and intermediate athletes. The movements, though incredibly strenuous, are less advanced, and the weights are lighter than in regional competitions. An elite athlete might get some multiple of a regular person's reps or rounds. But regular people can participate in the exact same event and see their performance ranked against other athletes in their region or globally. A forty-two-year-old woman can see how she stacks up against other forty- to forty-five-year-old women in the Mid-Atlantic states. A young gun can see he's in the top two hundred out of thousands in his region. People can see how they improve from year to year. And they usually do, because a year of training buys gains, and each year's crop of rookies is larger and less experienced than the last. The Open democratizes athletic competition in an unprecedented way. It is a global amateur league.

In 2011, 26,000 people registered to compete. In 2012, that figure more than doubled to 69,240.[1] In 2013, 138,000 people in 118 countries took part—triple the number of people who run the New York City Marathon. According to the *Guinness Book of World Records*, the largest footrace in the world was run by 116,086 people, completing three simultaneous runs (3K, 5K, and 10K) in Manila, in 2010.[2] The Open has that number beaten handily.

The Open operates largely on the honor system, with the onus on local judges to uphold standards, even if it means telling friends that their squats aren't deep enough or their arms didn't completely straighten, and therefore their reps are invalid. People call no-reps on their peers, even on their coaches, with a stern but pained expression that says, "This hurts me more than it hurts you."

Theoretically, it would be possible for a fraudulent affiliate to qualify an athlete for regionals. But regionals are where the honor system of the Open gives way to RFID (radio-frequency identification) chips that verify finishing times down to a fraction of a second. Performances are videotaped, and judges count reps for athletes they've never met. It would be obvious if a competitor didn't measure up at regionals. If there was evidence that any affiliate had massaged an athlete's qualifying results, both the gym and the athlete would be excommunicated from CrossFit. The potential costs are high. And the benefits are scant. It doesn't make sense to cheat one's way into regionals, only to come in dead last, under a cloud of suspicion.

In 2011, the top-five finishers in the 2010 Games were pre-qualified for the Games. One of them, Rich Froning, was trying to live down a mortifying flame-out. In 2010, at age twenty-three, he'd come out of nowhere—specifically, his dad's barn in Cookeville, Tennessee—to win sectionals, then the Central East regionals. He was one of those rural kids who'd been doing hard physical work all his life, either out of necessity or as a form of discipline.

Like a lot of boys, Rich dreamed of growing up to play baseball. In high school, he was a two-time all-region second baseman. He was even recruited to play baseball at a small college. But when he got there, baseball felt like a job. The joy went out of it. After a few weeks, he transferred to Tennessee Tech, to study exercise science and work as a firefighter. As a student firefighter, Rich alternated between class days and firehouse shifts that required him to move heavy weights as quickly as possible, in sobering circumstances. He saw houses in cinders and dead children.

Rich's exercise science course was taught by the university's full-time strength coach, Chip Pugh. Pugh was a CrossFit devotee—he'd played Division I football at the same university as Josh Everett. After college he'd worked in the campus ministry before getting a job as a football strength coach. He'd help athletes get stronger in the college weight room. If they were looking for inspiration and guidance, he'd do his best to help them grapple with, or stumble through, life decisions and spiritual questions. It was an unorthodox form of ministry but, Pugh says, "I have always considered myself an unorthodox minister."

When Pugh moved to be the full-time strength and conditioning coach at Tennessee Tech, Everett called him to pitch CrossFit. Before long, Pugh was fired up about it. He used videos and articles from the CrossFit website in his class. Rich sat in the back of the room watching the videos, thinking he might have to try this out. He started hitting daily WODs in the barn with his cousin Darren. Within a year, he was an absolute beast. From sectionals to regionals to the CrossFit Games, he dominated the field. He was on fire, right up until the final twelve minutes of the Games.

The Games' first year in a bona fide sports arena was 2010, at the Home Depot Center in Carson, California. To heighten and preserve the element of the Unknown and Unknowable, CrossFit HQ used the architecture of the stadium to enforce cultic secrecy among the competitors. Before each event, athletes were sequestered in a locker room underneath the stadium floor. They couldn't hear anything announced over the loudspeakers. They weren't allowed any contact with the outside world. All they could do, in the lead-up to each WOD, was watch athletes being called out for each heat, and then measure the time before the next group of athletes was summoned. The longer the lag, the longer the workout was going to be. As each set of athletes walked through the tunnel from the locker room to the floor, they were were still, literally, in the dark. Their names would be announced in the arena. Emerging into daylight, they caught a first glimpse of the gauntlet they'd be running. They heard a description of the task. Seconds later, they heard the signal to start.

The final event of the Games was a trio of WODs, each with a time limit. The first was three rounds of 30 push-ups, rope-climbing over a wall, and 21 squats with a 95-pound barbell held overhead. After describing the WOD, Dave Castro immediately yelled, "Three, two, one, GO!" For a confused split second, the athletes stood there before realizing, oh Jesus, we have to go *now*, and diving onto sizzling black rubber mats to do push-ups. Rich Froning was the only athlete to finish the last set of overhead squats, with five seconds to spare before the 7-minute time cap.

Seconds later, Castro announced the next WOD: three rounds of 30 toes-to-bar (grab a pull-up bar, hang vertically, and touch toes to the bar—it's a fairly brutal abdominal exercise) and 21 ground-to-overhead lifts (clean and jerks or snatches) with a 95-pound barbell. Again, there was an immediate "Three, two, one, GO!" The time limit was 7 minutes. No one finished. But Rich was handily in the lead. He could finish a few places behind his closest competitor and still win the Games, the twenty-five-thousand-dollar first prize, and the title of Fittest Man on Earth. It seemed certain that he was going to come out of nowhere and win it all, like Jason Khalipa. It was so close, he could almost taste it.

As the athletes labored to catch their breath, Dave Castro announced the final phase of the three-WOD finale: 5 wall-burpees (a push-up, then a jump and scramble over a 6-foot wall) and three 20-foot rope climbs, three rounds with a 12-minute time cap.

Rich hadn't climbed a rope in his adult life. He'd climbed ropes as a kid in his dad's barn. When he used his feet, his dad told him, "That's the sissy way. Use your arms."[3] As a kid, Rich had been able to muscle his way up the rope using just his arms. But now he weighed 190 pounds, and his arms and shoulders were smoked from three days in the red zone.

At the signal, he barreled through the push-ups and wall climbs, then ran to the rope. He jumped onto it and couldn't hold on. He jumped onto it, flailed, and dropped to the ground. Again and again. He looked to see what the other athletes were doing. Well-practiced and agile competitors were hooking one foot under the rope and clamping down on it with the other foot. The trapped length of rope functioned as a ladder rung, and they used their legs to push themselves up. But Rich was too exhausted, and his mind was too fogged to formulate a concept of how to do it.

Wiry Chris Spealler, all nimbleness and speed, was shimmying up his second round of rope climbs. Graham Holmberg, who trained at Rogue Fitness and looks like a blond surfer, glanced sidelong at his adversary and realized, *I'm going to be the champion of the CrossFit Games because this dude can't climb a rope.*

Rich was stuck. He dipped his hands in chalk, hoping for more purchase on the rope. He looked up to the top of the rope and leapt, kicking his legs the whole way up, until he tapped the bar with his left hand. One successful rep. One climb done. His left hand barely made it back to the rope before his arms, shoulders, and both burning hands declared mutiny and would have nothing further to do with the rope. Adrenaline surged in his blood as he fell eighteen feet. His heel hit the ground first, then his rear end. His head slammed into the chalk bucket, as if to punctuate the epic fail.

With three and a half minutes left on the clock, Spealler alighted from his last rope climb, two minutes ahead of the next-fastest competitor. Graham was on his final round. As Rich recalled in *First*, a youthful memoir of his Games career, what ran through his mind was that every rep still counted. One rope climb might make the difference between win, place, and show. "I'm going to figure this out," he thought, "I've got twelve minutes to fight with this rope."[4] In the end, he muscled his way up the rope a second and third time, then dived to the ground for a single push-up and wall climb before the clock ran out. The finish put him in second place for the Games, behind Graham and ahead of Chris Spealler.

The medics checked him out. Rich had his foot x-rayed. Nothing was injured, although his ego was badly bruised. "That verse from Proverbs about pride going before a fall?" he wrote. "I experienced that."[5] Over the course of three days, his own expectations had soared from "make my family proud" to "*I can win this.*" Victory had seemed inevitable. And then it slipped from his grasp, literally. The triumphant arc collapsed, and his aspirations curdled into graceless pique. As the silver medal was placed around his neck, Rich admits, he had to fake a smile.[6]

After the Games, Rich went to Michigan, where most of his relatives lived. He'd grown up in a large Catholic family with thirty-one first

cousins. Twenty-five of them were boys. On one of the cousins' family land in Michigan, they would all play a game called King of the Dock on a wooden platform in the middle of a pond. In this cutthroat aquatic version of King of the Hill, no one could hold the top spot for long. "The numbers always won out," he remembers. "Anyone who was beginning to establish a lasting presence on the platform would face an onslaught of a hastily put-together alliance of cousins intent on ending his reign."[7]

Two of the boys who'd flung Rich off the dock were gone. They were brothers. When Rich was a junior in high school, his cousin Matt Hunsucker had died at age fourteen in his parents' basement. Shotgun accident. Matt's older brother Donnie, just a few days older than Rich, had died a few years later. He was on his way home from a friend's house, in the dark hours of an icy Sunday morning—he'd promised his mom he'd go to church with her. He fell asleep at the wheel, skidded off the road, and hit the only tree in a roadside field, driver's side first. He was twenty years old. Rich's first two tattoos, on his shoulder blade and his right tricep, were in memory of his cousins. Their brother Darren was Rich's CrossFit training partner. After his big brother died, it seemed better for Darren to move down to Cookeville to be with Rich, who'd been close to Donnie, and who could act like an older brother.

On the same five acres where he'd played King of the Dock with all of them, Rich practiced climbing a fifteen-foot rope dangling from a tree. He'd watched online videos about how to do it. It wasn't hard to learn, when he was freshly rested. But that made him feel even worse about having lost. The chink in his armor had been trivially easy to mend. It was so frustrating. And the prospect of training like hell for an another year seemed overwhelming, because it was all or nothing. If Rich was going to compete, it seemed imperative to win. Bring home the gold, or go home as a two-time also-ran. If he couldn't take the podium, the effort to get there seemed pointless.

This is the dilemma of elite athletes whose identities are defined by their performance. Victory makes you a god. Conversely, defeat makes you worthless. So it's all on the line, in every training session, every qualifier, every competition. Success is winning. Not winning is failure,

and the social consolation of "We're proud of you *anyway*" and "You did your *best*" is almost worse than disappointed silence. Victory validates all sorts of borderline and over-the-line behaviors and rationalizations. And defeat implodes all sense of self-worth.

It never ends well. Every elite athlete, sooner or later, loses. Every elite athlete, sooner or later, can't compete anymore at the highest level. And then he's got the rest of his life to either live in the past or redefine himself.

At the tender age of twenty-three, Rich started asking himself some of the big questions: Who am I, why am I here on this earth, what defines me, what will people remember me for if I die, and so on. The uncomfortable answer was CrossFit. As far as anyone knew, Rich was an elite CrossFit competitor. That's how he spent his time. It's how he ran his life. It was all he talked about. It had been the axis of his daily existence. Looking back, he says, "I'd made CrossFit into something of an idol."[8]

Back at Tennessee Tech, Rich was working as Chip Pugh's graduate assistant. He trained athletes in the morning. Then he'd hit a strength WOD in the college weight room. After that, he cracked open the Bible and read his way through the New Testament, chapter by chapter, in the weight room.

Every so often, he'd poke his head into Pugh's office and ask a question about what he'd just read, if something didn't match what he'd heard or needed to be unpacked. He wasn't interested in going to church or participating in any organized religion. "He was trying to get away from that," says Pugh, reprising his role as weight-room minister. "He was searching for the truth, not what someone else thinks."

Earlier in the year, Pugh had started a a devotional blog for Cross-Fitters. CrossFit Faith, now known as Faith Rx'd, was a daily "spiritual workout" for CrossFitters who wanted to take the same approach to Christianity as they did to fitness: adopt a daily mindset and burn through some brief, high-intensity task in a community that's incredibly cohesive but not hierarchical.

"CrossFit is meant to be done in a community. And the same thing

with spirituality—we're meant to be in community." Pugh observes.[9]
But at the same time, people are turned off by the institutional politics, scandals, and church-committee bickering of religious institutions.
"That's why you're seeing a surge of these non-denominational churches
that are just autonomous," he says. "They operate the way a CrossFit
gym does. We do it our way here and love it. There's no body above us,
telling us what to do."

One day in the spring of 2011, Rich asked Chip about being baptized.
It seemed to him that there was a difference between being baptized as
a baby and the accounts of baptism he was reading in the Bible, about
mindful adults consciously affirming their faith. "I think I want to do
that," he told Pugh. "But I don't want to do it in a church. I want to do
it in a river. Could you do that?"

"Sure," said Pugh. "In Scripture, baptism doesn't have to be done
in a church. People just do it when they're ready to do it." So they took
about thirty friends and family members down to Rock Island State
Park. Chip Pugh baptized Rich in the rapids of the Caney Fork River.
And then people swam and had a party, and the young guys reverted to
their daredevil selves. Rich went in search of the biggest cliff he could
dive off and keep his skull somewhat intact.

"It was huge," says Pugh, laughing, and then, in the next breath he
says, "I knew he was going to win the championship. I didn't have any
doubt. I said, 'Rich, you're going to win the championship this year!'"

Rich shrugged it off genially and said, in the happiest and most honest way, "I don't care." His mind was different. Statements about how
he'd perform in the future, positive or negative, didn't trigger the same
response. The emotionally charged touchstone of self-worth had been
moved to a more stable spot that didn't depend on his ability to climb a
rope, or how much weight he could lift. And, paradoxically, this made
him a better athlete.

People are confounded when a football player puts Bible verses in his
eye black or kneels to pray in the end zone. To non-believers, it seems
like a kind of spiritual flamboyance or pushy proselytizing when athletes
publicly acknowledge God as the central pillar of their game plan. What

these spectators rarely consider is why this spiritual orientation is so effective, on and off the field—why it works, and feeds on itself.

Instead of "I'm the king of the world if I win, and a failure if I lose," and the crushing pressure that entails, the spiritually rewired athlete's internal logic is this: I'm a child of God; that's my primary identity. God loves me regardless of what happens in this competition. God has given me these talents, these amazing gifts, and it's my responsibility to use them as best I can, to perform and succeed to the utmost of my ability. But it's not for personal glory, or to feed my towering ego. Rather, every burst of speed and power is a testament to a higher power whose love transcends any kind of earthly success. The competitive results are not part of that higher reality. But the *effort* is. The leap toward perfection of effort, a kinetic hymn, is a connection to God. It's sacred, the way prayer is sacred. And at the same time it is exquisitely concrete. It has mass, speed, position, trajectory, in the *now* of a throw or a catch or a weight that needs to be lifted. It's where physics meets the soul.

This transcendent frame of reference doesn't take away competitive pressure. But it takes away the emotional pressure that degrades performance and locks an athlete up. Faith eliminates a lot of psychic gear grinding and inefficiency. For a well-prepared, well-trained athlete, it's a winning formula. And it was a winning formula for Rich Froning in July 2011.

THE FITTEST MAN
ON EARTH

FRONING GOES TO THE 2011 GAMES WITH A BIBLE VERSE TAT-
tooed in Celtic letters along the right side of his torso: Galatians 6:14,
a reminder not to boast about anything except God. Bible verses are
scrawled on the tops of his shoes: Galatians 2:20 on the right and Matthew 27:27–56, about the crucifixion, on the left. It keeps him focused.

The competition does not begin particularly well for him. The first
event is a 400-meter ocean swim, plus hundreds of push-ups, pull-ups,
squats, and two 1500-meter runs on the soft Santa Monica beach—a
splashy version of "Murph" in the sand. Smaller, faster athletes, Chris
Spealler and Navy SEAL Josh Bridges, have a field day with it. Rich
places twenty-sixth. The previous year, he would have been devastated
by such a disastrous start, he recalls. But he distinctly remembers thinking, *"If I finish 15th or 16th, my CrossFit competing days might be over. But I'm
okay with it."*[1]

The ocean swim takes Mikko Salo out of contention—the first wave
that breaks over him crashes into his ear and ruptures his eardrum.
Somehow, he completes the swim, vomiting into the sea three or four
times along the way. By the time he stumbles onto the beach, staggering
for balance, he can barely see the rig where he's supposed to do pull-ups.
He spends the rest of the Games in the stands, watching the rivals he
intended to beat.

"I put everything in my life to be in these Games," he says, ever the

stoic Finn. "Trained so hard, focused on the Games, I was well prepared. I was in the best shape of my life, and then this happened. Now
I realize that CrossFit isn't everything in life. It's an important part of
life. But I believe this makes me stronger. There is always a way to look
positively at things. You have to find things and be prepared for next
time. . . . I'm the predator who's chasing the guys who will win and be at
the podium this year. Those are the guys who I'm hunting next year."[2]

At the elite level, CrossFit competition includes Marines who've shot
their way through the back alleys of Baghdad and the gullies of Afghanistan, and tough sons of bitches from the Nordic steppes who've been
trained from childhood to endure pain, cold, and an extremely limited
fish-heavy diet without complaint. These competitors draw on their own
traditions and histories to put their athletic careers in context. Perspective on life is not reserved for born-again Christians.

But Scripture delivers the goods for Rich. After the swim, he tackles
every event of the Games with focused ferocity. He doesn't win every
event. But in the Games, an athlete doesn't need to win every event to
take the podium. The way different competitors' strengths and weaknesses stack up, anyone who's consistently in the top ten, across the
board, is in the hunt for first place. And Rich is nothing if not consistent.

The fourth WOD includes 15-foot rope climbs. Lots of them: 5
ascents, then 5 clean and jerks with a 145-pound barbell. Four rope
climbs, then 5 clean and jerks at 165 pounds. Three rope climbs, then 3
clean and jerks at 185 pounds. Two rope climbs, then 2 clean and jerks
with 205 pounds. One climb, then 1 clean and jerk, at 225 pounds.
The final heat is packed with fast rope-climbers: two track and field
stars and Bridges, a Navy SEAL who climbs up and down ropes for a
living. Khalipa is in the heat, but no one is particularly daunted by King
Kong's ability to get up and down a rope. Graham Holmberg, last year's
champion, has to realize that the dude he beat last year has learned how
to climb. As the athletes' names resound over the PA system, people
cheer. These names are now familiar, celebrated. The announcer re-
serves extra boxing-match fanfare for "the only athlete to compete in all
five CrossFit Games. The one, the only, Chris Spealler!!!"

Chris Spealler is a freakin' squirrel on the ropes. He is on Rich's heels until the barbells start getting difficult for his 142-pound body to propel up and overhead. He finishes his second 205-pound clean with perfect technique and races to the last rope. But Rich is already down, and closing in on the last lift. He split-jerks 225 pounds over his head, for a total time of 43 minutes and 57 seconds.

As Spealler's 225-pound bar lands hard on his shoulders, he shouts as if the impact of the bar has forced air and sound from his chest. He quickly gathers himself and gets the bar overhead. The whole stadium applauds, because it is a mystery how he does this. Everyone *knows* that Spealler can lift proportionally huge amounts of weight. But when you see him do it, it's always startling. It's visually improbable. So it seems like magic.

Spealler crouches down in a squat to recover and strips off his wrist wrap. Rich comes over to shake his hand. "Good job, brotha."

"You too," says Spealler. "How do you like climbing rope?"

"A little better." Froning smiles.

Much of the Games is a study in trade-offs between speed and power. In a WOD dubbed "The Killer Kage," athletes have to go hand-over-hand across a 100-foot-long set of monkey bars that Bill Henniger's stunt equipment riggers have constructed overnight. But that same workout includes sets of 7 front squats with a 225-pound barbell. Jason Khalipa slows down on the monkey bars and finishes twenty-second. On the other end of the size continuum, Spealler blazes across the monkey bars, but the load on the barbell, 158% of his body weight, drags down his pace, and he finishes twenty-sixth. Rich comes in sixth.

The next WOD, "The Dog Sled," is the same: three rounds of double-unders (speed and agility) and overhead squats (strength and muscular endurance), followed by three rounds of handstand push-ups (favoring smaller athletes) alternating with a sled push (385 pounds for 40 feet—an exercise favoring oxen). In the third heat, Chris Spealler runs out into the arena with his jump rope, to the customary rousing applause. Khalipa runs out, massive and buzz-cut. They're in adjacent lanes, and seeing them side by side, it really seems bizarre that these two athletes are competing in the same sport, in the same event. They're 70 pounds apart. It's like a fantasy face-off between movie monsters or comic book characters. Who would win: Superman or the Hulk?

Spealler whips through the double-unders in fifteen seconds flat. Then he falls behind Khalipa on the squats. Khalipa powers through the squats, and starts handstand push-ups ten seconds before his lithe adversary, then Spealler catches up and passes him with gymnastic speed on handstand push-ups. Spealler runs over to the sled. He puts his hands on it and digs his feet into the ground. His whole body is pushing against the sled. It doesn't move. He repositions his hands, and puts all the force he can generate with his 142-pound body against the sled's 385 pounds. It does not move.

Khalipa, built for heavy push, is moving forward, gaining.

FINALLY, SPEALLER GETS DOWN, LOW AGAINST THE SLED, HOOKS his arms around the handles so his biceps are pushing against the column handles most athletes are gripping. He puts his hands down on the sled's base and twists his neck around so that his head, his right temple, rests against the sled's stack of seven red 55-pound bumper plates. He pushes with his legs, with his arms, with his head pressed against the weight, and the effort carves furrows into the contours of his handsome face. But the weight moves slowly forward, and it keeps moving until it reaches the first stop mark. Spealler walks back to the wall to do his second round of handstand push-ups and erases larger athletes' gains against him. Then he goes back to the sled to struggle and push and be overtaken. Then back to handstand push-ups, to move faster than anyone else. And back, finally, to the sled, to suffer and to push the weight, seemingly by sheer force of will. He finishes in six minutes flat, twelve seconds ahead of Jason Khalipa.

In the final heat, Rich finishes second to Josh Bridges, but he is well ahead of Bridges overall. Heading into the final event, he is in first place again. The field has been cut to twelve competitors.

The final event is probably the most diabolical WOD in the history of the Games. It seems to have been designed as a form of mental torture. If there are enforced workouts in prisoner-of-war camps somewhere in the world, they must look like this WOD, which is aptly named "The End": 20 calories on a C2 ergometer, 30 wall ball shots, 20 toes-to-bar, 30 jumps onto a 24-inch box, 20 high pulls with a 108-pound kettle bell, 30 burpees, 20 shoulder-to-overhead lifts with a 135-pound barbell, and rope-pulling a 465-pound sled. Competitors have 3 minutes to get as far as they can into this beastly chipper of a workout. Three minutes, flat out, go as hard as you can. This is the time domain that invites a visit from Pukie the clown. It's a miserable interval. Graham Holmberg gets into the kettle bell swings when the clock hits three minutes, to win this event. No one finishes.

After the 3 minutes are up, the athletes get 60 seconds of rest. Then they have to do the same workout *again*, as a separately scored event, this time in 6 minutes. So: repeat the thing that just made you feel like you're going to die, and then some more. With full awareness of how awful that first few minutes is going to be.

This is when a vivid image of Someone Else being crucified really comes in handy. "When I think about how miserable He was going through that for us," Rich says, "what I'm going through ain't nothing." Rich is in his element, in this grinding test of physical endurance and mental fortitude. He stares down the Bible verses on his shoes during the sled pull.

Time is called. The athletes have 60 seconds of rest. Then they start the same workout *a third time* as a separately scored event, this time all the way through, for time. The athletes get back on the rowers. It's Sysyphean. Except every time they get to near the top of the hill, the hill gets higher. At this point, score-wise, Rich has already won the Games. But the format of the event does not exactly lend itself to a victory lap. So he sets about the business of finishing. Which means pulling the sled. No one has gotten to the sled yet. It's massive, and has to be pulled across the length of the tennis court, which is not a slick surface. Rich is out of breath. He is mentally and physically spent from the intensity of the first two rounds.

They all are. In this last round, the most striking thing about these elite competitors is how slowly they seem to be moving. They're doing burpees at roughly the same pace that soccer moms manage at 9:15 a.m. after they've dropped their kids off at school. The superheroes have been drained and drained and drained until the only strength they still have is residual. Their dregs look a lot like our best efforts.

Rich loops his arm around the rope attached to the sled and goes grimly to work. He finishes in 14:10, a minute and five seconds behind Spealler. But it's over. He's got the prize, the title, the money. His primary emotion is the same as anyone's after a WOD: relief. It is so exquisite, when the weight has been lifted, just to be done.

CORPORATE KOOL-AID
Reebok Gets Religion

"THEY TOOK THE BIBLE VERSES OFF MY SHOES," FRONING groused. Reebok was working up a limited Rich Froning edition of Nanos, the company's CrossFit shoe. The Froning Nanos were a charity fund-raising item for the Cookeville Fire Department, and their namesake wanted the shoes printed with Bible verses that had helped him power through the Games. The shoe samples that came back from Reebok did not have any biblical references on them. Someone in Reebok's marketing department had decided, without anyone else's opinion or consultation, to nix the religious references. It's the sort of thing that regularly happens at publicity-minded global corporations. Anything controversial is buffed out, and the edges softened, between concept and production, to make a finished product palatable to the mass market.

By the time the Froning Nanos went on sale, the Bible verses were back on the shoes. The marketing person who took the Bible verses off the shoes is, according to the company, "no longer with the Reebok brand."

In more ways than one, Reebok had gotten religion, starting with Matt O'Toole, the company's president. Coasting into middle age, O'Toole had been a typical out-of-shape exec buffeted by the demands of a high-pressure job and hands-on modern parenthood. The day runs out. The pants get tight. His father-in-law had exhorted him to "start a streak"—just pick some strenuous activity and do it every single day.

So O'Toole started running, and ran every day for nine years, until the repetitive impact of three thousand runs brought his streak to a creaking halt. He couldn't do it anymore. It was just too painful. Doctors evaluated his misaligned spine and multiple herniated discs and recommended surgery. In any case, long-distance running, the mainstay of busy people who want to keep their fitness formula simple, was off the table.

So the next question was: how to avoid becoming a fat middle-aged guy without spending hours in a gym or ending up in spinal traction. A neighbor described CrossFit and sang its praises. "That doesn't seem to make sense," thought O'Toole. "I can't even move right now." A month passed, and the same neighborhood friend mentioned there was a free introductory session at CrossFit New England, Ben Bergeron's box in Natick, Massachusetts.

If this neighbor was a typical CrossFitter, it would have been fairly apparent that these helpful reminders and suggestions would not abate until O'Toole dragged his beat-up body to the box and gave it a whirl. With his injuries, he couldn't do much of the introductory WOD. But he did what he could, and stayed to chat with Ben and Heather Bergeron, a CrossFit Games competitor and a superb coach in her own right. In the world of CrossFit affiliates, this was the equivalent of attending a cooking lesson with James Beard and Julia Child and hanging out afterward to swig sherry.

It was a crazy stroke of fortune that a top executive at Reebok was recruited by his neighbor into one of the greatest CrossFit boxes in the world. "I was totally blown away after just a couple of weeks by the environment, the community," he says. "There were all these people who were so outgoing and wanted to share their experience. I found myself going just to hang out. I was getting more functional from my back injury, and I was coming into work every day telling people about it."

When the office CrossFit proselytizer is a C-level executive, the Kool-Aid starts getting sprinkled into the plumbing of an entire organization. O'Toole's colleagues were soon roped into visiting CrossFit New England as well. He was convinced that CrossFit was "the aerobics of the twenty-first century," but coed, and with longer legs. A steady drumbeat of CrossFit advocacy reverberated through the offices of Reebok brass. "This is the most significant change in fitness that has happened in decades," went the pitch, "and it's at its very beginning. All the signs are, these guys have broken the code, and we need to be there."[1]

This evangelism came at a timely and turbulent moment for Reebok, because the company had just lost sponsorship of the National Football League to Nike. There weren't going to be any more NFL stars splashed across billboards as Reebok superheroes. But that was fine with O'Toole. He was was leaning hard on Reebok to pivot away from name-brand endorsements, "the sex end of sports." He invited Greg Glassman to Reebok's Massachusetts headquarters. Over dinner, he gave his testimony as a CrossFitter, and described the existential reboot he was trying to pull off at Reebok.

"For a long time," he said, "big athletic brands have been singing the praises of elite athletes and elite teams as a way to market our products. But on a per capita basis, fewer people are actually exercising. We're creating a nation of spectators and fans."

In the branding business, the assumption is that regular people want to be celebrities, so the best way to sell fitness gear is to slap a logo on celebrity athletes. But CrossFitters didn't seem to care about celebrity athletes. They were rabid purchasers of footwear and apparel. But the athlete they wanted to be, their aspirational ideal, was a fitter version of themselves: the athlete they'd be in six months or a year, or next week when they bagged a PR on a deadlift. The version of themselves that could do a muscle-up or twenty consecutive double-unders. Not some 260-pound linebacker or quarterback under the stadium lights.

What if Reebok were to shift its weight from "the sex end of sports" to whatever magic was motivating CrossFitters to lay themselves out four times a week? What if the perceived benefit wasn't the aura of some celebrity jock (with all the reputational liabilities that entails). What if the promise of the shoes was a chance to be totally engaged and totally present, to give it your all, every time you put them on, so that you can be a better version of yourself.

O'Toole's rhetorical train kept rolling at full steam, as born-again stories often do. On the product side, he observed, a lot of footwear from companies like Reebok and Nike involves technology, a spring in the heel, a conspicuous air pocket, or some other ostentation that visually suggests a mechanical boost to make you jump higher or run faster. The design implies that this magic gizmo will somehow make Joe consumer more like the elite athlete in the shoe companies' advertisements. But what if this aesthetic mirage is unnecessary? Maybe all people need is a basic product that's ergonomically correct and built around the way a body moves. Something functional, without the bulbous pumped-up heel foundations that vamp on a display shelf.

There were were hallelujahs all around. Glassman and O'Toole's "amen, brother" dinner started at six in the evening. It ended at two in the morning. Business particulars were broached the following day. A few big corporate bets were put on the table. One was the design of the Nano, which is now Reebok's hottest-selling shoe, not just among Cross-Fitters, but across the board. Another was Reebok's agreement, after a prickly set of negotiations with CrossFit HQ, to sponsor the CrossFit Games and manufacture a line of CrossFit gear, for which HQ would receive a royalty.

While it was clear that Reebok and CrossFit were in some kind of global brand tango, there were some highly charged discussions at Reebok about how large a role CrossFit was going to play in the future of the company. "In the athletic industry," O'Toole says, "we have lots of arrangements. You never really single one out and say this is the one. This is it. This is the one we're going to do in big, big way."

But in fact, CrossFit was the One, as impolitic as that may have been within the corridors of Reebok HQ. As if to underscore the point that Reebok had gone all in, the face of its world headquarters in Canton, Massachusetts, was reclad in a perforated screen that spelled "3-2-1 . . . GO" in numbers and letters two stories high. A fringe movement, the pirate brethren of fitness, had captured an actual navy.

One of the admirals, now flying the Jolly Roger, was Don Hassel-beck. A former pro football player who'd managed Reebok's relationships with NFL players for a decade.[2] To replace his roster of NFL stars, he was given a list of fifty CrossFit athletes with instructions to pick their brains, since Reebok's product designers knew nothing about the functional requirements of CrossFit gear. Hasselbeck invited the CrossFitters to headquarters and asked each of them to bring a bag packed with everything they wore during a CrossFit WOD. Dutifully, Reebok's new sponsored athletes brought their backpacks and duffels and dumped out the contents for show and tell with Reebok's product developers. The pile on the table was an exotic stew of niche brands like Innov-8, lululemon, Rogue, and Life AsRx. There wasn't a single Reebok item in it.

Some of the gear, on first sight, perplexed Reebok's designers. "Whoever thought that people would want to work out wearing knee socks?"[3] Hasselbeck asks. "But then you hear why they wear knee socks. You look at their shins and you design products so that people don't look like they were injured by a weed-whacker when they've been working out."

Every item on the table was critiqued and dissected, down to the placement of seams and labels. In most fitness activities, these minutiae don't matter—it's more a question of style than function. But the intensity and variety of CrossFit movements can quickly render the misplaced details of garment construction into a nagging annoyance or an outright wardrobe malfunction. Squats, handstand push-ups, and rope climbs each carry their own sartorial risks, in addition to functional imperatives for range of motion, elasticity, compression, heat dispersion, and stability. And that's not even counting sports bras, which are a whole other realm of complex and conflicting requirements.

Reebok may have gotten more design feedback from elite athletes on that one day than they received in decades of sponsoring NFL athletes, who are exquisitely well insulated by their agents. "With the NFL," says Hasselbeck, "you had some access. But you never had real access. You could talk to the trainers, some of the equipment managers. But you couldn't sit down with Peyton Manning and have him tell you what your shoe felt like." Unlike pro ball players, even the most exalted CrossFitters were happy to talk at length and in granular detail about what made a pair of shoes or shorts worth buying. If the feedback would make better products for other CrossFitters, they'd explicate gear and apparel for hours.

ANOTHER SERIOUS DIFFERENCE BETWEEN REEBOK'S NFL SPON-sorship and its CrossFit sponsorship was that when Reebok was sponsoring pro football, Reebok employees were not playing flag football out on the lawn. But when Reebok put its chips on CrossFit, CrossFit became the official corporate fitness program. In May of 2011, Matt O'Toole and Bill Holmes, Reebok's vice president of human resources, sent an e-mail to every employee on the campus. Everyone was expected to attend an all-hands meeting on the lawn, during which all attendees would be expected to engage in a CrossFit workout. Seven hundred and fifty people showed up to do push-ups, squats, and burpees. Not synchronously, in the style of North Korean dictators' birthday pageants, but at their own pace, as intensely as they could.

"The magic happened on that day," says Holmes. "That was the catalyst for change within our company. People saw that we were serious about fitness, that we were going to walk the talk, that we were going to actively participate. People of all ages, as well as people of all fitness levels, came together on a sunny day in May, and that started to change the culture."

"I've been at this company eighteen years," he says. "I look at my job as to help inspire, motivate, and engage a workforce. I have never, ever, ever seen anything that inspired, motivated, or engaged a workforce like this fitness program. . . . The covenant between the company and the employees has been strengthened through fitness."

In less grandiose terms, the deal is that Reebok gives employees paid time to work out, and roughly 40% of the workforce shows up several times a week to gut out a WOD at the company's 12,000-square-foot über-box in Canton. In the converted warehouse, now called Reebok CrossFit One, a seemingly endless whiteboard is covered with dry-erase thought-bubble annotations describing employees' personal fitness goals. Above the warehouse bay doors are "Rules to Live By," declaring that "fit people can change communities, schools, villages, and eventually the whole world."

THE BOX IS STAFFED BY SIX COACHES, INCLUDING TWO CROSS-Fit New England coaches recruited for their skills and tribal DNA—a former Marine and a British female soccer pro. As one of them leads a pack of Reebokers through a lunchtime WOD (twenty kettle bell swings, twenty burpees, five rounds), he cues participants to keep their arms straight and swing the bell high. "Stay virtuous" is the phrase. He doesn't yell it—this isn't some globo-gym boot camp where trainers bark at people. He just speaks the words. But the cue has a powerful effect, because when you hear that word during a workout, it implies in one breath virtuosity, the high level of technical skill that good athletes possess, and virtue—moral excellence.

As everyone recovers and makes their way back to the showers, the door they walk through has a motto stenciled above the lintel: "How you do anything is how you do everything." In other words, the spirit in which you tackle a WOD is a manifestation of the spirit in which you tackle your work. Snaking up on a push-up and cutting corners on a project are of a piece. Intentionally overstating rounds or understating times on the whiteboard would be a violation of personal honor that transcends the confines of the gym. Dedication to technique and execution, even it it means using less weight or going slower, breeds strength and excellence in the box, and likewise in the cubicle.

"How you do anything is how you do everything" enforces the discipline of leadership by example. Your boss's boss is expected to gut it out beside everyone else. If it doesn't look like he's giving the WOD his absolute effort, well then, that sends a message. If the chief of a division is a barely articulate puddle after twenty minutes, her decades-younger underlings don't have much of an excuse not to give it their all. Corporate group WODs are humbling for everyone. But higher-ups, by virtue of their advanced age, are generally behind the eight ball athletically, compared with junior employees. When a vice president struggles with a fraction of the new hire's barbell weight, and both get the same kudos, it shakes up the corporate hierarchy.

"If you go to a WOD, you might be partnered up with the chief marketing officer and one of the security guards," says Hasselbeck, who's met more coworkers in two years of CrossFit than he had in the previous twenty years at the company. "The designers, the developers, the marketing and sales people. We go to the box, and then we all come back here. We see each other in the hallway, in meetings. Barriers have been broken down. If you used to want to get something done in the legal department, it was impossible. Now it's not—you see each other in the twelve o'clock WOD, you suffer through it. You talk. You can work together."

"The common thread binding us together is the desire to fulfill our potential and have fun while we are doing it," declares Reebok CrossFit One's banner, hung high overhead. "For the committed, this is the path to a more healthy, happy, and productive life."

For the committed.

Most organizations give lip service to collaboration—sharing information across divisional boundaries, and such. It's another thing when you can call almost half the employees in the company, who don't work with you or report to you or vice versa, and ask them to do something, and they'll actually do it. This is why CrossFit tends to take on the quality of an insurgency when it gets a corporate foothold, or when coworkers discover they have CrossFit in common. They're more committed to each other than non-CrossFitters are to each other. In the "3-2-1-GO!" network that cuts up and down and diagonally across a large organization, obstacles get moved. Dominoes get lined up.

This is a network in which former athletes join forces with women who've lost significant amounts of weight. If you take all former athletes in an organization and thirty women who look like they could stand to lose thirty or forty pounds—the women who know everything about everyone and where the bodies are buried—and you fuse them into a cohesive network that can move and act in a coordinated way, it's pretty easy to see how you could flip an organization. Even a big, sclerotic one. It wouldn't take 40%. Maybe 10%, if that included someone at the top.

Michael Cordano, the president of HGST, realized this. And the prospect tantalized him. Unlike a lot of Silicon Valley firms, HGST isn't young or sexy or new. The company was formed when Hitachi's disk drive division bought IBM's disk drive business. A Japanese company, fused with the IBM pocket-protector culture whose lineage dates back to the1950s—it doesn't get any more hierarchical and conservative than that. And these people are old. The average age of an HGST employee is fifty-one.

Cordano had been doing CrossFit for a couple of years, at one of Jason Khalipa's boxes. And he could see that the tectonic plates of his industry were moving, that customers were shifting their information storage from onsite devices to "the cloud." If HGST was going to survive and thrive, it needed to become part of the cloud computing world. But that would take new talent, and a new way of thinking, and neither of those things is easy for a fifty-something workforce to integrate and adopt.

Cordano struck a deal with Khalipa: HGST would provide the real estate and pay for full-time trainers and affiliate fees. Khalipa would operate and manage two CrossFit boxes onsite at HGST. For CrossFit's most irrepressible entrepreneur, it was catnip. Instead of building bigger boxes, he could in-source boxes to companies run by Silicon Valley executives who were already working out at his gyms and were just as fired up as Reebok's Matt O'Toole. Unlike running a regular affiliate, even an archipelago of boxes like Khalipa's NorCal CrossFit, this was a business model that would scale. And if anyone was going to find an affiliate model that scales, it'd be Jason Khalipa.

IBM had built a 20,000-square-foot Nautilus gym at HGST's manufacturing and operations site. Cordano and Khalipa cleared out 6,000 square feet of it and covered it with rubberized floors, Rogue rigs, and bar racks. Cordano expected the younger and fitter employees to jump on board. But a sizable contingent of overweight fifty- and sixty-somethings figured they wanted to do what the cool kids were doing. They dropped a boatload of weight and started walking around with a bit more swagger. They could brag to their kids, or in some cases their grandkids. Their doctors' eyes were bugging out at the improvements in their blood panels.

"We're in the middle of a thoughtful, active transformation of the company," Cordano says. "We want to use CrossFit to break down the organizational silos. People are meeting people they would otherwise not be meeting on the job. You can hear people talking about it, and you can see them changing physically."

"You're all the same in there," he says. "You're suffering together." North of 10% of HGST's Silicon Valley employees hit a WOD at least three times a week, within eight months of the box opening. It's double that at HGST's office in Minnesota. ("Wintertime in Minnesota." Cordano shrugs. "I guess that's motivation.") An HGST CrossFit box has opened in Boulder, and Khalipa is prospecting corporate outposts in Thailand, the Philippines, Malaysia, and China. Even HGST employees in Japan are angling for a box (although admittedly, a visiting contingent of Japanese HGST employees surveying a CrossFit WOD clearly considered it to be insane).

Not everyone at HGST, or Reebok for that matter, has abandoned their companies' vestigial globo-gyms. But the cardio machine dead-enders are surrounded by dramatic evidence of fitness gains among the people who used to be next to them on the elliptical machine. If you're walking down the hallway and see someone who lost seventy pounds, that's a visual reference. You may want to stick with your elliptical, but Janet over there has lost seventy pounds and hasn't been that weight since since she was in high school. She got off the elliptical.

At a certain point, fitness starts to snowball, because the results are so dramatic and because the intensity of CrossFit forges esprit de corps that makes it easier for people to change their behavior. Healthy options—Paleo and Zone meals in the cafeteria—are within easy reach at Reebok and HGST.

But healthy options have been within reach for decades. Like most corporations up against the wall of escalating health costs, Reebok has been pushing wellness programs for years: smoking cessation, health-care assessments, biometric screenings for high cholesterol, high blood pressure, and diabetes. Reebok is self-insured—it's large enough to spread the financial risk of health catastrophes (car crashes, cancer cases, severely premature babies) across a large employee population. It saves on premiums that would be paid to an outside health insurer. But it also has to absorb the cost of every pill and procedure that's covered by its in-house corporate insurance policy. Even marginal reductions in health spending can translate into millions of dollars.

So the impetus to improve employee health is there, and has been there all along. But pleas about cost savings don't get people to change their behavior. Neither do voluntary assessments that are supposed to scare people straight. The people who'd be most scared don't show up for the assessments, because they know the assessments will tell them things they don't want to hear. And the people who show up, unless they're told they're going to keel over within a year, figure they can make marginal changes and be fine.

It makes you wonder whether the conventional corporate drive toward "wellness" isn't just ineffective, but also a huge missed opportunity. The reigning assumption in the world of HR managers, large insurers, and policy wonks is that changing behavior is hard, so people need to be nudged toward healthy behaviors by making that change seem easy and palatable. "Gamify" it. Give people points for reading informative online articles about nutrition. Count pedometer steps. Make the healthy choices seem just a little bit different than the choices that result in chronic disease. Make the change seem smaller, so that people can follow a bread crumb trail of small adjustments to a better life without really changing their perspective. There are a lot of snazzy mobile apps and candy-colored motivational posters that push this approach. There are a lot of single-serving snacks with low calorie counts, sold as healthier-but-you-wouldn't-know-it. They're packed with sugar, so they end up making people hungrier and fatter.

The sheer numbers associated with chronic disease, the magnitude of the medical and financial iceberg, make a mockery of this approach. The toll of the seven most common chronic diseases, in costs and lost productivity, was \$4.2 trillion in the United States in 2012, up from \$1.3 trillion in 2003.[4] Chronic diseases account for more than 65% of corporate health-care costs. In a single year, there were almost 0.5 million new diabetes diagnoses for Americans ages twenty to forty-four, and 1 million new diabetics aged forty-five to sixty-five. Those are just the people who felt bad enough to see a doctor. The Centers for Disease Control estimate that 79 million Americans are pre-diabetic, which means their bodies are teetering on the edge of a disease that leads to blindness, kidney failure, nerve damage, and limb amputations if it isn't controlled.[5] Those people can be pulled back from the brink to some kind of normal future if they decide to make some significant changes in their lives. Unfortunately, 65% of employers in a large 2011 survey cited the difficulty of motivating employees to change their behavior as their top health-care challenge.[6]

Maybe the answer isn't trying to get there by inches. Maybe the answer isn't HR wheedling employees into changes they're told are easy. Maybe the real opportunity is to say: We're going to try something crazy difficult, something really intense. Everybody who steps up to do it is going to feel like they're about to die, albeit for fifteen minutes, twenty minutes, tops. Strong people and not-so-strong people will see one another's heroic efforts. And in the end, we'll be more than faster, more powerful, harder to kill, and generally more useful.[7] We'll be a group of people that knows it can do crazy difficult things.

Reebok's CrossFit logo is a big equilateral triangle pointing up—the Greek letter *delta*, the mathematical symbol for change. If the wellness nudgers can't save us, if comfortable solutions won't make us strong again, maybe intensity—the willingness to get comfortable with discomfort—is the only thing that will really make a difference.

FORGING ELITE GEAR

Rogue Up-Armors the Box

MEANWHILE, BACK IN COLUMBUS, BILL HENNIGER'S SQUAT RACK and pull-up rack factory has expanded by three orders of magnitude. By the end of 2012, what began as a 500-square-foot workshop for Ian Maclean to weld gymnastic rings has exploded into 160,000 square feet of fabrication space, with another 100,000 square feet of warehouse and offices and two hundred employees. Like a CrossFit affiliate that's grown from one guy leading WODs in his garage to a hangar-size über-box, the operation is entirely bootstrapped. It has no outside investors, and carries no debt.

Postal and freight trucks back up to the warehouse to collect packages that range from a single jump rope to a new CrossFit affiliate's full arsenal of equipment. In the world of e-commerce, there are companies that ship envelopes and boxes weighing ounces or pounds. There are other companies that ship orders weighing tons. There aren't a lot of merchants who ship both kinds of orders on a single day, within twenty-four hours of those orders being placed. For workers on the warehouse floor, any given day is a constantly varied combination of pick, pack, and load, alternating between large- and small-item areas. As packers scan items into shipping boxes, a computer display projected onto the wall counts their reps. Henniger programmed the app as a kind of warehouse whiteboard. He's figuring out how to scale workers' scores, depending on what kind of items they're moving.

Packing might seem mundane, but Rogue puts an inordinate amount of money and time into it. "To ship this stuff and not have it explode when the UPS guy grabs it is a whole separate process," says Henniger.[1] Metal is heavy, and fitness gear is oddly shaped. There are lots of points and edges that can destroy a corrugated box when weight shifts in a truck. Henniger doesn't want Rogue products arriving like that. He wants the rigs and racks and bars to be tucked in and safe en route to their destination, and to arrive in pristine condition. Which is touching, considering how much abuse CrossFit equipment absorbs in the normal course of use.

This company spends a fortune on cardboard. Rogue makes its own custom boxes with specially designed cardboard inserts for structural stability and support. "We might have twenty dollars in a box, with all the inserts and pieces. Cardboard's expensive. A whole gym's worth of stuff, when they unpack it, they're standing on a thousand dollars of cardboard." Henniger sighs, "I wish I could tell them to go build something with it."

He rues the cost, but takes a sheepish satisfaction in the obsessive design of Rogue's packaging. It's the same sheepish satisfaction that new parents take in exorbitant, over-engineered strollers and car seats. He wants to give his precious cargo the absolute best.

As Henniger conducts a tour of his factory, he brims with pride. He points to the ventilation system that sucks air from fourteen welding tables through tuba-size funnels into a series of Willy Wonka pipes overhead. "Most welding shops are dirty," he says. "Ours isn't. I put in a whole system to pull out the dust so these guys have clean air to breathe." He leans over and sweeps his index finger across the floor. It comes up spotless. Henniger smiles, and casts his gaze across a continent of polished concrete. "You can see it shining," he says. "We have a Zamboni going around the floor *all day*." One can only imagine what kind of Christmas morning moment must it be for a thirty-something guy to take delivery of *his own Zamboni*.

Each of the factory's welding stations can make any piece of equipment Rogue manufactures. "We don't have single-purpose machines where the guy pushes the green button," Henniger brags. "There's five hundred jobs you can put on these tables." On the welding floor, no one works on one kind of job for more than half a day before switching to a batch of something different. If you don't vary the task, he says, "you wear people out."

Blue sparks cascade over the metal seams of a powerlifting rack. With one small movement, a welder flips the whole apparatus quickly around to work on the other side. "They call that the Rotisserie," Henniger says, describing the ingenious spinning jig that allows a two-sided welding job to turn like a chicken on a spit. "These guys made it themselves." The dazzling light of another MIG welding station illuminates a triangular cross-section of Rogue's "Dirty South" pull-up bar, which gives athletes multiple bar heights at a single station.

Henniger saw the original version of the bar at the CrossFit Games' Southeast regional qualifier, a throw-down for the baddest boys and girls in Alabama, Georgia, Florida, and South Carolina,[2] aka "The Dirty South." The Dirty South director, "Johnny Mac" McLaughlin, had welded the multi-height pull-up rig himself, and it was a solid solution to the problem of moving heats of male and female athletes through a competition without wasting time or space. Henniger asked if Rogue could make the bar and pay McLaughlin a royalty on it. "He's a good guy." Henniger shrugs. "If you read stuff about open-source communities, if someone brings something good to life, if you involve them, it works better." Royalties on CrossFit garage welders' cool ideas range from a dollar to twenty dollars per piece. Fifteen percent of the company's profit is distributed to hourly employees, "every quarter, like clockwork."

Most of Rogue's welders were hired in an economic downturn that cast a pall across huge stretches of the industrial Midwest. They were hired for their skill, but also for their attitude. Rogue hired guys like Ian Maclean, who learned to machine in a garage, and guys who made their own motorcycle parts. They had high school degrees and day jobs in factories and fabs. But on their own time, they liked to solve mechanical puzzles with tools and fire. Unlike debt-burdened college graduates with bachelor's degrees in identity politics, Rogue's recession-era hires can actually make and fix and build things.

"We look for people who can change their own oil. That's almost more important to us than engineering degrees," Henniger says. "We need people who have worked and *will* work. We're definitely a blue-collar company." With a lot of know-how and "git 'er done" work ethic on the fab floor, a new piece of equipment can be designed and built in a single day. In the lead-up to the CrossFit Games, Henniger says, "I'll hear from Dave Castro at 9:00 p.m. on a Sunday, and we'll weld it up on Monday." The rigs and equipment for the Games' surprise finale events are built at Rogue's old fab shop, separate from the main factory. Only four people are allowed into it. Guarding the secret of the Unknown and Unknowable is clearly pirate-adventure thrill for CrossFit's armorer. Running Rogue is a grade-school boy's fantasy. Every day, Henniger gets to work on double top-secret missions and play with fire and robots and lasers.

Rogue has two robot welding arms, which get assigned welding tasks that will take more than a week of continuous work. The jigs that position rig parts for assembly are designed to pop out of the welders' tables and click into the robots' tables. Building the jigs, with their ingenious array of nubs and pegs that keep separate pieces perfectly seated, is skilled work that usually falls to Josh Polcyn, Rogue's shop foreman and master welder. Polcyn also programs the robots. Training an articulated mechanical limb to weld a bracket for a pull-up bar, he physically guides the robot through a coordinated sequence of steps, punctuated by programmed instructions to apply a precise amount of heat in a specific amount of time. Refining subtle missteps with a coach's eye, Polcyn may take the better part of a day to train the machine to perform the proper movement pattern.

Certain rig parts fall into the robot's domain for liability reasons. The J-shaped brackets that hook into a rig and support the weight of a loaded barbell, for instance, are held in place by a single steel pin. A robot superheats each pin and bracket for precisely two seconds to ensure a rock-solid weld. A person can't manually trigger a precise two-second weld a thousand times in a row. That's not what people are good at. It's what robots are good at, whether they're welding pins into brackets or cutting the holes those pins hook into. Rogue's laser cutter is 150 feet long and slices perfect discs out of 24-foot square steel columns. Each tube spins like it's on the welders' Rotisserie as the laser perforates front and back-facing sides.

This is how Rogue counterbalances Chinese factory wages. "They have cheap labor—a guy's sitting there drilling something a thousand times. We don't do that," says Henniger, in a tone of voice that combines nativist working-class pride with design snobbery. Because the laser cuts more cleanly than the puncture holes of a Chinese mandrel, and won't wear out. And because it can delicately slice out Rogue's name and logo on a squat rack. And because it's a laser.

But for all the sci-fi manufacturing techniques at his disposal, what still puts the light in Henniger's eyes is the elemental quality of metal. He can rhapsodize about steel the way a sommelier expounds on the mineral qualities of soil and how sunlight on a south-facing slope in the Loire will affect the quality of the grape. The tempering attributes of a forge oven, and the timing of temperature fluctuations, or the quenching process that inundates a steel cylinder in oil—all these things affect the metallurgic properties of a weightlifting bar.

Neophytes might not appreciate the differences, but top-notch Olympic weightlifters can immediately suss out the whip of a bar, the way it bends down slightly on a fast lift, then springs back to straighten. Competitive Olympic lifters will use that whip when they catch a heavy clean. They time their drive "out of the hole" with the rising momentum on the ends of the bar, to harness the spring. Only elite Olympic lifters are technically proficient enough to time their movements to the whip of the steel. But they'd know in a heartbeat if it wasn't there. Powerlifters, on the other hand, require rigidity in a bar that's used for a 500-pound back squat. A CrossFit bar needs to a balance of both. It won't be the best bar for either sport. But it will support elite performance on a snatch or a deadlift.

It also needs to not break.

Given the sheer number of times a CrossFit bar is dropped from overhead, keeping the bar from breaking is an engineering challenge in and of itself. The metal sleeve that holds plates on most barbells is kept in place by a bolt or a snap ring. When bars crash to the ground, in the way that makes CrossFit strength WODs so uniquely satisfying, the impact and vibration of the bumper plates tend to jiggle out that bolt or loosen the snap ring. The barbell sleeve comes off. If this occurs in the middle of an Olympic lift, it's not pretty, and it's potentially dangerous. Rogue's bars have a stopping washer to keep that from happening. The test models of these bars were sadistically loaded, dropped, and pummeled to validate the improved sleeve design.

This level of over-engineering, seldom seen outside of Germany, is driven by two kinds of necessity: the first is the brutalizing physics of what CrossFit does to gear. The second is the customer's financial constraints. CrossFitters cobbling together a garage gym or a new box don't have oceans of money to spend. But they'll pay a fair price for a quality barbell if they know it won't break.

"I still want the normal guy to be able to purchase our equipment. It shouldn't be a $1,000 bar no one can afford. You should be able to buy it for your garage and have it last forever," Henniger says. He lines up a series of what he calls "bad bars"—ranging from $200 to $1,200—alongside Rogue's standard $290 barbell, and points out every flaw or evidence of sloppy construction in his competitors' products. "If you put our bar against a $1,000 bar, our specs are as high as a $1,200 bar. It debunks the myth that you need to charge $1,200. I want a lot of people to have them."

When you see a Rogue bar next to a bunch of other bars, it stands out in subtle and not-so-subtle ways. It projects an aura of quality. It makes bars costing twice as much look tinny. Part of this is the finish. Rogue has its raw steel cylinders ground and polished to a fine finish, so coatings don't reveal any imperfections. They use more expensive coatings, higher-quality chrome and zinc that clads the steel in bright silver or all-business black. Rogue's most expensive bars are coated with satin chrome, which is four times as expensive as any other coating. It has a matte finish that's less forgiving of surface imperfections than a black or shiny surface treatment. Its velvety smooth sheen communicates the precision of its manufacturing, the same way a MacBook Pro does. Henniger claims it gives a lifter more feel on the bar.

But the feel of a bar mostly comes down to the knurl—the diamond-shaped pattern of troughs that allows a lifter's hands to gain purchase on the steel. As with the whip of a bar, there are differences between the ideal knurl of an Olympic lifting and that of a powerlifting bar. Powerlifters girding for a deadlift appreciate an aggressive knurl, with deeper troughs and sharper points on the tiny diamond islands between them. Olympic lifters favor a more passive knurl, with shorter, smoother projections and more troughs per square inch, a "fuller" knurl. Rogue's knurlmeister, Nick Garcia, is the final arbiter of knurling perfection on Rogue's barbells. He plays the same role as a Sam Adams expert beer taster who taps a new brew, shakes his head, and says it has too much hops.

The knurl-forming process, he says, "is the machining equivalent of magic." The diamond pattern is produced by two knurling wheels that cut intersecting troughs in opposite directions. Each wheel is like a tractor plowing furrows in a farm field—when it moves to an adjacent strip of field, it needs to fall into the exact same groove in the area of overlap, or the tracking will be off. For that to happen on a knurling machine, the wheels have to match perfectly. A discrepancy of two-thousandths of an inch can create double-tracking, which compromises the grip value of the knurl. Knurling wheels sold as identical typically vary by five-thousandths of an inch.

In Henniger's worldview, "sloppy knurling" is worse than cut-rate manufacturing. It's actually an insult to the lifter. The virtuosity and beauty of a great lift deserves elegance and perfection in the steel. So Henniger has Nick Garcia go through boxes of knurling wheels with a caliper micrometer, to make sure they're matched to within a thousandth of an inch.

"It's an incredible mathematical process," Garcia says of all the factors that must combine to produce a perfect knurl: the diameter of the wheels, the diameter of the material, temperature, oil percentage in the turning tool's coolant, and the metallurgic properties of the material. "This is where math meets reality," he says "It's intensely mathematical. But at the end of the day it's a piece of metal that you lift. It's a Hegelian synthesis." It's a safe guess that Nick Garcia is the only factory machine operator in the United States who uses the phrase "Hegelian synthesis" to describe his work.

But there's something else about the knurl, when you see how much obsessive attention goes into it. When you sample the whole sensory range of those tiny diamonds, aggressive and passive, full and sparse, a sharp particle of truth lodges in the back of your mind and stays there, digging at you, until you realize what the pattern in the knurl is whispering to your palm.

Henniger talks about the feel of a great tool, a vintage wood plane or your grandfather's wrench. But those aren't the types of implements that get knurled. There are knurled surfaces that meet the tips of your fingers: the dials and knobs of audiophile sound systems, thumbscrews, and the barrels of expensive German mechanical pencils. But the knurled surfaces that meet the palm of your hand are meant to be gripped or moved with force. The knurling is there to keep the palm from slipping when a surface becomes slick with water, sweat, or blood. Knurled surfaces that meet the palm aren't just tools. They're weapons. The handles of kitchen knives are smooth. Hunting knives are knurled. Gun grips are knurled. Riot baton grips are knurled.

In the flash of violent effort it takes to jump a bar from floor to overhead, the central nervous system fires electricity into large muscles. The torso pulls quickly under loaded steel. As the bar moves up, its knurled grip is telling the nerve endings in your palm that it is a weapon. And your nerve endings believe it, because this is how good metal weapons feel in the hand.

REGIONAL COMPETITION
Nailing Colors to the Mast

OF THE THIRTY TEAMS THAT QUALIFY TO COMPETE AT THE 2012 Mid-Atlantic regional competition, only three will go on to the CrossFit Games. CrossFit Oldtown goes into the competition ranked fifteenth, the middle of the best. It's a fun place to be, because there's no heartache and there's no shame. The chances of the team barely missing a ticket to the Games are slim to nil. And unless something goes badly wrong, the team won't end up in the bottom quartile. The Oldtowners have practiced all the regionals workouts, and their goal is to do better in competition than they have in training.

Held at a 75,000-square-foot field house in Maryland, regionals is an annual gathering of the Mid-Atlantic tribes. It's a chance to see familiar faces from across state lines, check out the latest gear at the vendor booths, and admire a pageant of impressive tattoos and more-hardcore-than-thou team T-shirts:

"CrossFit Intense: Making You Harder to Kill."

"CrossFit Outlaw: Locked and Loaded."

"Beast Academy: Invoke Your Inner Athlete."

"Team CFOP," from Oyster Point, Virginia,
"I WILL FIGHT UNTIL I CANNOT BREATHE."

Several of the elite female competitors are former gymnasts, but they have jettisoned the distinctive quality of a young female gymnast: a bottomless desire to please, to charm the audience, make Mommy and Daddy proud, and earn a coach's hard-won praise. In their CrossFit incarnations, these athletes are adult females who can throw around some serious weight between rope climbs and chest-to-bar pull-ups. Their shoulders are strapped with RockTape to increase circulation. The black lines of the tape trace the contours of each muscle, a schematic overlay of each beautiful shoulder. As a punk rock kiss-off, these feral gymnasts weave ribbons and smear streaks of glitter into their hair and wear sparkly eye shadow. The cognitive dissonance between the ribbons and the glitter and the muscles and the badass attitude is electrifying.

Nicole Gordon and Christmas Abbott spot each other from across the warm-up area. They're on competing teams but rush to say hello and hug like sorority sisters. Christmas is gearing up for the WOD that scares and thrills her the most: a ladder of one-rep maximum lifts, snatching a barbell from ground to overhead inside of fifty seconds, with ten seconds to transition between bars.

At "Three, two, one, GO!" Christmas dives into a funnel of focus. In the first unfurling of this moment, the task is simply to leave the noise and motion of the crowd behind, to power down every signal that is not kinesthetic and proprioceptive: feet, spine, breath, grip. Her only awareness is hands on the bar and tension in her hamstrings, as all her body's springs are loaded. And then, in one gun-trigger instant, force ripples up legs, through a powerful extension of her hips, as the bar becomes weightless and her body drives underneath it to rise again with the weight overhead. A judge signals the rep. The crowd comes back into focus. The noise comes back on. There are emotions—a smack of satisfaction, the acknowledgment from a teammate. The buzzer sounds a ten-second transition to a heavier bar and the next moment, when everything but her body's signals will be mute.

Almost everyone in the stands has snatched a barbell. Not necessarily with the same weight, but with the same movement pattern. As Christmas walks up to the 135-pound bar, her teammates mentally project themselves into her setup for the movement. But she doesn't see them. In competition, she's in a completely different world. "A lot of people get distracted by the crowds or other teams or people beside them," she says.[1] "I don't see any of it. I'm in the eye of the hurricane. The more chaos is going on around me, the calmer I am, and the more focused and driven I am. If it's quiet, I don't have that same focus. I thrive on the chaos."

Christmas weighs 115 pounds, and her previous personal record on a snatch is 133 pounds. She sets, pulls, and fails, then quickly moves back to give her partner a stab at the lift. Her partner fails as well. On her second attempt, Christmas nails the lift and moves on to the 140-pound bar. Her awareness of anything that is not her body or the barbell is powered down now. The world is still. It's time. She crouches down, and pulls 140 pounds over her head. She's never done this before. It seems effortless.

There is a roar of applause. Her teammates go crazy. CrossFit Oldtown's girls cheer. The neurochemical pleasure of success ricochets between them.

Four members of the CrossFit Oldtown team—Melissa Lopes, Grace Chung, Adam Murphy, and Kevin Hare—went to regionals last year. Mike "Koz" Koslap, a videographer for CrossFit HQ, has local competition experience, although this is his first time at regionals. Thirty-six-year-old Laura Novotny is a rookie. She knows she wouldn't even be on the team if Oldtown's strongest female athlete wasn't seven months pregnant.

Laura's brow furrows under her bangs, which are dyed red from her natural blonde. Her green eyes are wide, and she's doing what she's beaten herself up for doing her entire life: obsessing about what could go wrong. At home, she's got two little boys and a husband whose career as an Army logistics officer means relocating every few years. She copes with chaos and flux by getting into her own head—gaming out all the problems in advance. But the demands of this competition are on the edge of her capability, and perhaps beyond her capability. She can't make the math work, and it's freaking her out.

She's been wringing her hands over CrossFit WODs for two and a half years. Looking at her, it doesn't seem logical that a woman who looks like Laura should be in the least bit nervous about an athletic performance. Laura has an optimal CrossFit body: five feet eight, strongly defined shoulders, and V-shaped back tapering down to strong legs and righteous ass. A mermaid tattoo unfurls down the length of her spine.

Below the flare of the mermaid's tail is a brittle star, the species Laura studied as a marine biology grad student in Hawaii. Drenched in salt spray and light off the water, she raced outrigger canoes twenty-five miles across the Kaiwi Channel from Molokai to Oahu. She did biathlons, running and paddling, and lifted weights in the off-season. Pulling oars through the water, or swimming and diving beneath it, she constantly tested her strength against the ocean. She was powerful in the water, beautiful in motion, in her element.

Once she left the ocean for a military base in Germany, and then the landlocked winters of Illinois and the Washington Beltway, all of life's grown-up circumstances converged to sap strength, grace, and beauty from her body. When the first trimester of her pregnancy got a little rocky, the doctor told her not to run. So she sat at her desk all day, then got home so hungry that she'd wolf down half a box of crackers while cooking dinner. By the time her first son was born, she weighed 200 pounds. Her husband bought her a treadmill. While the baby napped, she trudged away on it and wondered why it was so goddamned impossible to get under 160 pounds.

It was impossible because she was four months pregnant, on her way back to 200 pounds. She didn't own a single piece of clothing that fit, not even sweaters and coats. For a while she wore maternity clothes. But when she didn't have the baby with her, people would ask when she was due. She capitulated and bought clothes four sizes larger than the clothes she wore when her husband fell in love with her. Boarding airplanes, she could see a bow wave of tension and dread flip to relief as passengers realized the fat lady was not going to wedge herself in next to them. Every armrest was a clammy reminder of how badly her body had devolved.

Her husband's fit Army friends made her feel like an inferior life form. One female officer would rave about the adventure races she ran with her fiancé. She'd rhapsodize about riding bikes, running, paddling canoes, and finishing exhausted, euphoric, and filthy.

"That sounds so awesome," Laura sighed. "I would love to do that."

The woman's face fell, and she shook her head.

"Oh," she replied, "it's *so hard*."

The pity, the patronizing concern, hit Laura like a baseball bat to the head. It hurt, because the worst thing about being fat wasn't how she looked in the mirror, or that she could barely lift a thirty-six-pound stroller to load it into the back of her car. It was the way this lumbering, lumpen body engulfed and imprisoned the siren of her former self. Laura had almost resigned herself to the encasement and begun to accept it as herself.

The pain of being pitied jolted her memories of cutting through the Kaiwi Channel and, before that, of sprinting across a high school track. A recollection of being strong and fast and beautiful shook her into a ferocious fitness binge.

She ran. Monday through Friday, Laura showed up to work at 5:30 a.m. in her workout clothes. When the sun came up, she ran. Some days she ran five miles. Some days, ten. She trained for the Marine Corps Marathon. She dropped almost fifty pounds. But she couldn't shake off the last twenty. Running in Washington, DC, there were always traffic lights. It was hard to measure performance. And it was frustrating to put in all those miles and with no measurable improvement.

It was around this time that Harold Doran's CrossFit proselytizing became more persistent and annoying. At the same company where Harold ran statistics on standardized test scores for math and reading, Laura was responsible for statewide student science assessments. They'd go on business trips together, and at the end of afternoon meetings Harold would race out to hit a 5:15 p.m. WOD at some CrossFit box he'd located nearby. He'd arrive at social dinners with ripped calluses from countless pull-ups. And he kept insisting that she try it. Like most Cross-Fitters trying to recruit their coworkers, he spoke with the passion and persistence of a door-to-door missionary in the moment right after the door does not slam shut.

"Laura," Harold kept telling her. "You've *gotta* try this."

"You're insane," she replied. "Look at yourself. You're bleeding."

It was intriguing. But, Laura thought, *That CrossFit stuff is hard. I need to get in shape first, and then I'll go. I need to lose thirty pounds first. I need to finish the marathon.* But then the marathon was over, and the running wasn't working, and the year was winding down.

In January 2010, Laura walked into CrossFit Oldtown and did an intro class. The benchmark WOD for beginners was a 500-meter row, twenty push-ups, thirty air squats, and ten pull-ups, which she did by jumping up from a stack of plates. She finished in eight minutes and staggered over to where Harold was sitting with a few Blue Room veterans, shooting the breeze after their Saturday morning WOD. It was surreal, seeing tightly wound Harold with his shirt off, smiling and cracking jokes. But in Laura's fugue of flatline exhaustion, everything seemed to be melting around the edges.

"Are you okay?" they asked. "Do you need to sit down?"

Laura was completely unprepared for the intensity of moving through repetitions of full-body movements as fast as possible. Despite all the running—the long, slow distance five days a week—she had had her ass handed to her. And now, if she didn't come back, she'd have to go into the office and face Harold. So, she decided, it was time to suck it up and just go. She went through the Foundations course that Jerry, and most box owners, require for the uninitiated, to teach them how to lift bars and swing kettle bells correctly, so they don't end up hurting themselves.

After Foundations, Laura went online every night to see the next day's WOD. Then she'd lie awake in bed, thinking "Oh my God. How am I going to do that?" She torqued her back, rounding up on a deadlift. Her body was changing, but it hurt. Fat doesn't feel like anything when it melts off. But muscles, when they are broken down and rebuilt every day, are like a toddler's teeth pushing up through the gums. There wasn't much of Laura's body that didn't ache on any given day. But every time she broke a record, for time or weight, there was progress. In

July, when Jerry ran a CrossFit Total for everyone in the box—one rep max for back squat, deadlift, and strict shoulder press—she stacked up pretty well compared to the other women in the gym.

At the end of the year, Jerry ran a Hopper competition. All the movements and weight loads were written on pieces of paper and fished out at random to determine the WOD. What came out of the bag was ninety-five-pound thrusters and over-the-bar burpees (a push-up, jump over the barbell, repeat until done). She could just barely do that kind of weight on a thruster.

"Do I scale this?" she asked Jerry. "Do I do this? What do I do?"

He sized her up in a second. "You do it."

It took Laura thirteen minutes to finish the thruster-burpee WOD—she was still chipping away at it after everyone in her heat had finished. But she ended up placing third out of all the women in the box, because all but three of them had scaled down the weight. Only she and two other women had done the workout as prescribed.

Okay, she thought. *I'm going to be able to do this.* Once she decided that she could thrive, and even dominate the leaderboard on heavy metcons, it was a matter of showing up ready to attack the workout. Month after month, her times went down. Her loads went up. She rang the brass PR bell. Her spirit was ringing with the intensity of the experience.

On a microscopic level, that intensity triggered a chemical cascade that flowed through her blood, signaling her body to build muscle and burn fat. Weight-bearing movements made her bones denser and heavier. Repetition of movement under load, the balancing and counterbalancing of weight, built muscle memory and coordination. In metallurgy, there is a heat process called annealing that alters the microstructure of a material, and these microscopic structural changes alter the material's strength, hardness, and response to tensile stress. The ritual intensity of a WOD is a kind of annealing process. The microstructure of the human body changes, in ways that alter its fundamental properties, and the mental control system for those capabilities.

As Greg Amundson observed in the early days, it's not so easy to distinguish between physical capacity and mental toughness. The ritual of movement executed at high intensity, the development of muscle memory, is a process of binding muscle fibers to neural circuitry. And differences in neural circuitry are reflected in, and caused by, cognitive changes—this is the basis of cognitive behavioral therapy for anxiety, depression, and addiction. In a physically intense, ritualized effort, it's impossible to tell what is mind versus body versus spirit. When a gymnast vaults, or a sprinter rockets to the 100-meter mark, or a CrossFitter tackles "Fran" to the ground (or vice versa), these distinctions are not relevant, and perhaps they are not even real. They are real only for spectators.

As the structure and functionality of Laura's body changed, so did its outward appearance. The last twenty pounds of baby fat were replaced with almost as much muscle. More fundamentally, the annealing intensity of three hundred WODs transformed Laura into a firebreather. She's come full circle from pulling an outrigger paddle to jumping up a steel bar.

When it came time for Jerry to pick the six athletes who would compete at regionals, it was obvious that Laura was one of only three women who could hope to finish the brutally heavy WODs that CrossFit HQ had programmed to cull the competition herd.

But in the moments leading up to her competitive debut, Laura is unsure of herself. Putting up good numbers on the leaderboard in your local box is one thing. The work capacity required for CrossFit Games competition, even at regionals, is another.

In the athlete warm-up area, Melissa, Grace, Adam, and Koz file into the corral for WOD #1, an alternating sequence of 20 two-person deadlifts (two people, one bar, 455 pounds for the guys, 315 pounds for the girls) and 20 handstand push-ups. The corral's metal parade barriers split each team into a lane about two and a half feet wide and eight feet long, a kind of rodeo bullpen for elite athletes. Melissa hates the corral—it makes her claustrophobic.

"All right, Oldtown," Jerry growls with Marine Corps gravel in his voice. "Have some friggin' fun!"

Melissa and Kevin slap each other hard, once on each cheek, for luck.

Slap! Slap! Slap! Slap! "Yeeeeaaaaaahhhh!" It's a ritual they've worked up, based on some dubious sports research on the adrenaline spike produced by a hard shock immediately before running onto the field. Also, they're the goofballs in the group, and they perform better when their hard-core attitude is leavened with slapstick. They grin as they sprint into battle. The team finishes the WOD fifteenth out of thirty, knocking two minutes off their best time in the gym.

Rudy Nielsen, the head coach from Outlaw CrossFit, a notoriously hard-core box seven blocks down the street from CrossFit Oldtown, comes to needle Jerry about not being on CrossFit Oldtown's team. Jerry had the option to join the team at regionals. But in so doing, he'd risk an injury that would torpedo his prospects in the individual Masters competition, for Games athletes over forty-five. Rudy knows this. But insults are his way of bonding. Where others see abuse, he sees tough love. Rudy gets results from athletes who respond well to being denigrated at maximum volume while they train.

"These guys have their time," Jerry answers, "just like I have mine." Rudy leans over and confides, coach to coach, "I honestly hate this. There are so many moving parts. If one mistake happens, you're done."

The second WOD is a relay: Adam, Kevin, Melissa, and Laura each have to crank out 1000 meters on a C2 rower; do 25 one-legged squats with the non-grounded leg extended straight out ahead (otherwise known as a pistol, because the body takes that shape, with the floor foot and body as a grip and the leg straight out ahead as the barrel); and 15 hang cleans with 225 pounds for men and 135 pounds for women, which exceeds body weight for all of them. The guys get through the relay, although Kevin pauses between his hang cleans instead of stringing them rapidly together. Kevin is immensely strong, so when he gets lazy it drives Jerry nuts. "Touch and go!" he barks, "Come *on*, Kevin! Touch and GO!"

It's Laura's turn. Out of the corner of her eye, she sees Melissa is finished with the pistols and waiting for her to finish the hang cleans. *I'm holding her up*, she thinks, and this apprehension latches onto her nervous system. She jumps up the bar from hips to shoulders, but her body isn't synchronized. The bar tilts hazardously down from right, her stronger side, to left, and she fails. The bar drops. She goes to the chalk bucket, claps off the dust, grips the bar, and struggles it up to rest on her shoulders once, then again. On the next jump, she fails and throws the bar down, angry at herself. The fatigue of the rowing and the pistols has taken its toll, and the bar feels so much heavier than it did in training. She chalks up again, sets her shoulders, grips the bar with tension in her whole body, jumps, and barely gets under it. She fails again. She keeps going back to the bar, staggering under it, until all fifteen reps are done. Melissa finishes like a pro, and the team comes in seventeenth for the WOD in 22:01. They run to Jerry on the sidelines afterward. "I had to rest too much," Laura says. She is on the verge of tears.

He shakes his head and holds her gaze. "You were perfect."

As WOD #3 looms, Laura is trying to figure out how she's going to complete even one round of one-armed ground-to-overhead lifts with a 70-pound dumbbell (it'll be 100 pounds for Kevin). Imagine squatting down to pick up a can of soda, then jumping up and raising your arm straight overhead to hold the can of soda up like the Statue of Liberty's torch. Now imagine that can of soda weighs 70 pounds. The WOD is six rounds of these staggeringly heavy lifts done with alternating arms plus a 100-meter sprint. Each partner has to complete ten dumbbell snatches (one round) and the sprint before the other can start, and if either can't complete ten snatches on the first round, the team will be eliminated from competition. By design, this WOD is a gating function. It is meant to weed out teams that can't shoulder even heavier loads at the Games.

Laura has tried to train this WOD. The best she's ever been able to do with her weaker left arm is three lifts, and it took her twenty minutes. The cutoff for WOD #3 is twelve minutes for both partners. There is a very real chance that Laura will fail to complete a single round and DNF (Did Not Finish) on her first set of dumbbell snatches. She is afraid of failing, of letting down the whole team, her friends, and Jerry. She's afraid of going back to the box and facing dozens of people who'll know she's the one whose failure took CrossFit Oldtown out of contention.

"How do I do this?" she asks.

Jerry has to give her an answer. He has to tell her how to walk into the arena to do something that she's never done, that she's repeatedly tried and decisively failed to do, in front of people she loves and a thousand strangers. He must prepare her for an oncoming blow that will almost certainly bring her down.

"There's going to come a time," he says, "when you start to miss. Here's what you do: when a negative thought starts creeping into your head that you can't do this, just stop, look around you at the crowd and all the energy coming at you. Soak that up and use that. There is no better venue to snatch a 70-pound dumbbell."

In other words, it's a good day to die.

The clock starts, and Kevin nails his first set. Laura steps up to a dumbbell that's half her body weight. She is facing away from Jerry and everyone she knows, but she can hear them screaming her name as if their voices can buoy the weight. She leans over, grabs the dumbbell with her right hand, and jumps it high overhead. Alternating arms, she gets nine lifts—three more than she's ever been able to do—before the judge calls a no-rep on the tenth. Jerry is screaming, "NO doubt about it! Punch through this thing! PUNCH THROUGH!!!"

Laura's last lift defies logic and gravity, and seems more effortless than the first. She barrels through the sprint with both arms in the air, and as she races back from the halfway point, her face is blazing with pure joy. Melissa sees the light in Laura's eyes and starts to cry. After Kevin finishes his second set, Laura does four lifts in quick succession. She fails on the fifth. She fails again. Then something clicks. She starts jumping the load more efficiently, keeping the dumbbell close to the center line of her body. It's getting easier for her, not harder. Everyone from Oldtown is yelling their heads off as she finishes the round. On the final set, after failing twice, she completes a fifth lift before the buzzer sounds. She's done twenty-five 70-pound dumbbell snatches in half the time it took her to eke out half a dozen in the gym. She needed to do thirty and another sprint to finish the whole WOD, but no one cares. By finishing the first round, she has kept CrossFit Oldtown in the game.

Jerry is ecstatic, yelling, "I've never been so excited about DNFing a WOD in my life!" He hugs her. "You found a whole new level."

THE BALLAD OF
JERRY HILL

I love people who harness themselves, an ox to a heavy cart,
who pull like water buffalo, with massive patience,
who strain in the mud and the muck to move things forward,
who do what has to be done, again and again.

—MARGE PIERCY

BY THE END OF THE 2012 MID-ATLANTIC REGIONAL COMPETI-
tion, three teams have been cut and one has withdrawn. CrossFit Oldtown ends up ranked where they began, the middle of the best. They
won't go on to the Games. In 2011, when Jerry was competing with the
team, they finished seventeeth at regionals—they've raised their ranking without him, which is an achievement.

This year, Jerry is competing as an individual. At forty-five, he's old
enough to compete in CrossFit's turbo-geezer division, the Masters.
Forty-five to fifty is the youngest age category in 2012 (although the
Masters is extended to forty-year-olds in 2013). The age brackets move
up in increments of five years. The weights and rep schemes are downscaled versions of the same Games WODs performed by the younger
competitors. Jerry goes into the Games ranked number one in the Masters division, based on his performance in the Open.

Being an elite athlete at forty-five is different from being a twenty-four-year-old who can spend all his time training, eating, sleeping, and playing video games with quick recovery time and no family commitments. But even so, there are very few high school or college athletes who could hold a candle to the Games' forty-something competitors. They're just that fit.

Unlike the younger Games athletes, Masters competitors don't go to regionals. The number of categories for women and men in each age division would make those competitions too long and logistically unwieldy. So the top-twenty competitors in each Masters age category go directly to the Games. Their beat-up bodies are given a reprieve from peak performance between the Open's spring scrimmage and the summer Games.

Going into the Games, Jerry Hill is the man to beat. On day one, he ties for fifth in the first WOD, a one-rep max shoulder-to-overhead, and bolts too hard out of the gate in the second WOD. It's a triplet— four rounds of rope climbs, shuttle runs, and five front squats with 185 pounds, which is 20 pounds more than he weighs. He holds his breath to stay tight on the front squats, and by the time he finishes the first round unbroken, his blood pressure is jacked up and he's in oxygen debt. That leaves nothing in the tank for sprints and rope climbs. Bad pacing is a rookie mistake and a damaging miscalculation that sends him tumbling down the leaderboard.

On day two, he's back on his game, finishing second on a snatch ladder with a 195-pound lift, matching his personal record. He's in third place overall, on track to move into second place in the penultimate WOD, a chipper. After the chipper is a muscle-ups WOD he knows he can kill. There's an open window to first place, if he can just run the Saturday afternoon gauntlet, which will narrow the field from twenty contenders to twelve.

THE CHIPPER IS TEN 275-POUND DEADLIFTS, 20 PULL-UPS, thirty 24-inch box jumps, 40 kettle bell swings, 50 double-unders, and back down the sequence, 40 swings, 30 box jumps, 20 double-unders, and 20 deadlifts. Chippers are generally linear, moving from one set of movements inexorably to the next without repeating. But sometimes they climb up a numerical pyramid and back down, and when this happens it always seems like a sadistic Christmas carol, "A Partridge in a Pear Tree" with box jumps, double-unders, deadlifts, and so on. In December at CrossFit Oldtown, there is always a Twelve Days of Christmas WOD on this theme ("Five Golden Ring Dips"), and anyone who's survived one of these yuletide chippers gets flashbacks every time they hear the melody.

In the stands, forty people from CrossFit Oldtown are wearing blue T-shirts emblazoned with the word "Freakshow" and a comic-book rendering of Jerry's grinning face silk-screened on, like in *V for Vendetta*. The T-shirts have been worn for two days in the sun and heat. As Jerry walks into the arena, cheers rise from a small sea of blue cotton polyester, and so does the aroma of true fan loyalty. Jason Cox, Jerry's wild ginger-haired Marine buddy, the first guy to join him under the bridge back in Philly, has flown out to surprise him. So now, it's time to gun the engines.

"Three, two, one, GO!" Jerry grips the bar for his first 275-pound deadlift. In the next split second he drops it, as if it's given him a powerful electric shock. His right hamstring, which he pulled three weeks earlier, has blown out. He stumbles back. Forty people have worn their voices hoarse with cheering. But now they can't make a sound, or move. They stand there, stinking and stunned.

Jerry turns away from the bar like he's going to leave, because he's in serious pain and can't load one of his legs at all. He looks at his squadron of supporters, then turns around, picks up the bar and contorts his body to finish the ten ugliest deadlifts in history using only one leg. The announcer is clueless about what has happened and is grasping for words to provide color commentary: "A . . . very interesting style of technique that Jerry Hill is using with those deadlifts . . ."

The CrossFit Oldtown gang is in shock, watching this. Part of it is the heartbreak of seeing Superman stripped of his powers. The guy who never struggles is struggling. All anyone has ever seen of Jerry is super-human performance—he is a true firebreather. But now, the people who hold him in awe don't know if he can even finish the workout, and it's clear that he doesn't either. At this point, for him, it's just about finishing, the way it is for regular people, every day at the gym. It is a crushing feeling, for the Oldtown tribe, to realize that their leader is just like them now.

Except, he's not. After a moment's pause, Jerry jumps onto the pull-up bar and, because pull-ups don't require any leg power, turns into Superman again, cycling through rapid, perfect pull-ups that no one in the stands can even approximate. He lets go of the bar, hits the ground, and limps to the box. He stands in front of it, then takes a jump with the one good leg, lands, and windmills his arms for balance at the top. He jumps over and over with the one leg onto the box.

Jerry picks up the kettle bell, takes one swing, and walks away. Forty people are screaming, "Come on, Jerry!" Anna, his nine-year-old daughter, is yelling "Come on, Daddy!" The whole CrossFit Oldtown tribe is yelling at the top of its lungs. "We love you, Jerry!" Everyone wants him to be unstoppable, even wounded and in pain. It has taken a near-crippling blow to bring him down to this moment of agony they all face in the middle of a miserable CrossFit WOD: the riptide of temptation to stop, pulling against the will to go forward. Seeing their indefatigable coach in the trough of hesitation seals the pack into a moment that doesn't include the other competitors, or the other spectators. Everyone who belongs to CrossFit Oldtown knows that whatever happens next will change the story of who they are.

Jerry looks at his face printed on forty blue shirts, and he knows it too. He walks back to the kettle bell and grimaces through forty swings. He does fifty double-unders on one foot in forty seconds, another set of one-legged box jumps, then flies through the pull-ups and back to the deadlifts with the whole gang chanting JE-RRY, JE-RRY, JE-RRY through the last seven lifts.

Jerry ends up finishing second-to-last in fourteen minutes and change. No one at the box, it's later established, can beat this time with two good legs. He disappears into the athlete's area for a few minutes. When he comes back, the Oldtown posse swarms him.

"Who won?" he asks.

"We don't know," someone says.

Someone else adds, "We don't care."

"After a couple of those box jumps," he says, "I just started to figure out how to do the workout on one leg, and just load that one leg. I was kinda liking the one-leg thing after a while. I kept asking the judge how much time I had—I went back thinking I could catch a couple of these guys. It was like a Monty Python skit."

He pulls up the hem of his shorts on the hurt side and unravels a two-inch-wide, five-foot-long black rubber Reebok mobility stretch band that's wrapped around his upper thigh. The logos make it look like a trendy brand-name tourniquet.

He knew, going in, that it was not likely to end well. He hasn't pulled weight from the ground or run in three weeks. Laura Novotny is the only one besides Jerry's wife who doesn't seem shocked by this.

"He was in a lot of pain going into this," she says. In the lead-up to the morning's event, as Jerry prepared to face the WOD, she could tell that something was wrong, and had taken him aside. He told her that his leg was tight, that he was hurting. There was nothing left for either of them to say. She hugged him. It was a good day to die.

But this is the awkward thing: Jerry has so much comeback momentum, in terms of score, that this fiasco has only dropped him back to fifth place. The top-twelve contenders go on to the next day's first workout, which is two minutes to do as many muscle-ups as possible. Jerry can win this. The top-six finishers in the muscle-ups WOD go on to the final event, which is three rounds of thirty wall balls plus a 315-pound sled push. Jerry is shaking his head. "I don't want to take someone's spot who has a shot at it. I sucked it up for this WOD. I figure, if I tear it or whatever, the season's over. I don't want to go out there and repeat this—you think I can push a 315-pound sled with one leg?"

He turns to Jason Cox. When they were in the Marines as twenty-somethings, they challenged each other to see who could put the biggest dent in a newspaper vending box by tackling it, or in a wall locker using only their heads. "Bubba, what happened to us?" Jerry asks plaintively. "We never used to get hurt."

Jason cackles. "You're going to finals." Jason has known Jerry longer than any of Jerry's crew, and realizes that the college outfielder in Jerry won't be able to resist a moment on the field with a stadium full of people cheering. It's too good a moment to miss, even hobbled by injury.

Freddy Camacho, one of the Masters competitors, comes out with his girlfriend. "That was an inspiration, dude." Ron Thomas, another Masters competitor, walks up with his five-year-old daughter. "Jerry, my daughter wanted to meet you." She's hiding behind him, and he pulls her forward. "This is Jerry Hill. Shake his hand." This is the sort of thing parents used to tell children in front of astronauts.

The next morning, Jerry wakes up to the pain in his leg and breaks down in tears. He goes to the stadium and holes up in the athletes' tent. He's not sure he's going to limp out and do the muscle-ups. There's no physical reason he can't blast through them. It just seems pointless to progress from the muscle-ups to a wall ball–sled push WOD he can't possibly complete.

Sean Mulcahy and Kevin Hare, two Gonzaga College High School teachers whom Jerry recruited as CrossFit Oldtown coaches, subvert the Games' security and sneak back into the athlete tent, to see where Jerry's head is at. Sean is a former Marine who went head-to-head with Josh Everett and Greg Amundson on "Fran" back in the day (he was squashed like an extremely valiant bug).

Sean meets Jerry's gaze, Marine to Marine. "It doesn't have to be either/or—either you go out there and fail and be embarrassed or you don't go out at all," he says.[1] "I think there's another option. You came into this thing seeded as the top athlete in your division. I'm pretty sure if you hadn't gotten injured, you would have been right up there. There are so many people here behind you. You can still go out as a champion. You can go out there and do a couple of wall balls. Just do the first movement—we're all going to be sitting right there going nuts and cheering. You can just turn around and acknowledge the crowd and let the crowd acknowledge you back for being a champion and giving it your all. That's the way to do this. If you don't go out there, you're not going to get that recognition that you deserve. And you're not going to give us all an opportunity to recognize you. It's not just about you. It's about the community too. There's a lot of people that came to see you and are here to support you."

The athletes file out onto the field. Jerry is with them. He demolishes the muscle-ups and ties for first with the guy who ends up first overall. The CrossFit Oldtown gang howls that he was robbed of his last rep at the buzzer. On the final WOD, he does a few wall balls, expecting them to hurt like hell. But they feel surprisingly good. He walks out to the prowler sled, loaded up to 315 pounds. This is his finish line.

He touches the handle of the prowler, as if to make friends with a stout black dog. "I'll be back," he tells it.

He turns to face the crowd and waves good-bye.

THE MAN IN THE ARENA
Carson, California, AD 2012

IN THE GAMES INDIVIDUAL COMPETITION, THE FITTEST ATHLETES on earth are piling their energy onto a three-day bonfire of human work capacity: a triathlon and obstacle course at Camp Pendleton, track sprints, a one-rep-max ladder of ground-to-shoulder lifts, a ridiculously heavy version of the Masters chipper, a fireman-style sledgehammer event, and a final trio of benchmark Girls: "Elizabeth" (cleans at 135 pounds and ring dips, 21-15-9); "Isabel" (30 135-pound ground-to-overhead snatches); and "Fran" (21-15-9 thrusters and pull-ups) with no break in between.

By the last day, it is obvious that Rich Froning is unbeatable. In a scoring system that awards 100 points to the winner of most WODs, with a descending number of points awarded down the leaderboard, Rich finishes 114 points ahead of his closest competitor. Numerically, he could sit out the last WOD and still win the Games. People are in awe of him. But they don't relate to him, because he makes it look easy. They've done versions of what he's doing in the arena. They know it's not easy. They know they can never be Rich Froning. He's a demigod.

"You may not see another Rich Froning for another hundred years when his time has come and gone," says Chris Spealler.[1] But he's wrong. Every year, the number of CrossFit athletes expands exponentially, and the competitors get better. Within a decade, some other demigod will surpass Rich and become King of the Dock.

It is Spealler whose kind we'll never see again. Every year, the Games events get heavier and heavier. The loads get larger. Spealler has gotten larger—in 2012 he tips the scale at 151 pounds, positively beefy compared with the 129 he weighed in 2007. But his strength gains, and the strength gains of the smaller athletes, have been outpaced by the sheer load a Games athlete is expected to lift and carry.

The CrossFit gods are not malicious. But they are curious, maybe even greedy. They want to know how much energy they can extract from the fittest specimens of humanity they can find, over the course of a few days. And every year, it's more.

On day two of the 2012 Games, the last workout is 8 medicine ball cleans (pulling the ball, with a powerful jump, from the ground to shoulders); a 100-foot medicine ball carry; 7 handstand push-ups on parallettes (bars raised off the ground, which standardize the arm width of handstand push-ups and also make them more difficult); and another 100-foot medicine ball carry, back across the stadium to the starting point. Three rounds. The medicine ball is 150 pounds.

Chris Spealler weighs 151 pounds, and at thirty-three he's getting old for this. This isn't the downscaled Masters. It's the big leagues, and the loads are crushing. In the final heat, Rich goes in ranked first. Spealler is in the number twelve spot, the last of the best. At "Three, two, one, GO!" he pulls a 150-pound ball up and over his shoulder seven times. On the last clean, he keeps the ball on his shoulder and begins walking down the field. He finishes the handstand push-ups, hoists the ball up to his shoulder, and traverses the length of the stadium again. He does this over and over.

As he hoists the big black sphere to his shoulder for the last carry, a rattling roar rumbles up from the crowd. It is the loudest applause of the Games, even louder than when Rich wins. And there's an undertone of yearning it it, because almost everyone in the stadium has carried a weight that seemed as heavy as themselves—a 45-pound plate held overhead, or a couple of 53-pound kettle bells, one in each hand—and everyone has dropped the weight before they got to the line. But Spealler is carrying a weight that's literally as heavy as he is, and he isn't dropping it. The medicine ball stays on his shoulder, length after length. And everyone wants to be that sort of person.

He is so much smaller than the other athletes that it's clear this ordeal must be more difficult for him than it is for everyone else. It may not be—he's just as superhuman as any Games athlete, and outperforms half of them. But to see Spealler next to athletes with thirty or forty more pounds of meat on them creates a bridge between these superhuman feats and the familiar struggle, the ritual sacrifice of energy that is the essence of the sport.

Perhaps it is the essence of any sport. If you peel away the modern mass-market spectacle that sport has become, and the history of sport, to its root—the genesis of sport—there's ritual sacrifice. In the oldest chronicles of sport that we have, from ancient Greece, sport is sacrifice. It is the sacrifice of human energy. In the first Olympics, the ritual veneration of Zeus, the footrace began at the far end of the stadium. The athletes tore forward to a finish line at the footsteps up to the statue of their preeminent god. It was the winner who carried a torch to the top of the steps. At the altar, the torch was lowered to light a fire, not for the view of the crowd, but to consume the burnt offering of an animal. The champion himself was dedicated, although not literally sacrificed, to the god as well. His athletic performance was also an offering. It was energy, exertion, wattage, offered up alongside the animal. That athlete with the torch at the foot of the statue would recognize and understand what Rich Froning is doing in the arena in Carson, California.

The theory of sport-as-sacrifice, argued convincingly by University of Illinois classics professor David Sansone in a provocative monograph, *Greek Athletics and the Genesis of Sport*, is that human beings developed sacrifice as a cosmic pay-it-forward strategy: you give something up so that your people can have that same thing in the future. When this ritual developed among hunter-gatherers, it involved the sacrifice of a hunted animal, so that there would be more animals to hunt in the future. In this ritual, two things were sacrificed. One was the animal. The other was the energy of the hunt, because it took a lot of work to kill that animal and haul it back home.

When hunter-gatherers became farmers, they kept the ritual of blood sacrifice. They had animals—cattle, sheep, and goats—at the ready. They didn't have to hunt them. But the fullness of the ritual was defeated by this very convenience. "It is not only that the life of the beast must be 'taken' in order for the hunter to survive," Sansone notes. "The hunter must give of his own energy in order to get."[2]

It was at this point that athletics, things like footraces, became associated with religious festivals. The animal was sacrificed, and the race—the energy of the hunt—was laid down alongside it. The energy of the hunt, the element that was missing from the sacrifice of a domestic animal, morphed and evolved into athletic ritual.

"It became sport, which is itself a form of sacrifice," writes Sansone. "For only if sport is a form of sacrifice can we explain its ritual associations. There is no other plausible reason to account for the fact that the Hurons played a game of lacrosse in order to influence the weather for the benefit of their crops. It is only because they engaged in ritual sacrifice that natives of the Sudan hold wrestling matches at the time of sowing and harvesting. In Homer's *Iliad* the hero Achilles honors the death of his companion Patroclus with an elaborate funeral that consists of various kinds of sacrifice: hair offering; holocausts of sheep and cattle; libations of oil, honey, and wine; slaughter of horses and dogs; human sacrifice and athletic contests."[3]

Once the ritual expenditure of energy was decoupled from the hunt, it didn't especially matter how that energy was squandered. The rules and forms could proliferate a thousand ways, to accommodate the terrain and the materials at hand. The rules and conventions could morph and become subject to contention, debate, wagering, and technical innovation.

The ritual of sport, the sacrifice of a hunter's energy, persisted long after the practice of sacrificing animals gave way to less bloody, more symbolic religious traditions. Rituals have an incredible ability to persist, long after we've forgotten why they emerged to begin with. When people spill salt, they throw a pinch of it over their left shoulder—a Sumerian ritual that dates back to 3300 BC.[4] Christmas falls on the last day of the Roman Saturnalia—the date was chosen to celebrate Jesus's birthday by the fourth-century Catholic Church, which promised converted pagans they could continue to celebrate their holiday and sing in the streets the way they'd always done. Pagans who worshipped trees in the forest were brought into the fold with the assurance that they could bring the trees into their homes.

As rituals are drained of their intensity, their roots are buried in the sediment of years, centuries, even millennia. As the human movements that are *meant* to expend energy become easier, more comfortable, less intense—a leisurely tour through the Nautilus circuit, watching TV on the elliptical—sport becomes exercise. Without intensity, it's not a ritual. It's just a grind. Ritual becomes habit. The memory and meaning are lost.

But the roots of the ritual are still alive. And when the habits, for some reason, are re-endowed with intensity, they become rituals again. Because the root of the ritual, sport as sacrifice, is still alive inside us, it feels like a memory of something. It is a new shoot from an old root that makes a Hero WOD come alive. It's why, in a CrossFit box, you can be outrun or outlifted, but there's no way to feel defeated unless you slack off. The visceral sense of sacrifice, of giving all of one's energy up— underlies every WOD. Detonating all the fireworks means there will be more and bigger fireworks next time. Giving everything you have banishes regret.

This is why CrossFitters want to bring their families, friends, and neighbors to feed the caloric bonfire. It's why they cheer for the last athlete. It's why they suffer together, nationally, through "Fight Gone Bad," or CrossFit for Hope, or locally to raise money for friends felled by illness. They do this not because they've signed a contract or paid a fee, or out of guilt or obligation. CrossFitters give up their energy so that they, and their families, and their communities, can have it again in the future.

Sacrifice demands purity, and isn't worth as much without it. This is why people get so pissed off when athletes get busted for performance-enhancing drugs. If sport were merely a competitive quest for excellence, pharmaceutical augmentations would be considered an innovation, and their side effects would be considered the price of doing business. We would feel the same way about doped-up athletes that we do about doped-up musicians: it might make them better at what they do. It's part of the world they live in, although it's a shame when they overdose or die.

But if deep down, we know that sport is the sacrifice of a hunter's energy, then doping destroys the purity of the ritual, and that's what leaves us feeling robbed. It also spurs people to cheer for younger elite cyclists like Taylor Phinney, who conspicuously eschew not only banned substances but milder performing-enhancing measures like "finish bottles," the crushed-up caffeine pills and painkillers that riders gulp down in the home stretch.[5] The nutritional taboos of the Paleo Diet mesh perfectly with this mythos.

The living root of sport is why Jerry Hill does one-legged box jumps in the Games, coaching from the floor of the arena: no excuses. And it's why, when we see Chris Spealler carrying a 150-pound ball across the stadium, it seems like one of the great, for-the-ages moments in sport.

FIGHT FOR MIKE
A Box Takes Care of Its Own

WHEN JERRY CAME BACK FROM THE GAMES, WORSE FOR WEAR, one of his veterans was ailing. It was Mike Hart, the rugby player who'd stoked Blue Room's competitive spirit. He'd started coaching for Jerry and caught the competition bug. He'd won in the Masters category of a regional throw-down called the Mid-Atlantic Hopper. And then his double-unders winked out—the neurological knack of rhythm and timing was gone. Box jumps started to slow down. On a spring break vacation to Florida, he fell down on the tennis court. His legs hadn't done what he wanted them to do. His footing became unsteady.

By June, when he made good on his promise to join his brother, Joe, on a bike-run-canoe adventure race, he stepped off the bike midcourse. He was afraid he'd fall off and tumble down the side of a hill. He could run uphill. Footing on the downslope was precarious. He and Joe both laughed as he wobbled into and out of the canoe. The situation was ominous and frightening in an overarching way, but in the moment it was funny. Canoes almost always are. Mike laughed, but he didn't say much. He'd gotten quieter. Speech had become a disturbingly labored and deliberate effort.

Mike spent the next few months on a whirlwind tour of world-class research clinics. These were the sorts of places that get dramatized on TV, where teams of medical sleuths brainstorm to puzzle out rare and mysterious cases. At Johns Hopkins, which touts its *U.S. News and World*

Report ranking as the number one hospital in the United States, a crack diagnostics team brainstormed a long list of suspected pathologies and ran a battery of tests to narrow it down. When every testable candidate had been eliminated, they suggested Mike might have an autoimmune disease called Hashimoto's encephalopathy. This exceedingly rare condition is a once-in-a-career diagnosis, so it would have been a feat of medical virtuosity to correctly diagnose it. Unfortunately, the steroids that should have allayed Mike's symptoms didn't help.

The Mayo Clinic team were skeptical of the Hashimoto's diagnosis, but also concluded that Mike had an autoimmune disorder. His body had created antibodies to battle something foreign. But for some reason, the antibodies were attacking his brain. The problem was invisible. But by watching how Mike's body was trying to fight the problem, maybe they could figure out what was wrong. So they hooked him up to a blood-filtering machine for hours and removed all his antibodies. Then they watched to see the number and type of new antibodies that re-emerged. Mike's deterioration slowed, temporarily. The doctors were still in the dark. The treatments, which eventually included chemotherapy to kill the hyperactive antibodies, made Mike feel miserable (without the benefit of having done wall balls). He didn't get better. But his deterioration slowed.

Eventually, a rare disease specialist at the National Institutes of Health concluded that Mike had paraneoplastic syndrome—an invisible cancer that was undetectable in the body. It was so microscopic that no medical test could detect it. But Mike's body knew it was there, and his immune system was freaking out and eating his brain. There was no treatment for a cancer that couldn't be found. The only thing the medical establishment could do was promise Mike that they'd continue to run tests on him, in case the cancer decided to uncloak. For almost a year, he walked around believing he had invisible cancer, until a specialist at Memorial Sloan-Kettering Cancer Center said to scratch cancer off the list, without shedding any light on what had caused Mike's autoimmune system to go haywire. Mike drank a toast to not having cancer, and resigned himself to being a medical mystery, a walking embodiment of the Unknown and Unknowable.

He ditched the plasmapheresis treatments. He kept going to CrossFit with his brother and sister, and got his dad to join. For everyone else at CrossFit Oldtown, the Unknown and Unknowable was tomorrow's workout. For Mike, the Unknown and Unknowable was how much of his nervous system had been nipped around the edges since the last time he'd done the same WOD. Workout loads were going down from heavy to moderate to lightweight, and then to only bodyweight. The mission was simply to push his body as hard as it could go, with its corroded wiring, to make the system remember its repertoire of full-body movements.

In a way, finishing any WOD was like Sevens in the Snow, back in college rugby days: Mike Hart charging toward a goal, not knowing where the bounds were, and pushing forward as his body was slammed back in multiple unpredicted ways. There were no more PRs. There was no way to win the day. All that remained was to push forward in the scrum, as hard and as far as he could.

Forestalling defeat is different from fighting for victory. It requires a more tenacious effort. Everyone at CrossFit Oldtown saw this, and it sheared them of their excuses. If Mike could show up and give the WOD his all, what excuse did anyone else have to do less? He spurred the others by example, as firebreathers always do. Their presence makes people push to ignite the same fire inside themselves, by mimicry or osmosis.

When Mike was at the Mayo Clinic, the doctors told Joe they had a 70% chance of finding out what was wrong with his brother, and then a 70% chance of being able to treat him. "If I do the math right," Joe joked, "that gives him a 4900% chance of recovery, which I think is remarkable." On the whiteboard, next to the recorded results of particularly grueling efforts, people wrote "4900%," shorthand for "Those internal organs littering the floor? Those are mine." Also, a sign of solidarity: We suffer together; therefore we understand each other. We can do crazy difficult things together. Any WOD, when Mike was in the box, was a Hero WOD. It was just a question of when CrossFit Oldtown would formalize this and rally the whole pack, and all of its social networks, to his aid.

Mike's wife, a nurse at the local hospital, was leery. She was half of what CrossFitters jokingly describe as a mixed marriage. She wasn't part of the box, and she wasn't eager to make Mike a CrossFit cause célèbre. Her resistance was worn down by Mike's stack of medical bills, and by the sheer number of CrossFitters in Mike's large extended family. Even if she didn't think their "Fight for Mike" fund-raising idea would make much of a dent in the family's financial situation, it became pointless to oppose it. Resisting "Fight for Mike" was like resisting chocolate bunnies at Easter. Even if you do think chocolate bunnies are a meaningless feel-good ritual that doesn't affect anything, you can't stop chocolate bunnies at Easter. Too many people want them.

CrossFitters love fund-raising WODs—these events are a box's reflexive response to a crisis in its community. Fund-raising workouts are easy to plan. The venue is free. Cheap web services make it possible to set up a web page, complete with "Contribute" buttons and payment processing, in a matter of hours. It gives participants an easy way to express their support: pay the event fee, show up, pour out your energy, buy a T-shirt. But it also gives them permission to offer help. It's hard to know, when someone is in crisis, whether or when to volunteer support. But the minute the "Fight for Mike" web page went up, people knew it was okay to offer Mike a ride anytime he needed one, help with his kids, or anything that might make his life a bit easier. It broke the reticence to act.

Moral and financial support poured in from affiliates across the country and as far away as Afghanistan. On a cool October morning, boxes from all over northern Virginia sent athletes. Wounded warriors appeared from CrossFit Rubicon, where guys who've gotten their legs blown off in Afghanistan train to do one-legged deadlifts. These vets, with their high-tech prostheses and rippling muscles, are the most badass of the badass. Their presence at any CrossFit event renders it instantly legit. Even athletes from nearby Outlaw CrossFit, who rarely venture out of their pain cave of abusive coaching except to compete, showed up for Mike.

The street was closed. Eighties tunes blasted out the gym door. Simple Minds' theme song from *The Breakfast Club* blasted out the double doors of the box. Gen Xers who saw the movie as teens grinned when they heard it, realizing that any CrossFit box reprises the plot of the film, with a twist. All the geeks, weirdos, delinquents, and princesses end up becoming athletes.

Mike designed the WOD himself. Dubbed "The Unknown," it was a pair chipper, a series of movements to be completed by teams of two. In homage to Joe's 4900% remark, seven times seven was the numerical theme: 70 overhead squats (95 pounds for men, 65 for women); a 700-meter weight carry (45 pounds for men, 25 pounds for women, carried with arms straight overhead); 70 barbell snatches (95/65); a 700-meter walk carrying a heavy kettle bell in each hand (70 pounds in each hand for men, 45 for women); 70 walking lunges with a plate held straight overhead (45/25); 70 thrusters (95/65); and 70 front squats (135 pounds on the bar for men, 95 for women). After all that, each team had to draw a piece of paper out of a glass bowl—the Unknown—to determine their final set. You didn't know what was coming at you. But you had someone to share the load. Mike did a scaled version of the WOD with his thirteen-year-old daughter.

Commemorative WODs are odes of a sort. They tell a kind of story that is tied to movement. But this story is not for an audience—it's for the people who perform the movement. Only the people carrying the weight, struggling to get under the bar, moving under loads that make their shoulder muscles sizzle and fail, really understand the story. Only the people asking their partners to drop the weight understand how much easier it is to subject yourself to physical discomfort than it is to watch someone you love struggling to move. You want to let them fight their fight, pull their weight—it would be disrespectful, patronizing, not to let them do that. But you want to take weight, to be worthy of the other person's effort and fortitude. And the other person feels the same way.

CrossFitters are quick to talk about the push of competition. But what they'll endure in a partner WOD is on a different order of magnitude. The most intense event of any CrossFit competition is the WOD where one athlete has to do weighted movements while a teammate holds a stress position, typically a handstand against the wall or hanging from a bar. As long as one partner is executing movements that count as repetitions, the other partner is just trying to hold the stress position. If he drops off the bar, or out of the handstand, his partner has to stop making progress toward the total number of repetitions required by the WOD. Sometimes partners are allowed to choose when they switch positions. Sometimes they're not. But one thing is constant: an athlete lifting weight will not rest in front of a partner who's trying to breathe through the pain of a static stress position. And the person upside down against the wall knows that if he drops, the rep his partner is struggling to complete will not count. One person pays a physical cost for every second of the other person's effort. Knowing this doesn't make anyone stronger. It just boosts pain thresholds, and this drives performance.

About three hundred people, including rugby players from every Jesuit school Mike had attended—Bishop Ireton High School, Wheeling Jesuit University, and Loyola—showed up to do the WOD. Not just to "Like" him or his event on Facebook, or blog or tweet or contribute money, but to push themselves through a physical trial in one another's presence.

Physical presence matters. One morning of face-to-face commitment weighs more than weeks of virtual community. Social media was important, even necessary, to make Fight for Mike happen. Social media is important, even necessary, to the growth of CrossFit. But in the end, it's all about showing up face-to-face, as part of a geographically rooted community that's willing to do hard work. In the end, a good proxy for a person's social connectedness, the kind that matters in a crunch, isn't how many online friends you have. It's how many people will show up for you on a Saturday morning to do something difficult.

If Mike had just been one of the Oldtown veterans, the event's thirteen or fourteen thousand dollars' worth of entry fees and raffle ticket sales would have been the day's financial tally, and everyone would have counted it a success. But Mike had been working to strengthen his community, not just build his social network, his entire life. He was president of his high school alumni group. He was active in the Alexandria

Chamber of Commerce. He ran a Friday morning breakfast group for high school pals who worked in real estate and construction. They got together to swap gossip on city land use and find ways to help one another out. His family had been in Alexandria for generations and was deeply rooted there. The Washington Beltway is a transient place, full of out-of-town politicos and military personnel on rotation. But in cities like Alexandria, there are people who have parents and grandparents and dozens of uncles and cousins who know all the other long-time families. The Harts weren't upper crust. They weren't "society." But they had worked construction together, run local businesses, and rolled up their sleeves to help their neighbors for the better part of a century.

That's why, eight hours after the WOD, the local Toyota dealer threw a party at his sprawling suburban mansion, and a local restaurateur catered it for free. A local craft beer company, part owned by a member of the Friday morning breakfast club, donated the brew, and a local musician (and CrossFit Oldtowner) played the tunes. Dozens of silent auction items, from sports tickets to week-long vacation house rentals, were donated by friends-of-friends who were not physically intrepid enough to do the WOD. And the financial tally rose from an impressive five-figure sum to more than a hundred thousand dollars. That doesn't happen for a random dude at the box.

But it's not obvious that it would have happened, even for Mike, without CrossFit Oldtown. The box didn't create all the relationships that were brought to bear on that day. But it did catalyze a reaction that pulled support out of those relationships in a sudden and dramatic way. Perhaps there is social energy dissolved in communities that only ritual can precipitate—and some rituals are more powerful than others. Or, as Joe puts it, "Silent auctions are great, but to see people physically busting their asses is way better. You found out how amazing the people around you were, in the community you were linked into—how willing people were to help others. That may be the best single day I've ever had, short of my children being born."

Since Fight for Mike, Mike has continued to train at CrossFit Oldtown. He has gained lean body mass, and strength. He's ditched the walker, although he still uses a cane. He has clawed back his mobility. He does push-ups and pull-ups, and squats with eighty pounds of chains draped around his shoulders. On Memorial Day 2013, he did his own version of "Murph": a 2000-meter row, sixteen rounds of "Cindy" (5 pull-ups, 10 push-ups, and 15 squats), and another 2K row. It took him about an hour. Most guys pushing fifty would take longer. His speech has gotten a bit clearer.

No one fools themselves that Mike has reversed the course of his disease. But he has accelerated his adaptation to it. His muscles and nerves are finding ways to route around the damage. Even compromised systems can be made to function in a more robust way. It just takes a lot of work to force that adaptation, and that work requires an athlete's discipline and dedication. It may not be possible to train at this level, mentally or physically, as a patient. The work isn't a pill you can take. It's not something a caregiver can provide. Only someone who's an athlete in his soul, and is treated as an athlete and coached as an athlete, can do what it takes to hold the line.

OLD SCHOOL

The Original Firebreather
Goes Back to Basics

GREG AMUNDSON, THE ORIGINAL FIREBREATHER, WAS ALL
alone again. When Glassman moved to Arizona, he left the Santa Cruz
box in Amundson's care. Amundson ran it for a year until it closed,
then moved to Southern California to work for the Drug Enforcement
Administration.

"DEA was the real gunfighters, the guys that were really legit,"[1]
Amundson says. "A lot of guys that had worked the street for a long
time, that I would consider hard-core, they were warriors. They were
bad to the bone. They went into the DEA, which had the reputation of
being the knights of the round table . . . the stuff legends are made of. I
wanted to be on a team that was the best of the best."

Once he and his wife rented a house, they unpacked their CrossFit
gear into a 400-square-foot garage. The size of the garage had been the
house's selling point—it was about the same amount of space that Glassman had started with, in the jujitsu studio. They loaded equipment into
their car, drove to a nearby Navy base, and began performing CrossFit
workouts on the track in 115-degree weather, just in front of the base
globo-gym. After four of these field demonstrations, they'd recruited a
small group of intrepid souls, many of them Marines, to train with them
on Friday afternoons. To mix it up, they alternated between the track
and workouts at the on-base pool, some involving sets of fifty burpees

and fifty thrusters performed between 50-meter swims. It raised eye-brows among the lifeguards, but as long as people were gasping for air *outside* the pool, it wouldn't be death by drowning, so that was okay.

Amundson joined a boxing gym and a Brazilian jujitsu school, two more sources of CrossFit recruits. His wife found a local ranch where they could buy horse stall mats. Glassman had discovered horse mats back in Santa Cruz as a less expensive alternative to roll-out rubber matting. "There's something about a cement floor covered wall-to-wall in black horse mats that just fires me up," Amundson wrote in a *CrossFit Journal* chronicle of his mom-and-pop garage gym.[2] On the walls, they hung framed T-shirts from their favorite CrossFit affiliates, photos from their days at CrossFit HQ, a whiteboard, and a six- by ten-foot American flag. For a husband and wife, coaches at heart, it was a perfect pint-size box.

They tried to educate and inspire their athletes the way they'd been educated and inspired in Santa Cruz. They demonstrated the foundational movements and mechanics to novice athletes gathered in a circle. They also taught nutrition and emphasized the "between the ears" elements of CrossFit: goal setting, the discipline of incremental improvement, the frame of mind that makes it possible to push through metabolic misery and even embrace it. They bathed their athletes, many of whom had never considered themselves athletes, in the glow of constant acknowledgment and positive feedback. They introduced the term "relative intensity" to make clear that the goal of any WOD was to go as hard as possible with proper form—to build virtuosity before cranking up the load. In this way, the entire group could achieve intensity, even though the athletes varied widely in their capabilities.

No one paid. Athletes mopped up after workouts and donated equipment. The ones with carpentry and welding skills built equipment. Inevitably, the first couple of dozen athletes began to recruit their friends and family. Eventually, the Amundsons moved out of their garage and set themselves up as professional CrossFit trainers in a 1,300-square-foot warehouse. They knocked through the wall of that space into 2,800 square feet, then moved to a premier 14,000-square-foot facility in the Imperial Valley.

Amundson's name was plastered across one of the largest CrossFit boxes in the world. As an elite DEA agent, he was going undercover and busting Mexican drug cartels. He had the badge, the big career take-downs, and the fastest "Fran" time. He was the Man.

But it wasn't working out so well for his wife. She was managing the box, teaching CrossFit seminars, scrambling to hold down the domestic fort, and then getting chewed out by Greg, who came home from a busy day of taking down Mexican drug cartels and wondered aloud why dinner couldn't be ready at a reasonable hour. In the middle of 2011, after his twelve-year-old dog died of cancer and his mom passed away suddenly from a brain tumor, his wife told him she wanted a divorce.

Everything about his life that wasn't about being an elite badass was imploding. There seemed to be only one sane option: get the hell away from other human beings. Amundson took a leave of absence from work, bought an Airstream trailer, and leased a parcel of land in the mountains near Santa Cruz. For two months, he lived in the woods and rolled back the tape on the last fourteen years of his life as a SWAT team cop, Army reservist, DEA gunslinger, and husband. He wrote an after-action review of his marriage, *Your Wife Is Not Your Sister*, a self-critique so detailed and unstinting that it could have been subtitled *Confessions of a Knuckle-Dragger*. The book, lovingly dedicated to his ex-wife, is filled with recollections of moments when he thought he was justified but later realized his behavior was thoughtless, myopic, toxic. At the end of each chapter are concrete "Action Steps" to prevent fellow knuckle-draggers from repeating his mistakes. It's been well received in the law enforcement community.

At the end of his two-month woodland retreat, Amundson realized two things. The first was that it doesn't matter how much of a fire-breather you are if you can't cut any slack to the important people in your life. The second was that all his macho law-and-order jobs had defined him, and if he wanted to stop being That Guy, he couldn't work that kind of job.

He could have opened another CrossFit megabox. He could have opened an elite training facility for firebreathers gunning for the Games. He had enough stature in the community to do either of those things and succeed in a heartbeat. But in a way, that would have been more of the same: the triumph of the strongest, fastest, hardest dominant alphas. He didn't need more "HTFU." Or perhaps, the *H* needed to change from *Harden* to *Humble*. "Humble the F Up."

So he opened a tiny gym for non-elite athletes. He leased the smallest suitable space, about 1,000 square feet, just a little bigger than the Glassmans' original box and just four blocks away. One block in the opposite direction was the Brazilian jujitsu studio where Claudio Franca had given Glassman some mat space in exchange for training his fighters. The energy of the place felt familiar. It felt even more familiar when Amundson pulled some of the original Santa Cruz gear out of storage.

When Greg Glassman had closed the original CrossFit gym and moved its contents down to Camp Pendleton, all the original athletes kept something. Since Amundson was legally in charge of the box when it closed, he held on to a few more pieces of gear. But he kept only enough for his personal use: one of the horse mats, a rower, a set of rings, a barbell, kettle bells, some bumper plates, and one of the Iron Mind racks. "It was all the original athletes who had their hands on that gear," he says. "I kept what had my blood, sweat, and tears on it."

In July of 2012, without fanfare, he set up a pull-up bar outside the door of CrossFit Amundson. In board shorts and no shirt, he worked out every day in front of the place, doing pull-ups, squats, and sprints up and down the driveway. As rumors circulated that Greg Amundson, the original firebreather, was beginning to train athletes a short sprint away from the original gym, people showed up. If the box was closed, they slipped applications under the door. Half of them were strangers. Half of them were friends from the old days. Naomi Silva, who won the female Toughest Cop Alive trophy alongside Amundson in 2004, came back to train alongside middle-aged moms and graying athletes with creaky shoulders. John Shepard showed up to remind his old partner from Santa Cruz sheriff days that neither of them was twenty-two years old anymore. Five of the jujitsu black belts who enrolled were white belts at Claudio Franca's place when Glassman started training at their dojo. None of them pay. Law enforcement officers get a discount. Everyone else pays about half of what a typical CrossFit box charges for unlimited monthly membership.

Amundson decided to take the first hundred people who showed up, regardless of their fitness levels. Within three months, he had his hundred and capped the membership. Fifty more were allowed to work out twice a week, and the rest were on a waiting list. Although anyone in the community can attend a free class on Saturday mornings, there are no plans to expand. Scale destroys the essence of the endeavor: to reclaim and invoke the magic of CrossFit's founding days.

CrossFit's original violation of conventional business wisdom was to abandon the globo-gym model that profits from members who don't show up. But the mega-CrossFit boxes that have emerged in the wake of CrossFit's success are about scale as well: how many people can you move through constantly varied, high-intensity functional movement in a warehouse. CrossFit hangars run by luminaries like Jason Khalipa, Tanya Wagner, and Christmas Abbott, or the Black Box in Manhattan, have hundreds of athletes moving in twenty- to forty-person groups in staggered starts (in CrossFit NYC's case, on $200,000 worth of three-inch-thick, impact-absorbing NeoShock flooring).

The more people belong to a box, the less it feels like a family. That's not what the original CrossFit gym was about. "That gym was a family," Amundson says. "It was a community." In the new old-school place, Amundson knows everybody. "Nobody slips through the cracks. If I don't see somebody, I call them.

"It feels the same," he says. "True CrossFit."

Amundson's let his hair and beard grow out. It gives him a bear-like, almost cuddly appearance, in contrast to the sharp, clean-shaven jaw and shaved head of his early photos. His times and weights have not devolved from youthful high-water marks—they've gotten better. He's very conservative in his training, striving for tiny improvements at the margins. He gets to the box at five in the morning and leaves at nine at night. He spends the whole day interacting with athletes, setting goals, teaching private classes, or leading an advanced class where he works out as well.

"My business model is love and support," he says. "I've known for a long time that you can be the world's best trainer, know all the cues, be a Games athlete, but in the end none of that matters. What people care about is being loved and supported in their own goals and dreams. That's what I got from Glassman. That was what was so unique about how Glassman taught. He really cared about his athletes and wanted to help them. He tutored me in math—I'd go over to his house. I was applying for the Army and needed higher test scores, so he tutored me in math."

At least once a week, someone will come to CrossFit Amundson to see the closest thing there still is to Greg Glassman's original CrossFit gym. If they're from overseas, they add their names to an international banner with signatures from ten countries. "I know it's not in operation anymore," they'll ask, "but can you take me to the original space?" Amundson drives them down to what's now a computer repair shop and shows them where it all happened, and tells them about it. There's even a tour company now, WOD Tours, that runs trips to a string of hallowed CrossFit destinations. Extremely fit pilgrims from Australia and New Zealand land in San Francisco and visit Kelly Starrett's box, thence to Khalipa's CrossFit NorCal, down to Annie Sakamoto's gym ("home of the original 'Nasty Girl'!") and a morning session "with the original firebreather," Greg Amundson.

Even regulars at CrossFit Amundson jostle over the relics. There's always a scuffle over who gets to use the storied old barbell, as if it had been used to slice off Grendel's arm or slay St. George's dragon.

The WODs reprise Amundson's daily battle with whatever the Glassmans had to throw at their original crew. Literally, he wrote down all the WODs, day by day. He was very disciplined about taking notes and keeping records, and he kept all his journals. For the first year, CrossFit Amundson's programming was a day-for-day re-enactment of whatever the WOD was exactly ten years before. Three times a week, CrossFit Amundson's WOD comes from the original liturgy. Other days, there's something new. And if it seems like people are getting overtrained, or the WODs are too consistent, Amundson will pile people into a twelve-passenger vehicle dubbed "The Epic Fitness Van" and go to the beach to run or do kettle bells or jump in the ocean and swim. On Tuesday afternoons, the Epic Fitness Van takes people out of the box to do some real-world outside activity—hiking or sailing or learning how to surf or paddle-board. He loves the van, and people love piling into it with him, even if they don't know where they're going, or what sort of Epic Fitness activity awaits them at their destination.

Unlike a lot of boxes, Amundson's has abundant natural light. Along the length of the exposed brick walls, at wall ball target height, white words are printed on a black background. The banner on the barn in Aromas during the 2009 Games was printed in the same white sans-serif typeface. The Games banner proclaimed, "The strength and value of CrossFit lies entirely within our dominance of other athletes. This is a truth divined through competition, not debate." Every competitor had to hit one of those words with a medicine ball ninety times on the first night.

Amundson's banner delineates CrossFit's ten attributes of fitness— Endurance, Stamina, Speed, Strength, Balance, Accuracy, Coordination, Agility, Flexibility, Power. And then, in continuous fashion, Courage, Confidence, Perseverance, Virtuosity, Resilience, Service, Faith. "Words that have a spiritual root in them," he says. "Those words are seen every day by the athletes, and words have a manifesting power. When you see those words in the gym, you're repeating those words in your mind, and that creates a higher level of consciousness and awareness."

This is particularly true when the visual mantra is ten feet up and has to be hit repeatedly with a twenty-pound wall ball. Language used within this space is circumscribed. No one's allowed to speak in the negative tense. Amundson never coaches movements by telling athletes what not to do. He believes that even if the error is presented as a caution or correction, the phrase still lodges in the athlete's mind, and that the athlete is so focused on the phrase that he unconsciously follows it as a direction. On a deadlift, most CrossFit coaches say, "Don't round your back." Two of those words, "don't" and "round" are negative. Amundson won't use those words. He'll say something like "Maintain your lumbar spine." If an athlete says, "I want to work a bit light on the deadlift because I don't want to get hurt," he can scale down the load. But he has to rephrase his request: "I want to stay light *to protect my back*."

Every athlete is required to keep a notebook and record all his workout results, but also responses to CrossFit Amundson's Question of the Week. "We're contemplating why we were brought to this earth," Amundson says. "What are we here to do?"

The questions are scrawled on the whiteboard before Monday's workout. They're all calls to action. "How can I contribute to the betterment of the world today?"

"How can I be of service to other people?"

"Who do I need to thank in my life today?"

Athletes write in their notebooks. Sometimes they team up in groups of two or three to discuss their answers. Then they start the warm-up and the workout, which is probably some couplet, triplet, or chipper designed by the Glassmans and performed by the original firebreathers ten years before, to the day.

A lot of the data in the athletes' notebooks is quantifiable evidence of progress. But some of it, by design, is intangible. "What's happening between the ears," Amundson says, "in the heart and spirit of the athlete—it's a combination of mind, body, and spirit. Everything is interwoven. The movements, we've been doing since the beginning of time. We've forgotten them, but our ancestors were deadlifting rocks to build homes. There is definitely something magical about intensity—pushing past your perceived limitations. It gives you a tangible reference point, and we judge ourselves from that new reference point forevermore. No pull-ups to five pull-ups becomes a reference point. The goal then is to continue to push those reference points in our lives further and further out into the horizon."

ACKNOWLEDGMENTS

Thanks to Sloan Harris at ICM—if I didn't have a literary advocate of his caliber who also did CrossFit, this book would have never come to light. Likewise, thanks to Rick Horgan at Crown, whose editorial coaching was valuable and much appreciated, and who gamely learned to do double-unders to validate my description of the movement. I am obliged to my astute first-pass readers, Betty Sue Flowers and John Fritz, for their thoughts and comments. I'm also grateful that this book project put me back in touch with two college professors, Pat Hoy and Gregory Nagy—brilliant teaching has a very long half-life. Thanks to Chris Nolan for taking such a great cover photo, and Matthew Longworth (a Marine—hooah!) for hoisting that Atlas ball at the Mid-Atlantic Hopper. Profound appreciation and respect goes to Chef Wallach of CrossFit Rubicon, the athletes and coaches at CrossFit Walter Reed, and the Working Wounded Games for showing us what real firebreathers can do.

Much thanks to everyone at CrossFit Oldtown for sharing their stories, to Dan Wilson, and to the athletes I interviewed in the course of this book: Laura Novotny, Nicole Gordon, Tanya Wagner, Sara Wilkinson, Christmas Abbott, Eva Twardokens, Annie Sakamoto, and Nicole Carroll—you ladies are the bomb. Thanks to Bill and Caity Matter Henniger for allowing me into your awesome factory, and to Josh Polcyn and Nick Garcia for sharing the secrets of robotic welds and the art of knurling. Thanks to Don Hasselbeck, Matt O'Toole, Bill Holmes, and Bryant Mitchell at Reebok, for their time and access to Reebok CrossFit One.

Thanks to Rich Froning, Darren Hunsucker, Dan Bailey, and the crew at CrossFit Mayhem for letting me shadow them during the lead-up to Mayhem's grand opening (I'll never forget the expression on Rich's face when a mom told him it was okay for him to sign her son's forehead in Sharpie). Thanks to Chip Pugh for his perspective on faith and the finish line. Thanks to Jason Khalipa, Chris Spealler, and Jill Spealler (it's a brave athlete who gives you his mom's e-mail address). Thanks to Greg Amundson for calling whenever he had spare time on the road. Thanks to Kelly Starrett for his boundless expertise on matters of mobility—his Mobility WOD website is an invaluable resource for anyone with less-than-perfect range of motion.

Heartfelt thanks to Greg Glassman, Dave Castro, Nicole Carroll (again), and the folks at CrossFit HQ, who generously shared their time and perspective. When I started this book, I was terrified of Dave's reputation as the big bad wolf of CrossFit HQ. Contrary to rumor, he was disarmingly open and eager to talk about points of controversy and contention in an even-handed way. I kept giving him opportunities to ditch me during the Open, at regionals, and at the Games, and he kept inviting me to tag along as he kept a thousand plates spinning. It made me appreciate the magnitude of his job, which is like pulling off a royal wedding, an outdoor rock festival, and a UN Security Council resolution, all rolled into one.

Last, but not least, I'd like to thank my husband, John Scott, for roping me into CrossFit in the first place. He started doing it after he ruptured a lumbar disc doing a stupid boot camp workout at the local YMCA that included jumping up and down while holding a forty-five-pound plate. "I know what ten is on the pain scale," he said afterward. "It's when you wish someone would hit your head with a brick and put you out of your misery." After a surgical procedure to slice off the piece of disc that was oozing out of his vertebra like jelly from a doughnut, he vowed to make his core muscles so strong that this kind of injury would never happen again. That led him to CrossFit.

A former high school lineman and heavyweight wrestler, he fell in love with it. He talked about it constantly, regaling me with the movements and rep schemes of his daily WODs. It was really boring to hear him go on about it every time we sat down to dinner. The jargon was unintelligible. The regimen sounded crazy. As the weeks went by, I realized that I sort of had to give it a shot. Because if I could get into it, maybe all this CrossFit talk would be interesting instead of indecipherable and tedious. For the sake of our marriage, I figured I had to try it, and hopefully like it. Or else I'd end up like a golf wife or triathlon widow.

So I tried it, and ended up loving it, despite the fact that, as an athlete, I'm neither a Lamborghini nor a diesel truck—I'm more of a Fiat. But after a few years of sprints, gymnastics, and Oly lifts, I'm an excellent example of what a person can accomplish with scant genetic endowment for sports. "Cindy" is my BFF.

Thanks to all the CrossFit athletes, competitors, and coaches who continue to inspire me. See you at the box.

GLOSSARY

Note: All the following terms (and more) are explained in comprehensive detail on the CrossFit website, www.crossfit.com.

AMRAP: "As many rounds as possible" in a fixed period of time—e.g., "a 20-minute AMRAP of 5 push-ups, 10 pull-ups, and 15 squats."

Below parallel: A squat position in which the crease of the hip (the angle formed by the torso and upper thigh) is below the knees.

Booty shorts: Workout shorts with a minimal inseam that blurs the line between exercise apparel and a swimsuit bottom.

Box: A CrossFit affiliate, so named because CrossFit gyms are fairly basic, unrenovated, and often industrial spaces.

Box jump: Jumping from the ground onto an elevated platform, typically a wooden box (alternatively, stacks of bumper plates, park benches, or picnic tables). Box jumps are typically onto a 20- or 24-inch box, although 30-inch box jumps are not unheard-of. For this reason, Rogue makes a Swiss Army–style box that measures 20 × 24 × 30 inches.

Bumper plates: Barbell plates encased in rubber. A barbell loaded with bumper plates.

Burpee: Diving from a standing position into a push-up, then jumping up and clapping overhead—an aerobically taxing movement, particularly for larger or taller athletes.

Butterfly: A pull-up technique whereby the athlete uses momentum from the hips and continuous rotation of the shoulders to rapidly cycle through pull-ups.

Chipper: A workout in which all repetitions of one movement are completed before progressing to the next movement, as opposed to a rounds-for-time workout, in which a sequence of movements is repeated multiple times.

Clean and jerk: Pulling a barbell from ground to shoulders, then propelling it overhead with arms extended.

Deadlift: Raising a barbell from the floor to hip level, with full hip extension.

Double-under: Jumping once while a jump rope passes under the feet twice.

EMOM: "Every minute on the minute"—i.e., doing a movement or series of movements every sixty seconds.

"Fran": CrossFit's most dreaded WOD, consisting of 21 thrusters, 21 pull-ups, then 15 thrusters, 15 pull-ups, then 9 thrusters, 9 pull-ups. "Fran" was one of CrossFit's original Girl WODs. The rep scheme, 21-15-9, is recognizable to any CrossFitter as the shorthand recipe for metabolic misery.

Handstand push-up: Kicking up to a handstand, usually against a wall, bending arms until the head touches the ground (or a designated target), then fully extending the arms. Handstand push-ups are made more challenging by requiring the athlete to grip raised parallettes or put his hands on raised plates. They can be made easier by reducing the range of motion (raising the head-touch target) or using large rubber bands suspended from a pull-up rig.

Hang: Holding a barbell at hip height at the beginning of a lift instead of raising it from the ground. Lifts from the hang reduce the distance a bar has to travel, but also eliminate the benefit of momentum generated by leg extension as a bar moves up from the ground.

Hero WODs: WODs formulated and named in honor of fallen soldiers, firefighters, or law enforcement officers.

Hopper: A WOD composed by drawing movements and repetition counts at random from a container.

HTFU: "Harden the fuck up"—a motto often used to describe the most challenging variation of a WOD with multiple scale or difficulty levels, and generally used as a more-badass-than-thou T-shirt motto. As CrossFit has become more mainstream, this phrase and general attitude have fallen out of favor.

Kipping: Using momentum from the hips to complete a movement or to augment power during a movement. Kipping is the CrossFit default for pull-ups, and can also be used to extend shoulder endurance on handstand push-ups. Kipping makes the body more efficient—a first principle of functional fitness. For that same reason, military trainers and old-school PE teachers disapprove of it.

Knee socks: Often worn, by men as well as women, during barbell WODs to protect the shins as a bar closely follows the vertical line of the body in a maximally efficient lift. Looking like a leprechaun is an acceptable trade-off when the alternative is bloody shins.

Masters: The "seniors" age division of a CrossFit competition—forty years old and up.

Metcon: A "metabolic conditioning" WOD that alternates strength movements with cardiovascular stress. For example, deadlifts and box jumps, or power cleans, double-unders, and pull-ups.

"Murph": A Hero WOD in honor of Navy Lieutenant Michael Murphy, killed in Afghanistan on June 28, 2005. "Murph" consists of a 1-mile run, 100 pull-ups, 200 push-ups, 300 squats (partitioned as desired), then another 1-mile run.

Muscle-up: An advanced CrossFit movement, wherein the athlete grabs a pair of rings overhead and pulls up to extend the arms straight down, with rings at hip level.

"Nasty Girls": A CrossFit WOD made famous in a video featuring Annie Sakamoto, Eva Twardokens, and Nicole Carroll. "Nasty Girls" consists of 50 squats, 7 muscle-ups, and 10 power cleans (135 pounds for men, 95 for women), three rounds for time.

Olympic lifts: The snatch and the clean and jerk.

Overhead squat: Raising a barbell overhead with arms fully extended, lowering the body into a full squat with hips below the knees, then rising to a full standing position.

Parallettes: Miniature parallel bars, usually about eight inches tall and two feet long, used for bodyweight exercises like L-sits, or to increase the difficulty of handstand push-ups.

Pistol: A one-legged squat, so named because the outline of the body looks like a pistol—the extended leg is the barrel, and the planted foot is the grip.

Power clean: Raising a bar from the ground to shoulders without landing in a squat.

PR: Personal record.

Rx'd: As prescribed—i.e., doing a WOD without modifications.

Scaled: A WOD that has been modified with the substitution of less advanced movements, lighter weight, or fewer repetitions.

Snatch: Pulling a barbell from the ground to overhead, with arms fully extended, in one uninterrupted movement.

Strict pull-up: A pull-up from a dead hang, with no kipping.

Squat clean: Pulling a barbell from ground to shoulders, landing in a full squat, and rising to a standing position with the barbell resting on the shoulders.

Tabata workouts: Named after a Japanese exercise physiologist, Tabata workouts employ an interval scheme consisting of 20 seconds of all-out effort alternating with 10 seconds of rest, repeated 8 times for a total of 4 minutes.

Thruster: Starting in a full squat with a barbell resting on the shoulders, then rising up to a standing position with the barbell overhead and arms fully extended.

Wall ball: A medicine ball, typically 20 pounds for men (14 pounds for women), thrown against a target on a wall (10 feet up for men, 9 feet for women, although women typically use a 10-foot target in competition). The ball is caught as the body lowers into a full squat, then explodes up to relaunch the ball to the target.

WOD: Workout of the Day, constantly varied.

RECOMMENDED READING

Amidon, Stephen. *Something Like the Gods: A Cultural History of the Athlete from Achilles to Lebron*. Emmaus, PA: Rodale Books, 2012.

Amundson, Greg. *Your Wife Is Not Your Sister (and Fifteen Other Love Lessons I Learned the Hard Way)*. 2nd ed. Los Gatos, CA: Robertson Publishing, 2013.

Bell, Catherine. *Ritual: Perspectives and Dimensions*. Rev. ed. New York: Oxford University Press, 2009.

Caillois, Roger. *Man, Play and Games*. Translated by Meyer Barash. Urbana: University of Illinois Press, 2001.

Culin, Stewart. *Games of the North American Indians*. 1907. Reprint, Mineola, NY: Dover Publications, 2012.

d'Aquili, Eugene, and Andrew B. Newberg. *The Mystical Mind: Probing the Biology of Religious Experience*. Minneapolis: Fortress Press, 1999.

Froning, Rich, with David Thomas. *First: What It Takes to Win*. With a foreword by Dave Castro. Carol Stream, FL: Tyndale House Publishers, 2013.

Green, Harvey. *Fit for America: Health, Fitness, Sport and American Society*. Baltimore: Johns Hopkins University Press, 1986.

Grimes, Ronald L. *Beginnings in Ritual Studies*. CreateSpace Independent Publishing Platform, 2010. First published in 1982 by University Press of America.

Huizinga, Johan. *Homo Ludens: A Study of the Play Element in Culture*. Boston: Beacon Press, 1971.

Plummer, Thomas. *Where Did That Member Go? Rediscovering the Lost Art of Member Service*. Monterey, CA: Healthy Learning, 2010.

Sansone, David. *Greek Athletics and the Genesis of Sport*. Berkeley: University of California Press, 1992.

Sargent, Dudley Allen. *Dudley Allen Sargent: An Autobiography*. Edited by Ledyard Sargent. With an introduction by R. Tait McKenzie. 1927. Reprint, Whitefish, MT: Kessinger Publishing, 2007.

Spivey, Nigel. *The Ancient Olympics*. New York: Oxford University Press, 2012.

Starrett, Kelly, with Glen Cordoza. *Becoming a Supple Leopard: The Ultimate Guide to Resolving Pain, Preventing Injury, and Optimizing Athletic Performance*. Las Vegas, NV: Victory Belt Publishing, 2013.

Taubes, Gary. *Good Calories, Bad Calories: Fats, Carbs, and the Controversial Science of Diet and Health*. New York: Knopf, 2007.

Tharrett, Stephen, Frank O'Rourke, and James A. Peterson. *Legends of Fitness: The Forces, Influencers, and Innovations That Helped Shape the Fitness Industry*. Monterey, CA: Healthy Learning, 2011.

Webster, David. *Scottish Highland Games*. Edinburgh, Scotland: Reprographia, 1973. More information on the Highland Games can be found at http://www.highlandgames.net/historical.html.

NOTES

UNDER THE BRIDGE

1. Jerry Hill, interview by the author. Hill's personal narratives about his childhood, days in Philly, and the Marines were related by him in March of 2012 and follow-up interviews through July of 2013, and by Jason Cox in an interview by the author in November of 2012.

INTO THE RED ZONE

1. Pat Sherwood, "Intensity (and Its Role in Fitness)," *CrossFit Journal*, March 13, 2009, http://journal.crossfit.com/2009/03/intensity-and-its-role -in-fitness.tpl.

2. Lon Kilgore, "The Most Powerful Human Being in the Entire Universe," *CrossFit Journal*, July 2007, http://journal.crossfit.com/2007/07/the -most-powerful-human-being.tpl.

3. Craig Angle, "Aerobic and Anaerobic Energy—Phosphagen, Glycolytic and Oxidative Phosphorylation Systems," Section One Wrestling (an online knowledge base for wrestling), http://www.sectiononewrestling.com/ documents/aerobic_anaerobic_energy_systems.html.

4. Tony Leyland, "Human Power Output and CrossFit Metcon Workouts, *CrossFit Journal*, July 2008, http://library.crossfit.com/free/pdf/71_08 _Human_Power_Output.pdf.

5. G. R. Hunter, L. A. Belcher, L. Dunnan, and G. Fleming, "Bench Press Metabolic Rate as a Function of Exercise Intensity, *J. Appl. Sports Sci. Res.* 2 (1988): 1–6.

6. Tony Leyland, "Rest and Recovery in Interval-Based Exercise," *Cross-Fit Journal*, April 2007, http://library.crossfit.com/free/pdf/56_07_Rest _Recovery.pdf.

7. R. J. Godfrey, Z. Madgwick, and G. P. Whyte, "The Exercise-Induced

Growth Hormone Response in Athletes," *Sports Medicine* 33, no. 8 (2003): 599–613.

8. G. R. Hunter, R. L, Weinsier, M. M. Bamman, and D. E. Larson, "A Role for High Intensity Exercise on Energy Balance and Weight Control," *International Journal of Obesity and Related Metabolic Disorders* 22, no. 6 (1998): 489–93, http://www.carnevalijunior.com.br/wp-content/uploads/2010/03/a-role-for-high-intensity-exercise-on-energy-expenditure-balance-and-weight-control-1998.pdf.

9. "'Weight Training' Reduces Fat and Improve[s] Metabolism in Mice," *Science Daily*, February 7, 2008, http://www.sciencedaily.com/releases/2008/02/080205121740.htm.

10. A. Tremblay, J. A. Simoneau, C. Bouchard, "Impact of Exercise Intensity on Body Fatness and Skeletal Muscle Metabolism," *Metabolism* 43, no. 7 (1994): 814–18.

11. Stephen Boutcher, "Review Article: High-Intensity Intermittent Exercise and Fat Loss," *Journal of Obesity* 2011 (2011), Article ID 858305. Originally published online November 24, 2010.

12. E. G. Trapp, D. J. Chisholm, J. Freund, and S. H. Boutcher, "The Effects of High-Intensity Intermittent Training on Fat Loss and Fasting Insulin Levels of Young Women," *International Journal of Obesity* 32 (2008): 1–8.

13. T. Wu, X. Gao, M. Chen, and R. M. Van Dam, "Long-Term Effectiveness of Diet-Plus-Exercise Interventions vs. Diet-Only Interventions for Weight Loss: A Meta-Analysis: Obesity Management," *Obesity Reviews* 10, no. 3 (2009): 313–23.

14. Huiyun Liang and Walter F. Ward, University of Texas Health Science Center, "PGC-1α: A Key Regulator of Energy Metabolism," *Adv. Physiol. Educ.* 30, no. 4 (2006): 145–51, http://advan.physiology.org/content/30/4/145.full.

15. Ian Janssen and Robert Ross, "Vigorous Intensity Physical Activity Is Related to Metabolic Syndrome Independent of the Physical Activity Dose," *International Journal of Epidemiology*, first published online March 24, 2012, http://ije.oxfordjournals.org/content/early/2012/03/23/ije.dys038.abstract.

16. Hunter et al., "A Role for High Intensity Exercise" (see n. 8).

THE MONKEY BARS

1. Greg Glassman, "The Story of 'Fran,'" video, http://www.youtube.com/watch?v=hAT6AFMiL14, 6:46, uploaded November 13, 2010.

2. Ibid.; lecture to Marines at Okinawa, April 22, 2009, *CrossFit Journal*, video, 19:15, http://library.crossfit.com/free/video/CFJ_Glassman_ OkinawaLecture1.mov. This video is part one of a five-part video series that appears here: http://journal.crossfit.com/2009/06/glassman-talks-at -okinawa.tpl.

3. Greg Amundson, "CrossFit HQ 2851 Research Park Drive," *CrossFit Journal*, January 2010, http://journal.crossfit.com/2010/01/crossfit-hq-2851 -research-park-dr-santa-cruz-calif.tpl.

4. Greg Glassman, "Seniors and Kids," *CrossFit Journal*, February 2003, http://library.crossfit.com/free/pdf/seniors_kidsFeb03.pdf.

5. Amundson, "CrossFit HQ" (see n. 3).

6. Jimmy Baker, "Coaching the Elderly—Introduction," *CrossFit Journal*, October 10, 2008, http://journal.crossfit.com/2008/10/coaching-the-elderly -introduction.tpl.

7. Tony Leyland, "Variable Resistance: Nature or Design?" *CrossFit Journal*, October 2007, http://journal.crossfit.com/2007/10/variable-resistance -nature-or.tpl.

8. Greg Glassman, "What Is Fitness?" *CrossFit Journal*, October 2002, http://library.crossfit.com/free/pdf/CFJ_Trial_04_2012.pdf.

9. Eugene d'Aquili and Andrew B. Newberg, *The Mystical Mind: Probing the Biology of Religious Experience* (Minneapolis: Fortress Press, 1999), 35–37.

RISE OF THE MACHINES

1. Dudley Allen Sargent, *Dudley Allen Sargent: An Autobiography*, ed. Ledyard W. Sargent, with an introduction by R. Tait McKenzie (1927; repr., Whitefish, MT: Kessinger Publishing, 2007), 151.

2. Ibid., 108.

3. Ibid.

4. Ibid., 149.

5. Ibid., 117.

6. Dudley Allen Sargent, *Health, Strength and Power* (Boston: Colonial Press, 1904), 5.

7. Ibid., 19.

8. Ibid., 36.

9. Ibid., 154.

10. Bainbridge Bunting and Margaret Henderson Floyd, *Harvard: An Architectural History* (Cambridge, MA: Belknap Press of Harvard University Press, 1998), 96.

11. Dudley Allen Sargent, Henry James Whigham, et al., *Athletic Sports* (New York: Charles Scribner's Sons, 1897), 20. Available on Google Books, http://books.google.com/books?id=80lAAAAAYAAJ&printsec=frontcover& dq=inauthor:%22Robert+Duffield+Wrenn%22&hl=en&sa=X&ei=rw AcUuvIJvPDsATFoYCoBA&ved=0CC4Q6AEwAA#v=onepage&q&f=false.

12. Ibid., 43.

13. Sargent, *Dudley Allen Sargent*, 211 (see n. 1).

14. Bruce Lanyon Bennet, "The Life of Dudley Allen Sargent, M.D., and His Contribution to Physical Education" (unpublished dissertation, University of Michigan, 1947), 93.

15. Ibid., 185.

16. Sargent, *Dudley Allen Sargent*, 211 (see n. 1), 175.

17. Bennet, "The Life of Dudley Allen Sargent," 236–41 (see n. 14).

18. Greg Glassman, lecture at Fort Hood, August 28, 2009, video, 9:07, http://journal.crossfit.com/2009/11/coach-glassman-at-fort-hood.tpl.

19. Ibid., "Finding the Fittest," video, uploaded January 24, 2011, 5:47, http://www.youtube.com/watch?v=ob0b0bvyMNg.

20. Sargent, *Dudley Allen Sargent*, 211 (see n. 1), 181.

THE ORIGINAL FIREBREATHER

1. Definition of *firebreather*, as given at http://www.firebreatherathletics .com/pages/history.

2. Greg Amundson, *Your Wife Is Not Your Sister*, 2nd ed. (Los Gatos, CA: Robertson Publishing, 2013), xi.

3. Anthony Pinizzotto and Edward F. Davis, "Offenders' Perceptual Shorthand: What Messages Are Law Enforcement Officers Sending to Offenders?" *FBI Law Enforcement Bulletin*, June 1999, http://www.valorforblue .org/Documents/Publications/Public/Offenders_Perceptual_Shorthand _FBI_Law_Enforcement_Bulletin.pdf.

4. Greg Amundson's descriptions of his sheriff days and early years of CrossFit are from a series of interviews in January 2013, with follow-up interviews through August 2013. Amundson's remarks are from these interviews unless otherwise cited.

5. Greg Amundson, "CrossFit HQ 2851 Research Park Drive," *CrossFit Journal*, January 2010, http://journal.crossfit.com/2010/01/crossfit-hq -2851-research-park-dr-santa-cruz-calif.tpl.

6. Greg Amundson's website, Firebreather Athletics, http://www .firebreatherathletics.com/pages/history.

7. Amundson, "CrossFit HQ" (see n. 5).

8. Greg Glassman, "Evidence-Based Fitness," *CrossFit Journal*, January 2007, http://library.crossfit.com/free/pdf/53_07_Evid_Based_Fitness.pdf.

9. Interview with Greg Amundson, January 2013.

10. Catherine Bell, *Ritual: Perspectives and Dimensions* (New York: Oxford University Press, 1997), 150.

11. Greg Glassman, "The Story of 'Fran,'" *CrossFit Journal*, December 24, 2009, video, http://journal.crossfit.com/2009/12/the-story-of-Fran.tpl.

12. Greg Glassman, "Benchmark Workouts," *CrossFit Journal*, September 2013, www.crossfit.com/journal/library/13_03_Benchmark_Workouts.pdf.

13. John Shepard's recollections are from interviews conducted in June and July of 2013.

14. Sergeant Adrienne Quigley, "Fit for Duty? The Need for Physical Fitness Programs for Law Enforcement Officers," *Police Chief*, September 2013, http://www.policechiefmagazine.org/magazine/index.cfm?fuseaction=display_arch&article_id=1516&issue_id=62008. See also: John M. Violanti et al., "The Buffalo Cardio-Metabolic Occupational Police Stress (BCOPS) Pilot Study: Methods and Participant Characteristics," *Annals of Epidemiology* 16 (2006): 148–56.

15. Greg Amundson, "CrossFit Law Enforcement Training Seminar," *CrossFit Journal*, January 26, 2012, http://journal.crossfit.com/2012/01/amundsonleolecture.tpl.

16. Interview with Greg Amundson, January 2013.

NASTY GIRLS

1. Speech at National War College, National Defense University, January 6, 2009, video, http://library.crossfit.com/free/video/CFJ_Glassman_WarCollegePart1.mov.

2. Greg Glassman's recollections in this chapter were recounted in a June 2013 interview.

3. A popular T-shirt reads: "My girl warms up with your PR [personal record]."

4. Lauren Glassman, CrossFit.com blog archive, post date December 4, 2005, http://www.crossfit.com/mt-archive2/000990.html.

CHRISTMAS IN IRAQ

1. Christmas's recollections of her childhood and experiences in Iraq are from a November 2012 interview.

2. *Defense Federal Acquisition Regulations Supplement, Part 237—Service Contracting, Subpart 237.71—Laundry and Dry Cleaning Services,* revised January 23, 2006, http://www.acq.osd.mil/dpap/dars/dfars/pdf/r20130710/237_71.pdf.

3. Ray Bily and Chazz Rudolph recounted their Iraq experiences in separate interviews in July 2013.

4. CrossFit Rockford has assembled the history and composition of the "Painstorm" workouts, available here: http://crossfitrockford.typepad.com/crossfit_rockford/files/Painstorm.pdf.

FALLUJAH, FOR TIME

1. Sam D., active-duty member of Naval Special Warfare, "A Soldier's Perspective on Functional Fitness," *CrossFit Journal,* April 2005, http://library.crossfit.com/free/pdf/32_05_Functional_Fitness.pdf.

2. Greg Glassman, Capt. Wade Rutland, and Capt. J. T. Williams, "AOFP/CrossFit Austere Program," http://www.crossfit.com/cf-journal/AOFP-Austere-Program_equipment.pdf.

3. James Decker, "Training in Austere Environments," *CrossFit Journal,* March 2006, http://library.crossfit.com/free/pdf/43_06_austere_training.pdf.

4. Brian Chontosh, "CrossFit for Combat Fitness," *CrossFit Journal,* August 5, 2009, http://journal.crossfit.com/2009/08/asep-lecture-another-speaker.tpl#featureArticleTitle.

5. Andrew Thompson, "Characteristics of a World-Class Trainee," *CrossFit Journal,* April 2008, http://library.crossfit.com/free/pdf/68_08_WorldClass_Trainee.pdf.

6. "The Little Gym That Could, Part 1," video, http://media.crossfit.com/cf-video/CFSC-pt1.mov; "Landslide: Operation Phoenix Part 2," video, http://media.crossfit.com/cf-video/CrossFit_Phoenix2Landslide.mov; "Operation Phoenix: The Final Chapter," video, http://library.crossfit.com/free/video/CFJ_Szoldra_OperationPhoenixFinal.mov.

THE BLUE ROOM

1. Newman's recollections in this chapter are from an October 2012 interview.

2. Jerry Hill described the early days of the Blue Room in a March 2013 interview, with follow-up questions and answers at CrossFit Oldtown (pre- or post-WOD) over a period extending through June of 2013.

3. Video, uploaded September 26, 2008, http://www.youtube.com/watch?v=2ynmLVRDAuc.

4. Interview with Harold Doran, March 2013.

5. Jerry Hill, blog post to *Jerry Hill's CrossFit Challenge*, September 11, 2007, http://crossfitchallenge.blogspot.com/2007/09/crossfit-hero-workout.html.

6. Jerry Hill, blog post to *Jerry Hill's CrossFit Challenge*, January 16, 2008, http://crossfitchallenge.blogspot.com/2008/01/epic-pain-boot-bull-keep-keel-crucible.html.

7. Jerry Hill, blog post to *Jerry Hill's CrossFit Challenge*, October 15, 2007, http://crossfitchallenge.blogspot.com/2007/10/nasty-girls.html.

8. Jerry Hill, blog post to *Jerry Hill's CrossFit Challenge*, February 25, 2008, http://crossfitchallenge.blogspot.com/2008/02/character.html.

THE FIREFIGHTER CHALLENGE

1. Thiel's recollections in this chapter are from a March 2013 interview.

2. Mike Warkentin, "Firefighter Combat Challenge and the Definitions of Fitness," September 2009, http://journal.crossfit.com/2009/09/challenging-the-definitions-of-fitness.tpl.

3. Lon Kilgore, "Putting Out Fires," *CrossFit Journal*, March 2007, http://www.crossfit.com/journal/library/55_07_putting_out_fires.pdf.

4. Ibid.

5. Christopher K. Haddock, Walker S. C. Poston, and Sara A. Jahnke, "Addressing the Epidemic of Obesity in the United States Fire Service: A Report Prepared for the National Volunteer Fire Council," http://www.nvfc.org/files/documents/Obesity_Study.pdf.

6. National Fire Protection Association, *NFPA 1583: Standard on Health Related Fitness Programs for Fire Department Members* (NFPA, 2008), http://www.nfpa.org/codes-and-standards/document-information-pages?mode=code&code=1583.

7. Centers for Disease Control and Prevention, "Fatalities Among Volunteer and Career Firefighters—United States, 1994–2004," *Morbidity and Mortality Weekly Report* 55 (2006): 453–55.

8. Mike Contreras, "The Fire Service and CrossFit: The Perfect Combination," *CrossFit Journal*, November 2006, http://library.crossfit.com/free/pdf/51-06-FireServiceAndCF.pdf.

9. Cited in Steven Levitt and Stephen Dubner's blog, *Freakonomics.com*, November 30, 2009, http://www.freakonomics.com/2009/11/30/bagel-danger.

10. Newsblaze.com, "Lawsuit Against Nintendo for the Ill Effects of

Their Wii Games," February 9, 2009, http://newsblaze.com/story/ 20090209062004zzzz.nb/topstory.html.

11. Denise Head et al., "Exercise Engagement as a Moderator of the Effects of *APOE* Genotype on Amyloid Deposition," *JAMA Neurology* 69, no. 5 (May 2012): 636–43, http://www.ncbi.nlm.nih.gov/pubmed/22232206.

12. The Editors of Harvard Health Publications, in collaboration with Dr. Michael Craig Miller, assistant professor of psychiatry, Harvard Medical School, "Exercise and Depression," excerpted from a special report entitled *Understanding Depression*, published online in 2013, http://www.health.harvard .edu/newsweek/Exercise-and-Depression-report-excerpt.htm.

13. Adrian Thorogood et al., "Isolated Aerobic Exercise and Weight Loss: A Systematic Review and Meta-Analysis of Randomized Controlled Trials," *American Journal of Medicine* 124, no. 8 (August 2011): 747–55, http://www .ncbi.nlm.nih.gov/pubmed/21787904.

14. Jim Bledsoe, "Rhabdomyolysis," *Sports Injury Bulletin*, http://www .sportsinjurybulletin.com/archive/rhabdomyolysis.html.

15. Stan Reents, Pharm.D., "Exertional Rhabdomyolysis," article posted to AthleteInMe.com, May 6, 2007, http://www.athleteinme.com/ArticleView .aspx?id=241.

16. Ibid.

17. Marta Lawrence, "Rhabdo Requires Prompt Diagnosis, Treatment," NCAA.org, posted April 21, 2011, http://fs.ncaa.org/Docs/NCAANews Archive/2011/april/rhabdo%2Brequires%2Bprompt%2Bdiagnosis,% 2Btreatmentdf30.html.

18. David Epstein, "Rhabdomyolysis Problem Is Real, and Not Unique to Haynesworth," *Sports Illustrated* online, posted August 25, 2010, http:// sportsillustrated.cnn.com/2010/writers/david_epstein/08/24/haynesworth .rhabdo/index.html.

19. Michael Russel, "Combination of Intense Drill, Heat, Dehydration, May Have Sent McMinnville Players to Hospital," *The Oregonian*, published online August 22, 2010, http://www.oregonianlive.com/news/index .ssf/2010/08/combination_of_intense_drill_h.html.

20. Dr. Michael Ray, "The Truth About Rhabdo," *CrossFit Journal*, January 2010, http://library.crossfit.com/free/pdf/CFJ_Ray_rhabdo1.pdf.

THE HOPPER

1. Interview with Greg Glassman, June 2013.

2. Dale Saran, "The First CrossFit Games," *CrossFit Journal*, August 2007, http://library.crossfit.com/free/pdf/60_07_CrossFit_Games.pdf.

CHRIS SPEALLER

1. CrossFit Games archive, "2007 CrossFit Games Hopper Workout," video, uploaded July 5, 2007, 5:27, http://games.crossfit.com/video/2007 -crossfit-games-hopper-workout.

2. Interview with Dave Castro at the 2013 Mid-Atlantic regionals, June 2013.

3. Russell Greene, "Chris Spealler: The Fire Inside," *CrossFit Journal*, November 2011, http://library.crossfit.com/free/pdf/CFJ_Spealler_Green.pdf.

4. Ibid.

5. http://crossfit.com/mt-archive2/001508.html.

THE AMAZON AND THE ENGINEER

1. Caity Matter, "An Interview with Caity Matter," *CrossFit Journal*, January 10, 2009, http://journal.crossfit.com/2009/01/an-interview-with-caity -matter-part-1.tpl#featureArticleTitle.

2. Athlete profile, Buckeysports.com, http://ohiostate.scout.com/ a.z?s=145&p=8&c=1&nid=1288076.

3. Dick Patrick, "Tragedy Doesn't Deter Ohio State's Matter," *USA Today*, February 18, 2004, http://usatoday30.usatoday.com/sports/college/ womensbasketball/2004-02-18-buckeye-courage_x.htm?csp=34.

4. John Porentas, "A Special, Special Day," TheOzone.Net, March 2004, http://www.the-ozone.net/hoops/03-04women/matter.htm.

5. Ibid.

6. Caity Matter, "An Interview with Caity Matter: Party 3," *CrossFit Journal*, February 2, 2009, http://journal.crossfit.com/2009/02/an -interview-with-caity-matter-part-3.tpl.

7. A vintage video of Jolie Gentry and two imposing male backup dancers doing the "Bear Complex" WOD can be found at http://media.crossfit.com/ cf-video/CrossFit_TheBear.mov.

8. Bill Henniger's remarks are from an April 2013 interview and an interview at Rogue's factory in May 2013.

9. http://board.crossfit.com/showthread.php?t=20487.

DARK HORSES

1. Tony Budding, "Capacity, Standards, and Sport," *CrossFit Journal*, June 2008, http://library.crossfit.com/free/pdf/70_08_capacity_standards_sport .pdf.

2. Looking to established multi-event competitions, such as the decathlon (http://en.wikipedia.org/wiki/Decathlon), isn't that helpful in designing a scoring system for new multi-event competitions, because multi-event Olympic scoring systems contain a lot of arbitrary calculus, weighting factors, and exponents, all subject to the decades-long bickering of international committees.

3. Jolie Gentry is so staggeringly kick-ass gorgeous in the 2008 Games, the sight of her beggars description. See http://games2008.crossfit.com/ Games08WomensThruster0920.html; http://games2008.crossfit.com/ athletes/return-the-favor-pat-interview.html.

4. At the same time as he is screaming his head off, Bill Henniger is holding a video camera. No image stabilization software will ever salvage the resulting video, but the soundtrack will melt your heart: http://media.crossfit .com/cf-video/Games08_CaityMatterRun.mov (video).

5. CrossFit Games archive video of Caity Matter's final reps in the 2008 CrossFit Games: http://media.crossfit.com/cf-video/CrossFitGames08 _CaityMatterFinalRepsCJ.mov.

6. *Every Second Counts*, directed by Sevan Mattossian and Carey Peterson (CrossFit Pictures, 2009). Viewable on YouTube: http://www.youtube.com/ watch?v=_NZyPHYIswc.

A CLYDESDALE LEARNS TO RACE

1. "An Interview with Jason Khalipa," video posted to *CrossFit Journal*, December 2, 2008, http://journal.crossfit.com/2008/12/an-interview-with -jason-khalipa-part-2.tpl.

2. Crossfit Milpitas, coach profile of Austin Begiebing: http://www .crossfitmilpitas.com/coach/1/austin-begiebing.

GLOBO-GYM

1. Anyone interested in a comprehensive history of gyms, exercise equipment, and the fitness industry would do well to read *Legends of Fitness: The Forces, Influencers, and Innovations That Helped Shape the Fitness Industry*, by industry veterans Stephen Tharrett, Frank O'Rourke, and James A. Peterson

(Monterey, CA: Healthy Learning, 2011). It is a comprehensive and well-written chronicle that spans more than a century.

2. Mark Huffman, "Bally's Customers Hope to Exercise Their Rights," *Consumer Affairs*, August 20, 2005, http://www.consumeraffairs.com/news04/2005/ballys.html.

3. New York State Attorney General's Office, "Consumer Complaints Lead to Health Club Sales Reforms," February 16, 2004, http://www.ag.ny.gov/press-release/consumer-complaints-lead-health-club-sales-reforms.

4. Texas Attorney General's Office, "Attorney General Abbot Charges Fitness Center Operator with Unlawfully Deceiving Texas Customers," June 8, 2010, https://www.oag.state.tx.us/oagnews/release.php?id=3350.

5. PR Newswire, "Gold's Gym Identifies February 7th as the 'Fitness Cliff' . . . the Day When New Year's Resolutions Begin to Fail," February 4, 2013, posted to Franchising.com, http://www.Franchising.com/news/20130204_golds_gym_identifies_february_7th_as_the_fitness_c.html.

6. Ray Algar, Oxygen Consulting, "2011 Global Low-Cost Gym Sector Report: A Strategic Investigation into a Disruptive New Segment." This report was sponsored by Precor, which manufactures gym cardio equipment, http://www.sportsthinktank.com/uploads/1319576881-2011globallow-costgymsectorreport.pdf.

7. Stuart Goldman, "State of the Fitness Industry: What's in Store for 2013," ClubIndustry.com, January 1, 2013, http://clubindustry.com/profits/state-fitness-industry-what-s-store-2013?page=2.

8. Nick Heil, "American Gladiators." *Outside*, January 2012, http://www.outsideonline.com/outdoor-adventure/first-look/American-Gladiators.html?page=all.

9. Spartan Race website: http://www.spartanrace.com.

10. Description of Tough Mudder obstacles can be found here: http://toughmudder.com/obstacles.

11. The relative ease of Muddy Buddy's obstacles, plus its pair-team rule, has earned it a reputation as the adventure race for chicks, and for less competitive dudes who want to see pretty girls, covered in mud, hugging each other at the finish line. The race's slogan, "Good Times + Crazy Friends = Amazing Memories," evokes girls' sleep-away camp—the last place many participants experienced the same combination of grime and glee.

12. Tough Mudder website: http://toughmudder.com/about/.

13. Spartan Race has a dedicated prize category for Fittest Box. Teams

must consist of at least four people, two of whom must be female, who all belong to the same CrossFit box and register under the affiliate name. The top-four finishers win points, depending on how fast they finish. The box with the most points at the end of the year, from all Spartan races, wins the grand prize. Spartan Race has even staged hybrid events that are half obstacle course, half CrossFit competition: see http://blog.spartanrace.com/spartan-race-and-wodstock.

14. Greg Glassman, "Pursuing Excellence and Creating Value," *CrossFit Journal* video, posted January 22, 2013, http://library.crossfit.com/free/video/CFJ_StatePolicySpeech3_Hayley.mp4.

15. Entrepreneur.com, Planet Fitness company profile, current to year-end 2012: http://www.entrepreneur.com/franchises/planetfitness/329333-0.html#.

16. Greg Glassman, "Unfettered Capitalism," video posted to CrossFit .com's blog on March 20, 2013, http://media.crossfit.com/cf-video/CrossFit_FreeMarketUnfetteredCapitalism.wmv.

17. Russell Berger, "CrossFit Affiliate Competition," *CrossFit Journal*, December 16, 2008, http://journal.crossfit.com/2008/12/crossfit-affiliate-competition.tpl.

18. CrossFit New England is in Natick, Massachusetts, a mere four miles from the Army's Soldier Research, Development, and Engineering Center (http://nsrdec.natick.army.mil). This military lab focuses on the "Soldier as System," which means anything a soldier carries, wears, or uses in the field. A huge amount of lab funding goes to battery innovation—specifically, how to reduce the weight of all the batteries a soldier is humping around to power all his equipment. Until this lab succeeds in its research mission, soldiers do CrossFit so they can haul these heavy loads quickly. The industrial park that houses CrossFit New England also rents space to an emergency medical services company that answers EMT calls across a big chunk of Massachusetts and New Hampshire. So emergency first responders are only a few bay doors down from their preferred mode of exercise.

19. Ben Bergeron, "The Deeper Side of Coaching," *CrossFit Journal*, December 2011, http://library.crossfit.com/free/pdf/CFJ_Coaching_Bergeron.pdf.

20. Ben Bergeron, "The Emotional Bank Account," video posted to *CrossFit Journal*, June 16, 2012, http://journal.crossfit.com/2012/06/emotionalbankaccount.tpl.

21. CrossFit New England website, "About Us," http://crossfitnewengland .com/about/.

22. Primatologists who study human evolution have pegged the primordial human social group to between 110 and 230 people. The seminal work on this subject is Robin Dunbar's *Grooming, Gossip, and the Evolution of Language* (Cambridge, MA: Harvard University Press).

23. Scott Shane, "Small Business Failure Rates by Industry: The Real Numbers," *Small Business Trends*, September 24, 2012, http://smallbiztrends .com/2012/09/failure-rates-by-sector-the-real-numbers.html.

24. This statistic was given by Greg Glassman, who concedes that calculating the five-year failure rate for affiliates required some judgment calls in the categorization of failure when boxes split or a military affiliate put his garage gym on hiatus. "It's hard—you have to make some rules up when you do this. You've got an affiliate and it splits up because the owners don't agree anymore and they form two new affiliates. A guy goes on deployment and has to shut the doors. Did it fail? Somewhere around 2%." Greg Glassman, "CrossFit—Health and Wealth," video posted to YouTube August 11, 2012, http://www.youtube.com/watch?v=M-gFFOf6CfQ&feature=g-u-u.

CAVEMAN KOSHER

1. "Welcome CFOT: Moving for Time, Our Inaugural WOD, and Finally Being a Family . . . ," *Katie's Mindless Ramblings* (blog), January 6, 2009, http://katiesmindlessramblings.blogspot.com/2009/01/welcome-home-cfot -moving-for-time-our.html.

2. Gary Taubes, *Good Calories, Bad Calories: Fats, Carbs, and the Controversial Science of Diet and Health* (New York: Knopf, 2007).

3. There is, in the taxonomy of dietary factions and subfactions, a distinction between the Paleo Diet and the Clean Eating Diet, which allows grains, dairy, and legumes in an unprocessed state. However, both factions refer to strict adherence to their own dietary restrictions as "getting clean."

4. A landmark study in the *New England Journal of Medicine* used social network analysis of the Framingham population to demonstrate that people with obese social networks are more likely to become obese themselves. See Nicholas A. Christakis, M.D., Ph.D., M.P.H., and James H. Fowler, Ph.D., "The Spread of Obesity in a Large Social Network over 32 Years," *N. Engl. J. Med.* 357 (2007): 370–79, doi: 10.1056/NEJMsa066082, http://www.nejm .org/doi/full/10.1056/NEJMsa066082. This finding yielded the sensational

new headline: "Obesity Is Contagious." The same mechanisms that propagate obesity through social networks can propagate leanness, especially if the social mores that create that leanness (i.e., dietary restrictions) are a defining element of the social networks themselves. One can almost visualize the body mass index of newly minted CrossFitters shrink as they link into the social graph of a CrossFit box and become enmeshed in that group.

CRUCIBLE

1. Nicole Gordon's recollections of her CrossFit experiences are from a series of interviews with the author, from November 2012 through April 2013.

2. Greg Glassman, "CrossFit Games: Coach on the '09 Format," video from CrossFit Games archive, http://media.crossfit.com/cf-video/ CrossFitGames09_Coach09Format.mov.

3. Greg Amundson, "The Chink in My Armor," *CrossFit Journal*, September 16, 2009, http://journal.crossfit.com/2009/09/the-chink-in-my-armor .tpl.

4. Much of the action of the 2009 CrossFit Games was captured on video, viewable on the CrossFit Games website (e.g., http://games2009.crossfit .com/thegames/mikko-and-speal-71k-friends.html). This account of the 2009 Games was assembled from exhaustive review of video footage of the Games (http://games2009.crossfit.com/thegames/index.html), as well as interviews with the participating athletes.

5. CrossFit's documentary filmmaker, Sevan Matossian, followed Mikko back to Finland after the 2009 Games, to get a perspective on his warrior-monk ethos. His famous never-lie-on-your-back remark appeared in Matossian's documentary *Sisu* (http://www.youtube.com/watch?v=sC-hvvs7mvA) and inspired a True Grit cadre of CrossFit athletes to eschew postworkout recovery on the floor.

6. Mike Warkentin, "Redeeming a Bad Run," *CrossFit Journal*, July 15, 2009, http://journal.crossfit.com/2009/07/redeeming-a-bad-run.tpl.

7. Mike Warkentin, "The Quick and the Deadlifts," *CrossFit Journal*, July 17, 2009, http://journal.crossfit.com/2009/07/the-quick-and-the -deadlifts.tpl.

8. "Nicole Gordon: Finger vs. Stake," CrossFit Games video archive, http://games2009.crossfit.com/thegames/sledge-vs-finger-bloodmatch.html.

9. CrossFit Games video archive, "Coach Burgener on the Snatch Event," October 12, 2009, http://games2009.crossfit.com/thegames/coach -burgener-on-the-snatch-event.html.

10. Carey Peterson, "The Chipper—Women's 09 Games," *CrossFit Journal* video archive, posted December 31, 2009, http://journal.crossfit.com/2009/12/part-19-the-chipper-womens-09-games.tpl.

11. CrossFit Games archive, "2009 CrossFit Games Men's The Chipper," video posted July 12, 2009, http://games.crossfit.com/video/2009-crossfit-games-mens-chipper.

12. Ibid.

13. Carey Peterson, "Life After the Games: The Tanya Wagner Documentary," *CrossFit Journal* video feature, posted January 3, 2010, http://journal.crossfit.com/2010/01/tanya-wagner-doc.tpl.

A GOOD CULT

1. Greg Glassman, interview with the author, July 2013.

2. Nicole Carroll, interview with the author: "60% [of a 33% response rate] in the post–Level 1 survey say that they're interested in being trainers or affiliates."

3. http://psychcentral.com/lib/mirror-mirror-in-the-brain-the-biology-of-how-we-connect-to-others/00011067.

4. http://www.manningpassingacademy.com/history.

5. *Every Second Counts*, directed by Sevan Mattossian and Carey Peterson (CrossFit Pictures, 2009).

6. Greg Glassman, interview with the author.

FAITH AND THE FINISH LINE

1. For detailed statistics on the Open's exponential growth, see the Tabata Times's year-over-year breakdown, "How Fast Are the CrossFit Games Growing? The Numbers Tell a Story," http://www.tabatatimes.com/how-fast-are-the-crossfit-games-growing-the-numbers-tell-the-story.

2. *Guiness Book of World Records* online: http://www.guinnessworldrecords.com/world-records/9000/most-participants-in-a-racing-event.

3. Rich Froning with Dave Thomas, *First: What It Takes to Win*, with a foreword by Dave Castro (Carol Stream, IL: Tyndale House Publishers, 2013), 84.

4. Ibid., 87–88.

5. Ibid., 91.

6. Ibid., 90.

7. Ibid., 12.

8. Interview with Rich Froning in Cookeville, TN, December 2012.

9. Interview with Chip Pugh, August 2013.

THE FITTEST MAN ON EARTH

1. Rich Froning with Dave Thomas, *First: What It Takes to Win,* with a foreword by Dave Castro (Carol Stream, IL: Tyndale House Publishers, 2013), 141.

2. Mikko Salo, interview with Rogue Fitness at the 2011 Games, video, http://www.youtube.com/watch?v=Vq_0RVTOwys.

CORPORATE KOOL-AID

1. Interview with Matt O'Toole, December 2012.

2. Football fans of a certain age will recall Hasselbeck's career as a tight end for the New England Patriots, the Raiders (in Superbowl XVIII), the Vikings, and the Giants. Football fans younger than a certain age will recognize the name of his son, Matt Hasselbeck, who was quarterback for the Seattle Seahawks in Superbowl XL and later signed with the Indianapolis Colts. Hasselbeck's other son, Tim, played seven seasons in the NFL and does commentary for ESPN.

3. Interview with Don Hasselbeck, October 2012.

4. Lauren Weber, "The Office Nurse Now Treats Diabetes, Not Headaches," *Wall Street Journal,* July 10, 2013, http://online.wsj.com/news/articles/SB10001424127887324867904578595913843743822].

5. "National Diabetes Fact Sheet, 2011," http://www.cdc.gov/diabetes/pubs/pdf/ndfs_2011.pdf.

6. Aon Hewitt, *2012 Health Care Survey,* http://www.aon.com/attachments/human-capital-consulting/2012_Health_Care_Survey_final.pdf.

7. "Stronger people are harder to kill than weak people and more useful in general" is one of weightlifting coach Mark Rippetoe's most oft-repeated epigrams. A not-safe-for-work compilation of Rippetoe's Wit and Wisdom can be found online at http://startingstrength.wikia.com/wiki/Wit_and_Wisdom_of_Mark_Rippetoe. Highlights include:

> "Mediocre athletes that tried like hell to get good are the best coaches."

> "The full squat is a perfectly natural position for the leg to occupy. That's why there's a joint in the middle of it, and why humans have been occupying this position, both unloaded and loaded, for millions of years. Much longer, in fact, than quasi-intellectual morons have been telling us that it's "bad" for the knees."

> "Trust me, if you do an honest 20 rep program, at some point Jesus will talk to you. On the last day of the program, he'll ask if he can work in."

FORGING ELITE GEAR

1. Bill Henniger and Rogue's machinists explained the mechanical ins and outs of Rogue's manufacturing and logistics onsite at the Rogue Fitness factory and distribution center, May 2013.

2. CrossFit's regional competition boundaries have shifted over the years—the Dirty South originally included Mississippi, Tennessee, and North Carolina, in addition to Georgia, Florida, Alabama, and South Carolina. More competitive regions are allocated a higher number of qualifying slots for the Games than less competitive regions. The Central East division— which includes Tennessee, Michigan, Ohio, Indiana, and Kentucky—sends three men, three women, and three teams to the Games, not counting Rich Froning. The continent of Africa sends one man, one woman, and one team to the Games. As CrossFit's athlete population grows and improves, the Games are periodically subject to competitive redistricting.

REGIONAL COMPETITION

1. Interview with Christmas Abbott, November 2012. Christmas's recollections and comments are from this interview and a subsequent interview in June 2013, with intermittent questions and answers via e-mail.

THE BALLAD OF JERRY HILL

1. Interview with Sean Mulcahy, March 2013.

THE MAN IN THE ARENA

1. "How Do You Beat Rich Froning?" video, http://games.crossfit.com/video/how-do-you-beat-rich-froning.

2. David Sansone, *Greek Athletics and the Genesis of Sport* (Berkeley: University of California Press, 1988), 63.

3. Ibid.

4. Michael Lemonick, "The Iceman's Secrets," *Time*, October 26, 1992, 66.

5. Shane Stokes, "Taylor Phinney Interview: Getting the Pill Culture out of the Sport," Velonation.com, October 16, 2012, http://www.velonation.com/News/ID/13076/Taylor-Phinney-Interview-Getting-the-pill-culture-out-of-the-sport.aspx#ixzz2begFKOzo.

OLD SCHOOL

1. Greg Amundson's recollections are from a series of interviews between January and August of 2013. Because of the time difference between Virginia and the West Coast, Amundson's calls would often come in at ten or eleven at night, when he was driving home. My husband, an ardent CrossFitter, got a thrill every time he looked at the phone's caller ID and handed it to me with the word "Amundson" in LCD letters on the handset.

2. Greg Amundson, "Garage Gym 101: How to Grow a Successful Garage Gym," *CrossFit Journal*, February 2010, http://library.crossfit.com /premium/pdf/CFJ_Amundson_GarageGym.pdf?e=1375216002&h=3f8ae 690372a74f2618220456f9ec89e.

INDEX

Note: Abbreviations "CF" and "WOD" stand for CrossFit and Workout of the Day, respectively. Named WODs are shown in *italics*.